MUSICAL PATHWAYS IN RECOVERY

'Music triggered a healing process from within me … I s[illegible] the joy of singing myself … and it helped me carry my recovery beyond the state I was in before I fell ill nine years ago … to a level of well-being that I haven't had perhaps for thirty years…'. This book explores the experiences of people who took part in a vibrant musical community for people experiencing mental health difficulties, SMART (St Mary Abbotts Rehabilitation and Training). Ansdell (a music therapist/researcher) and DeNora (a music sociologist) describe their long-term ethnographic work with this group, charting the creation and development of a unique music project that won the 2008 Royal Society for Public Health Arts and Health Award. Ansdell and DeNora track the 'musical pathways' of a series of key people within SMART, focusing on changes in health and social status over time in relation to their musical activity. The book includes the voices and perspectives of project members and develops with them a new understanding of how music promotes their health and wellbeing. A contemporary ecological understanding of 'music and change' is outlined, drawing on and further developing theory from music sociology and Community Music Therapy. This innovative book will be of interest to anyone working in the mental health field, but also music therapists, sociologists, musicologists, music educators and ethnomusicologists. This volume completes a three part 'triptych', alongside the other volumes, *Music Asylums: Wellbeing Through Music in Everyday Life*, and *How Music Helps: In Music Therapy and Everyday Life*.

Gary Ansdell is an experienced music therapist, trainer and researcher. He has published widely in the fields of music, music therapy, and music and health/wellbeing, and is co-editor, with the music sociologist Tia DeNora, of the Ashgate series *Music and Change: Ecological Perspectives*.

Tia DeNora is Professor of Sociology of Music, in Sociology, Philosophy and Anthropology at Exeter University, UK. She is the author of *Music-in-Action*, *Music in Everyday Life*, *After Adorno: Rethinking Music Sociology* and *Beethoven and the Construction of Genius*. She directs the SocArts Research Group at Exeter.

Sarah Wilson is an experienced music therapist who has worked in both medical and non-medical mental health settings. She is currently music therapist and Music Project Supervisor at SMART.

Music and Change: Ecological Perspectives

Series Editors:

Music and Change: Ecological Perspectives, is a cross-disciplinary, topic-led series for scholars and practitioners. Its aim is to explore the question of how, where and when music makes a difference. If music is a dynamic ingredient of change, what are the processes and mechanisms associated with music's powers, and how can ecological perspectives help us to understand music in action? Book proposals are welcome in any of the following areas: healthcare, social policy, political activism, psychiatry, embodiment, mind and consciousness, community relations, education and informal learning, management and organizational cultures, trauma, memory and commemoration, theories of action, self-help, conflict and conflict resolution, the life course, spirituality and religion, disability studies, palliative care, social criticism, governance, resistance, protest, and utopian communities.

Published titles in the series:

Music Asylums: Wellbeing Through Music in Everyday Life
Tia DeNora

How Music Helps in Music Therapy and Everyday Life
Gary Ansdell

The Passion for Music: A Sociology of Mediation
Antoine Hennion, translated by Margaret Rigaud and Peter Collier

Musical Pathways in Recovery
Community Music Therapy and Mental Wellbeing

GARY ANSDELL
Nordoff Robbins and University of Exeter, UK

and

TIA DENORA
University of Exeter, UK

with

SARAH WILSON
Music Therapist & Music Project Supervisor, SMART

Routledge
Taylor & Francis Group
LONDON AND NEW YORK

First published 2016
by Routledge
2 Park Square, Milton Park, Abingdon, Oxon OX14 4RN

and by Routledge
711 Third Avenue, New York, NY 10017

First issued in paperback 2017

Routledge is an imprint of the Taylor & Francis Group, an informa business

British Library Cataloguing in Publication Data
A catalogue record for this book is available from the British Library

Library of Congress Cataloging in Publication Data
Ansdell, Gary, author.
Musical pathways in recovery : community music therapy and mental wellbeing / by Gary Ansdell and Tia DeNora with Sarah Wilson.
pages cm – (Music and change: ecological perspectives)
Includes bibliographical references and index.
ISBN 978-1-4094-3416-0 (hardcover) 1. Music therapy. 2. Music–Psychological aspects. 3. Music–Social aspects. I. DeNora, Tia, author. II. Wilson, Sarah Ellen, author. III. Title.
ML3920.A79 2015
615.8'5154—dc23
2015024489

ISBN 13: 978-1-138-50488-2 (pbk)
ISBN 13: 978-1-4094-3416-0 (hbk)

Typeset in Times New Roman
by Apex CoVantage, LLC

Dr Williams would look at buildings, doors and windows, long and hard before he actually entered a place to meet people. Once I heard the fast-talking, very busy doc say this:

> I like to stop in my tracks sometimes, watch kids teasing and touching and daring one another; I'll see grown-ups tired and worn, or tough and ready to take on one more day, get through to the next one – and I'll think, there's me, taking it in during house calls, coming up with my medical pictures in my mind, like those artists do with their head and heart using the easel, and like photographers do in the same way with their cameras. So it goes for many of us: doctors with a stethoscope, an opthalmoscope, trying to figure things out, get the right picture, as do artists, painting or photographing, trying to get their kind of 'right picture'.

Robert Coles and Thomas Roma (2008).
House Calls with William Carlos Williams MD. Brooklyn, NJ: Powerhouse Books.

***

Stories always pose that question: what kind of truth is being told? Stories never resolve that question; their work is to remind us that we have to live with complicated truths.

Arthur W. Frank (2010). *Letting Stories Breathe: A Socio-Narratology.*

***

Inescapably, the world of mental health work is a world of stories.

Bradley Lewis (2012, in Rudnick).
'Recovery, Narrative Theory, and Generative Madness'.

Contents

List of Figures

Preface

This book is part of a larger book project or, as we have described it, a 'triptych'. In fine arts terminology, a triptych is a three-paneled work where the two side images fold into the central panel. So too here, where the side panels are, to the left, DeNora's *Music Asylums* (2013a) and, to the right, Ansdell's *How Music Helps* (2014a). We use the metaphor of triptych – pretentious as we fear it might seem! – to capture the ways in which this book, *Musical Pathways*, aims to *demonstrate*, to *show rather than tell*, what music does, and what can be done with music here, within a place called SMART, during this 10-year period.

Our aspiration is to keep to a minimum theorising about 'how music helps' and how musical asylums can be built and occupied (theorising was the task of the two 'outer' panels). Here, the aspiration is, as much as we can, to present theory through the events, musicking, words and deeds of SMART members (which of course includes us too). Perhaps inevitably, we will import resources from, as it were, 'abroad'. By this we mean that now and again we draw upon some concepts ready made from others and elsewhere (these you'll find occasionally in the boxes in different type throughout the text). But if this book is to be evaluated to our own standard, it will seek to ensure that those concepts 'fit' what happened and is happening in SMART; that they are appropriate and – where necessary – altered to fit what SMART members said and did.

'Trying to get the right kind of picture' (as the poet/doctor William Carlos Williams said) – this book is our way of trying to record, document, recall, narrate, portray, listen, understand and try to explain an extraordinarily complex scene that's been forever changing and developing over a period of 10 years. Obviously a near-impossible task, but we think one worth the effort. Our strategy to try to 'get the right kind of picture' has been to look, listen, talk to, sketch, model, imagine, reflect; re-look, re-listen, think, consult, re-listen, compare, contrast, formulate, check; re-look, reflect, re-listen … this done individually, and together in continual creative dialogue over many years. You can read more in Appendix A about the details of the methods we used for this, and our attitude towards method.

The SMART Music Project (which began life as the 'Chelsea Community Music Therapy Project' in 2005) was designed both as a very practical music therapy enterprise, but also as a research project. But from the beginning we were determined that this was research *with* people, and not 'on' them. We try to present the following account as a multiple and sometimes messy form of explorative conversation on the key insight that has emerged from our staying immersed long term in this musical community: how people find a place and a pathway in music during challenging times. There are ethical and personal issues that arise from this inquiry which we've tried to address as professionally and honestly as we can throughout the project and this account of it (again, see Appendix B for more detail on this and on how confidentiality is handled in respect of the text).

***

The book has an unusual, perhaps unbalanced shape, with a bulging Part I in 45 shortish sections that tell the story of the project and present direct evidence from a variety of different perspectives, and with a variety of different voices. Parts II and III are more conventionally shaped and present our reflections on the outcomes of the project, and what outcomes might mean within a concept of mental health recovery. Because, hopefully, we sketch all of the necessary background and context as Part I unfolds the story it's not necessary to introduce much in this Preface, save to make a note on the terminology for people and places. The overall geographical site that the study we report in this book took place in includes a large general hospital ('the big hospital' in this text), a smaller psychiatric medical setting ('the mental health unit' in this text), and SMART, the central venue for this account. In SMART people are 'members', whereas in the adjacent mental health unit they are 'patients'. We will keep to these terms in the text.

***

When we say that this project and book would not have been possible without the following people we're not merely following the polite convention of the Preface. It's literally true in this case: we would not have told the story of this project without the goodwill, generosity, encouragement, practical and intellectual help, support and inspiration of perhaps literally hundreds of people over the 10-year period. More specifically we'd like to mention:

- All the many members of SMART who have been involved in the different aspects of the SMART Music Project long term, or for a few months, or even for a few hours. They, and their musical and personal generosity have been the central inspiration.
- The long-term support and inspiration of Sarah Wilson, the other music therapist of the project (apart from Gary) – who joined the project in 2007 and still runs it in 2015. You will read about Sarah throughout the text, and she's also written a Coda herself that brings the story up-to-date. Although Sarah did not write the remainder of the text we feel that we have very much written this book *with* Sarah. It couldn't have reached this stage without her support and insights.
- Rob Szymanek helped us as a research assistant during 2005–7 when he was an ethnomusicology student at Royal Holloway, University of London. His practical help doing interviews was invaluable, but we're also grateful for the quality of his insights and the poetry of some of his evocations of

the work in his field notes and summaries, which are sometimes quoted in the text.

- During the 10 years of the project SMART has had three Chief Executives, and each has given generous backing and support for both the music project and its research arm (as have the Trustees of the organisation). In particular we have to give thanks to the current Chief Executive, Amelia Mustapha, whose unwavering support and belief in the project has kept it safe and sound over many years now. You will also read about Amelia and her wise thoughts about the project during the text.
- The consultant psychiatrist Dr John Meehan has been a supporter of music therapy in this context since 1999. He has been a clinical supervisor for both Gary and Sarah, and research advisor to the project, ensuring ethics compliance and at key points adding his unique professional and human wisdom to our understanding.
- Various colleagues in both music therapy and sociology have generously shared their thoughts about aspects of the research or the book, either informally or in more formal events arranged around this project during the last 10 years. In particular: Mercédès Pavlicevic, Rachel Verney, Simon Procter, Jane Davidson, Stuart Wood, Ken Aigen, Alan Turry, Brynjulf Stige, Cochavit Elefant, the SocArts Group at Exeter (in particular Rita Gracio Alberto, Pedro dos Santos Boia, Elizabeth Dennis, Trever Hagen, Mariko Hara, Rosie Mead and Simon Procter), Anna Lisa Tota, Antonio Strati and the members of the ESRC Seminar on Arts, Health and Wellbeing.
- We'd like to acknowledge the support of three organisations too: SMART, the music therapy charity Nordoff Robbins, Exeter University Department of Sociology, Philosophy and Anthropology.
- Heidi Bishop, music commissioning editor at Ashgate baulked only momentarily at our suggestion of a three-book triptych on music, health and wellbeing in 2009, and has since been incredibly supportive and helpful, including waiting rather a long time for this book, the last installment. We also thank the other staff at Ashgate for their professional handling of the whole project.

***

When we started thinking of the idea of a triptych of books one of the inspirations was the *Mérode Altarpiece* (Tia sent a reproduction of this to Gary who pasted it in one of his early notebooks). This work, painted around 1425 by the Master of Flémalle is seen to be revolutionary in both its form and content.[1] The central panel depicts the annunciation, with an angel visiting Mary. There are, however, two unusual aspects to the Master's treatment of this. Firstly, that it takes place in

[1] We draw here from the social anthropologist Michael Banner's account of this painting in his book *The Ethics of Everyday Life* (Oxford 2014).

a fully everyday setting that is particularised and specified à la mode c.1425 with furniture, candle stick and flowers (rather than in an abstract landscape setting as would previously have been typical). Secondly, Mary carries on reading her book whilst the angel visits (the only signs of something unusual happening being that the candle has recently gone out and the pages of Mary's books flutter). The key moment of the annunciation is depicted as both ordinary and extraordinary at the same time. This message is reinforced by the side panels. On the left two contemporary figures (probably the patrons of the painting) kneel quietly, observing and witnessing through a half-open door the mundanely transcendent event that's taking place next door. On the right hand panel an elderly craftsman in his workshop gets on with his work, seemingly oblivious to what's happening. As viewers to the whole triptych we are drawn into this intimate, exceptional moment, but reminded that it's happening alongside the mundane and everyday. The social anthropologist Michael Banner (2014) suggests that the moral point of this painting is to universalise the 'transcendent particular': the painter 'has presented the event of the annunciation as a real and regular moment, not as an exceptional one' (p. 33).

This message links to our attempt in the current text to 'get the right picture' of the SMART music project. This final book of our triptych is placed as the central panel, refracting the message that all three volumes convey about music, health and wellbeing: that the extraordinary constantly takes place within the context of the ordinary and everyday – if we take care to listen and look.

***

For all the SMART musicians, past and present, with admiration and thanks.

Part I
Musical Pathways

1. Bridget's Pathway Between …

Gary goes across to the Mental Health Unit to fetch the songbooks from the music therapy room and as he comes out he meets one of the patients, a middle-aged woman. She is slowly shuffling along the corridor towards the doors, which are secured. It's not someone he knows so he keeps a respectful distance, but the two of them converge at the door. The patient looks tense and anxious, and her body mirrors this state, her shoulders hunched, her movements inhibited and controlled. She pushes a buzzer, talks to the security guard and the door is released. Gary signs out of the building and the security man at the front desk says to this woman 'You've got two hours leave now, but don't go too far, and make sure you're back at four!'

Through the doors the woman turns left, and Gary maintains his distance. As they walk, separately, the short distance along a quiet side road towards a building on the periphery of this medical site, Gary realises that they are probably both heading for the same place. He can't help noticing as he walks behind this woman that she changes slightly as she walks free of the mental health unit. Her pace quickens a little, her shoulders seem to release, and she looks up for the first time, as if she's heading somewhere rather than just shuffling along a corridor.

The place they are heading towards is an older building with a homemade looking sign directing down to the basement of a two-storey Victorian structure (very different in style and feel from the modern medical facility we've just left 100 metres back). The sign says 'SMART' and indicates *SMART Cafe*. They go down the stairs, recently repainted in friendly, non-institutional colours (painted by a group of bankers doing volunteer work as part of a weekend bonding exercise). There is homemade art hung on the walls. At the bottom of the stairs the woman opens the door, holds it open for Gary – and someone calls, 'Bridget! Come and sit down and have a cuppa! It's great you managed it again!'. She smiles and sits down next to Lucy, a long-term member of SMART and *SMART Music*.

***SMART*, the place where it all happens**

SMART's website describes this organisation and its purpose simply and imaginatively:

> SMART has 2 doors, one that faces the mental health hospital, and another that backs on to the wider Chelsea community. You are welcome to visit us through either.

SMART was set up as a charity in 1985 by some forward-looking psychiatrists to help form a bridge for patients between a stay in hospital and life back in the community. It has been helping people ever since, in a unique way that combines respect, challenge and opportunity for people treading the often-difficult path to recovery between mental health services and everyday social and cultural life. SMART's mission states that 'the founders recognised the importance of meaningful activity and training as a way to rebuild lives, giving people purpose, confidence and skills. As the Charity grew it also recognised the importance of friends, music, laughter and fun'.

Part of this 'serious fun' has been the music project that this book follows, is connected to and seeks to celebrate. It started in 2005 after Gary had been working as a music therapist in the adjacent hospital setting for five years. As he handed this work over to another music therapist, Sarah Wilson, he was faced with a new and interesting challenge. One day on the street outside the hospital he met Robert, someone he'd done music therapy with on a one-to-one basis. Asking how Robert was now he got the answer: 'I'm fairly well now – but there's no music! That's one of the things that got me well again – and now I'm discharged from the hospital there's no music therapy!' (This disconnect is a common problem with acute services. Enhancing the links between in-hospital provision and supportive services in the community to help people stay well remains an on-going challenge due to funding shortages.) Gary asked Robert where he spent his time now, and he pointed to SMART, but said that there was no music there.[1]

Gary investigated and found that although there was no active music-making, there were many musicians – amateur, semi-professional and former professionals whose mental illness had stopped them from playing. There was a lot of *talk* of music, but no actual music being made. With the help of the Nordoff Robbins music therapy charity and the staff of SMART, Gary set up a weekly music session called simply 'SMART Music' in the cafe. Like the cafe, this session was open to anyone – members of the SMART community, members of the public just dropping in for a coffee. Over the next few years it found its shape, and its participants – musicians, music-lovers and those for whom music simply helped,

---

1 For more detail on the genesis/development of the project see Ansdell and DeNora (2012).

whether they were singing, playing or just witnessing because they happened to be in the cafe that day. SMART's website currently describes this group:

> Every Wednesday from 2pm to 4pm we host a jam session in our cafe that is open to all. Anyone can sing, play an instrument or simply sit and watch. All types of music is played: rock 'n' roll, blues, ballads, pop, songs old and new. Come down and enjoy tea, cake and good company.

Overall then, the project established a place outside of hospital where people in hospital and discharged from hospital could make music together:

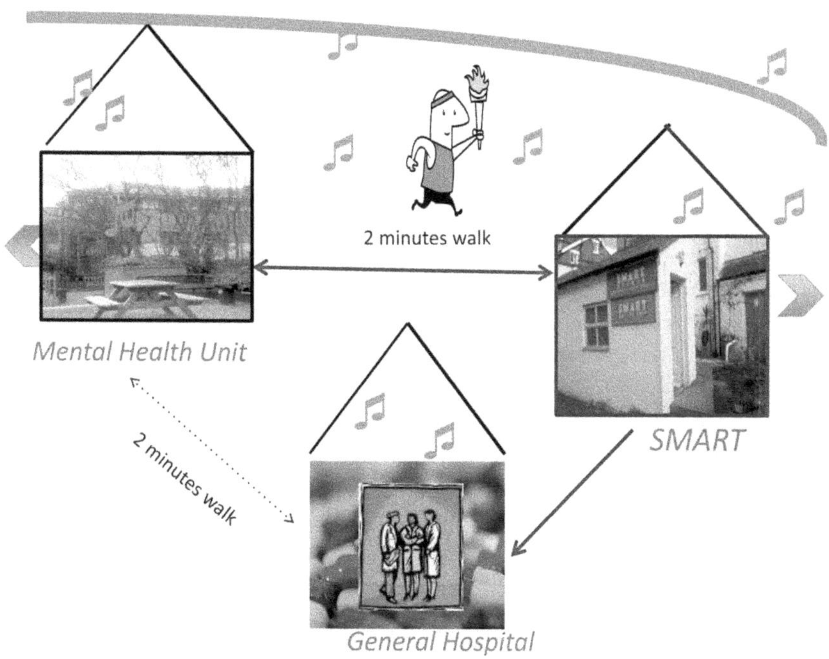

Figure 1 The site of the Chelsea Community Music Therapy Project

The SMART Music group is facilitated by music therapists, but is not explicitly named or identified as a music therapy session. It is more like a hybrid between a large music therapy group and an open mic session. The event has run from February 2005 to the present. In the summer of 2006 ethnomusicology student Rob Szymanek joined the team as a Research Assistant (he had been in SMART the summer before where he did fieldwork for an MA in Ethnomusicology). Rob produced further field notes and conducted interviews with all the core members at SMART. In 2007, music therapist Sarah Wilson joined SMART to develop and expand the music project, which by then had become a joint practical and research project supported by SMART and Nordoff Robbins, called the *Chelsea Community Music Therapy Project* (later renamed the *SMART Music Project*). In the second year of the project 39 members of the SMART community were interviewed by Rob – both those who did and did not take part in the music group. In 2008 Gary did a second round of interviewing, this time with a smaller group of key participants in the project, people who had begun to be thought of as 'pathway cases'.

Also in the second year, Tia joined the research arm of the project, visiting as and when she could. (An application to the Economic and Social Research Council was rated well but never funded.) Around 2009 Gary and Tia began to conceive of the book project (a 'triptych') of which this book is Book Three, the central panel of the triptych.[2] Tia's role was occasional (Gary did all the work of setting things up and he did the lion's share of collecting the data; Sarah took over from Gary as the Music Therapist in 2008).[3]

In what follows, the main narrative 'voice' we use to tell the tale is primarily a mix of Gary, Tia, Sarah and Rob – but it is also supplemented with the voices of SMART members and staff, and other commentators at key moments. We hope to convey the ethnographic feel of SMART and its participants, changing over a long sweep of nearly 10 years. Alongside this we will weave into the mix as appropriate various theoretical and conceptual matters, but through the unfolding of the descriptive narrative, and from the point of view of how people and creative musical practices led to changes – mostly for the better – at SMART between 2005–14.[4] Our narrative strategy is to refrain from attempting to insert ourselves and our impressions too far forward, but instead to follow the actors as they engage with music, objects, each other and the SMART space to build collective culture and identity and thus to pave pathways away from illness, and its habits and trappings. This type of journey is, we want to emphasise, by no means confined to these people, to people in a hospital or to people living with mental health conditions. The continuum, or the 'being between' health and illness is one on which all of us stand as we experience, as Kathy Charmaz (1997) memorably put it, our 'Good Days/Bad Days'. We hope therefore that there will be relevance for anyone in the stories that follow of SMART and its continually evolving 'music of changes'.

***

---

[2] DeNora, Tia (2013). *Music Asylums: Wellbeing through Music in Everyday Life*. Farnham: Ashgate; Ansdell, Gary (2014). *How Music Helps: In Music Therapy & Everyday Life*. Farnham: Ashgate. The 'triptych' forms a series of volumes in the Ashgate series *Music & Change: Ecological Perspectives.*

[3] For more overtly theoretical perspectives on this same material see Ansdell and DeNora 2012; Ansdell 2014a; DeNora 2013.

[4] The main research project was between 2005–11, with the peak in data-gathering during 2007–10. The narrative includes, however, a final update on how the project has fared up to the present time.

Overall, we found how much a relationship to music was a key resource for many members in their everyday attempts to keep themselves (and each other) well. We also found that this small community needed more than a weekly open music session: it had different sub-groups who needed specific musical resources and musical help. Amelia, a new Director of the charity said that what she wanted was the active nurturing of a *musical community* at SMART. Sarah worked with great skill and sensitivity in the following years to realise this aim, creating two further musical groups and identities at SMART: *SMART Singers* – a smaller closed group who work at learning and performing songs, and *SMART Band* – made up of experienced players who are supported in jamming, rehearsing and doing gigs. The three aspects of the music project have proved to be organically related and self-supporting. SMART has indeed become amongst other things a vibrant musical community since 2005. The two smaller groups have provided music for SMART's in-house parties and events; and have also performed externally for other audiences.

One key aspect of the project is how it created an informal 'musical bridge' between the medical services just up the road in the psychiatric hospital, and SMART. Gary knows many of the people at SMART from his time working at the hospital (1999–2005), and Sarah has worked at the hospital site as well as at SMART since 2007. For ethical reasons, for this study and this book we will follow people in their musical pathways only within and beyond SMART (and where their paths included the medical site, we will only talk about them from the physical and symbolic door of medical services).[5] It will be increasingly apparent, however, that one of our key discoveries through this long-term engagement with the SMART musical community and particular people from it, is that music accompanies people in their pathways in recovery, between states of illness and health, and between sites of treatment, care and support in unique and valuable ways.

***

When Gary followed Bridget to SMART Music that day it turns out that Bridget is taking part for the second time. She was encouraged by Sarah to use her two hours daily leave from the ward at the psychiatric unit to come down to SMART and join the music group. As Gary sits at the piano that afternoon he occasionally glances towards this woman, and sees her gradually thaw, as she shares a songbook with Lucy, and begins to sing. Once she looks up and shares a wary smile with Gary as he somehow catches and acknowledges her enjoyment in the music. In the tea-break Gary talks with Bridget, and she tells him that she's recently been overwhelmed with anxiety and agoraphobia, and had to be taken into hospital. Music therapy in the hospital was one of the few things there that had made her feel human again, but she'd been nervous about coming to SMART as any group

---

[5] For further details of our decision about method and ethics in regard to the research arm of this project see Appendix A.

of people usually terrifies her: 'What if I burst into tears in Starbucks?' she says. 'But here I feel I could, and nobody would mind'. She'd been relieved to find last week how friendly and informal the group was, and she'd come back today. 'It helps' she says.

***

Bridget's story here stands for many similar tales we report in this book, and for an overall pattern that our research has suggested for how music helps many people with mental health problems to start, develop and follow-through *musical pathways* – in both modest or profound ways. At one level Bridget traced a very simple pathway: from the corridor of the mental health facility to the conviviality and support of SMART Music. But more symbolically she also traced a pathway between being a patient ('make sure you're back by 4!') within a medical-model treatment where her primary identity is an illness identity, to a setting and event where her potential and actual health-identity is recognised, nurtured and celebrated through musicking.

Thus Gary followed Bridget in a real and concrete way that day: over just 20 metres and three minutes – and yet he witnessed modest yet real transformations in her physical, social and psychological being. This tactic of following, witnessing and then engaging-with through listening, attending-to, understanding and making sense of someone's experience is an exemplar of the larger research enterprise that is presented in this book. We (Gary, Tia, Sarah, Rob) have followed, traced and tried to faithfully represent the varying musical pathways of many individuals, group and occasions in this musical community. Sometimes these pathways extend over many years (up to 10 years to date), and over many different sites and circumstances. Pathways are often complex: they extend and lead onwards, but also sometimes turn back on themselves, get tangled and knotted, and in doing so encompass the full range of life in all of its joy, sorrow, conflict and courage. But whatever scale these musical pathways have covered, there are we think some key understandings that they communicate as a whole about the complex but vital inter-relationships between people, music, places, health states, wellbeing and the potential for 'musical flourishing' within challenging times and situations. They help illuminate what mental health can be; and how music can help in cultivating and supporting it.

Our research approach – 'gentle empiricism' – and the data[6]

As we write this book, the role of the arts in healthcare is coming under increasing scrutiny. We have described this change, and our responses to it, in other work, and in the two books of the 'triptych' that are associated with this one (Ansdell 2014; DeNora 2013a). We have outlined our respective understandings of 'delicate' or 'gentle' empiricism, an approach first outlined by Goethe in his scientific work (Ansdell and Pavlicivec 2010), and we have engaged in some of the ongoing debates over what counts as 'evidence' or 'effectiveness' of the arts in healthcare situations. We do not intend to rehearse those arguments all over again here. What we do want to do, however, is to hold our project work up to the mirror of prominent work that has sought to provide standards of 'rigour' in qualitative research in healthcare settings. In fact, we believe that qualitative research, and in particular the intimate form of enquiry otherwise known as ethnographic research, offers a very rigorous mode of knowing because it is the method most closely associated with ecological validity, with insuring that what is asserted is not only reliable (generalisable) and valid (correctly describing the phenomenon) but also the most truly representative of research participants' behaviours, interpretive practices and accounts offered in their everyday lives (DeNora 2013b). We have sought, in other words, to describe how music featured in our respondents' daily experience longitudinally across time, and how they used and related to music on their own, and on music's, terms. Thus we hope that the 'musical portraits' we offer below will bear strong resemblance to what was, and is still happening at SMART and among these music makers.

As we have mentioned, the research arm of the SMART Music project ran from 2006–11. The research team consisted of Gary, Tia, Sarah (who kept diaries for two years of her time working as the music therapist at SMART) and Rob (all described above). The aim was to document and develop a grounded theory of how music helps SMART participants – and mental health clients more generally – to create pathways away from illness. How does music offer resources for and encourage wellbeing, personal and social development, symptom management and – in a most general sense, flourishing? (Ansdell & DeNora 2012).

During the main six years of data collection, we gathered:

- 20 volumes (1500 pages) of **logs** of detailed field notes and analytic memos. These represented 200+ SMART Music Sessions, including Sarah's detailed logs of SMART Singers and SMART Band during 2007/8, with accounts of musical events. This data was reduced in 2013 to an analytic summary of 236 pages and was also coded according to the principles of modified grounded theory and its focus on emerging and recurring themes.
- 29 **interviews** (2006), with a further nine interviews of 'pathway people' (2010), also reduced to analytic summaries (2013).
- **audio-visual data** consisted of: more than 50 complete audio recordings of SMART Music Sessions (2005–11); four films of whole sessions and occasional

[6] See Appendix 1 for a more detailed account of method.

filming of events. A DVD compilation of audio/visual material was made with SMART members themselves in 2010.

The researchers also held informal conversations with staff, SMART members and others (visiting music therapists, other visitors, visiting staff from the hospital) who came into contact with SMART Music. They also discussed the data at academic and clinical seminars, with SMART's Chief Executive, the senior Consultant Psychiatrist attached to the Mental Health Facility and other music therapists at Nordoff Robbins. Gary and Tia have presented many aspects of the project (scrupulously anonymised) at a wide range of conferences, symposia and seminars.

In what follows we will draw upon the data liberally with the primary aim of sharing our findings and, simultaneously, our methods of data collection with readers, SMART members and ourselves. Our aim is to mostly 'show not tell', by which we mean that we hope the documentary materials will let you see what we saw, but not because you have to 'take our word for it'. Accordingly, the aim is to remain grounded, to ensure that our theoretical accounts take shape through the medium of specific examples, and to allow the stories offered to refract back on to the theoretical and conceptual frameworks that we offer in the two 'side panels' of our overall 'triptych' project on music, health and wellbeing. This central panel picturing the SMART Music Project is – as we hope to make very clear – 'where the action is'.

2. An Ethical Moment

There's a particular moment – an 'ethical moment' – when it becomes clear what it really is to study a project like this, at this place, with these people, and its relationship to the conventions and protocols of ethical scrutiny of research projects as currently understood at institutional and statutory levels. Several such moments happened fairly regularly during our time participating in, and studying, this project. They illustrate the particular dilemmas we faced and the ways we've tried to work creatively with them:

> Jeremy has his pen poised to sign the consent form for his second interview. But he hesitates, and looks distressed. Gary is puzzled – he's known Jeremy for many years, has his trust, and knows that Jeremy is supportive of the practical and research project overall, and wants to participate by sharing his views. Gary suggests that they stop and asks Jeremy what's happening. Embarrassed, Jeremy says that he suddenly had a flash-back as he was signing – to about 25 years ago when he was consenting to ECT. It had not been a good experience for him then ...

***

At the end of the main data-gathering phase Gary returns to SMART to do a final check so that the key participants know what will be happening in the final phase of this project: that the practical work will continue, but Gary and Tia will stop gathering data, and will now start the writing-up phase, then return to them for agreement on any specific material we use. Since the beginning of the project we've carefully informed members of SMART what the research arm of the project is, and what we're doing. With SMART Chief Executive Amelia, Gary and others have run public information sessions, and countless more individual briefings with those people who've turned out to be 'key informants' (who we call 'pathway cases'). This process has been (we think) scrupulous. People have received written participation information sheets, signed consent forms for interviews and use of material. We have a basic confidence that we've done our best, both formally, in terms of following the usual – and in this case intricate – procedures of 'informed consent', but also because we've tried to respect people's right to know what we're doing in real time, to recognise, and negotiate, any areas of discomfort. But, as we've often found, it's more complicated than simply being 'procedural'.

***

> Today I sit at a table and have coffee with three of the key participants, who have been involved since the beginning of the project. I tell them that the next week I'm doing a talk on how we've managed the research ethics of this project. '*What* research ethics?' says one of the members. I'm slightly stunned at this question, but luckily the other members prompt him. 'You know', they say, 'when Gary gets us to sign those forms, and you remember that talk about the project ... ?'. The other member looks a bit embarrassed, and says to me 'I'm sorry, I forget so much these days – it's the medication.' So I start again with the research ethics agenda, right then and there – five years after we first mentioned it – trying to tell these SMART members what we're doing, how, and why ... (Gary, Field-note Log, 21 July 2011)

These 'ethical moments' exemplified something of the true nature of trying to do 'good research' in somewhere like SMART over a long period of time, with some people who are experiencing more than most of us transitions in their mental states and cognitive powers, and for whom there are charged and idiosyncratic meanings attached to seemingly innocent institutional protocols. There were also events within the more formal process (the information meetings, negotiating consent) where confusions, conflicts, resolutions and new understandings were naturally part of the process. And indeed, this 'mess' as John Law (2004) calls it, is not dissimilar to what fieldwork in any setting is like – there are ethical moments to be grappled with anywhere, if we are willing to recognise them (our tick-box culture often directs our attention away from these forms of complexity).

Raymond Tallis (2013) writes of the 'messy ethics' of any clinical practice, where it's almost *always* a case of deciding what's best (rather than necessarily what's *good*, per se), and of arriving at a workable conclusion only through sometimes difficult consultation, negotiation and instinct. Overall the 'ethical moments' involved in our SMART research brought to our attention in vivid, and often uncomfortable, ways the true complexity of researching the project in honest but fair ways. It was not research *on* the project, because we too were part *of* the community after these years of immersion. Research, and its ethical dimensions is not, then, just a formal, procedural, institutional process – but also a practical-social process that is, and must be, negotiated face-to-face, in real-time and real-place, with us together; doing justice to the thing we're trying to understand together, and ensuring that we do justice to each other, and to the community as a whole.[7]

3. Eloise's Cymbal/Symbol

There is a regular to-and-fro between the hospital site and SMART. Different times of day, or day or week, people are on leave from the wards (as with Bridget, in the preceding pages), or visiting the wards (Gary and later Sarah, the part-time Music Therapists, Tia tagging along for special events held in the hospital), or else people on leave from the wards, heading 'back' after a few hours in the community. And as with people, objects also migrate.

Each week for the first few years setting up for SMART Music Sessions meant fetching and moving things between the hospital and SMART sites. This included songbooks (compilations of lyrics from frequently performed numbers, and colour-coded red, blue and yellow); a miscellaneous collection of percussion instruments such as shakers, tambourines and rattles (a giant beanpod, dried gourds ...), and a collection of more 'conventional' instruments such as two djembe, electric guitar and bass, and a small suspended crash cymbal.

As it happens, it is this cymbal that Tia carries over to the SMART basement on her first ever visit to the site in May 2006. As she enters SMART someone directs her to the front of the room. The cymbal goes *there*, just opposite the white, upright piano. The room is furnished with cafe-style tables and chairs that are arranged to face the front of the room – the improvised 'stage' area – which is where the piano and a microphone (for the singing of solo numbers) are positioned. As Tia sorts out the cymbal, a bit fiddly at first, someone else offers her a bit of instruction, but also a gentle word of caution – *Don't sit there, don't play that cymbal – that's Eloise's.* Eloise sits there and that's her instrument.

A model for a firm of haute couturier in her youth, now in her late sixties, Eloise exudes a certain, distinctly British, style. At SMART, with her grey hair pulled off her face by an Alice band, she is usually wearing (more on this below) a countrified woollen skirt and a quilted gilet. She looks, in fact, exactly like what she is – a lady of the gentry who married into the aristocracy. Perhaps she'd played an instrument

---

7 See Appendix B for a more detailed account of research ethics in relation to this project and book.

earlier in life, but here at SMART Eloise seldom sings, and always refuses to 'do a performance' by herself up at the mic. Instead she contributes entirely through this cymbal, both peripheral (just a bit of percussion, not requiring too much musical skill or even dexterity) but central too (right up in front and a visually conspicuous instrument). She animates the front row with a form of musical participation that is rich and varied, witty and exuberant.

This unusual performance builds during the early years of the project, and culminates many years later, triumphantly. From the first time that Gary's logbook mentions Eloise playing the cymbal, throughout this session in May 2006, and into the five following years that Eloise participated in SMART, Eloise's unique participation, with the cymbal and with SMART, undergoes change. This change comes about through many small adjustments and all of these take *time*. Time to develop, time to cultivate, time to become a staple feature of group musicking, time to become an iconic part of Eloise's identity at SMART. Within this long durée the many small steps draw Eloise closer into the web of collective culture at SMART and, of course, this drawing-in simultaneously allows Eloise to help make that culture, to furnish it with her signature way of being, her musical tastes and loves, her sensibilities.

For example, Gary's log reports on a musical conversation where mutual tastes are being discussed outside of the actual music making ('June 1, 2006: Rob and Eloise – musical exchange, they are beginning to swap CDs of African music – see Rob's field notes.'). So too, a certain amount of tinkering with musical 'mechanics' occurs, and it sets in motion a chain of social, musical and physical transformations – *in relation to the cymbal*. Initially, Eloise uses a drumstick to hit the cymbal, but this is too loud and conspicuous for Eloise, too domineering in the blend with other instruments in the group. Eloise has to take care not to play with too much force and this in turn constrains the physical strength that she could deploy while at her instrument. The next week when setting up, Gary substitutes a jazz brush for the drumstick, and the 'problem' is solved, the possibilities for physical exertion expanded. This freedom in turn allows Eloise to be more playful, more gesturally expressive within her playing. And with this her career as a musician within SMART is launched.

'Musical things' – the material culture of musicking

One of the findings of this project is how important 'musical things' are in relation to 'musical people' and 'musical situations'. Studies of music therapy have previously tended to overlook the importance of the material culture of social musicking (unless this was especially technical – such as adapted instruments for people with limited movement). Our observation, rather, was that the success and direction of the musicking in the SMART project was highly mediated by a range of very material facts concerning musical instruments and their ancillary aspects, such as sticks; scores and texts; notebooks; CDs; recordings and so on. These were not aspects to be glossed over as we rush to understand the 'real music'. Rather, these things – in what they afforded, and how they could be appropriated by people within this setting – actually *made* the musicking, and its success (or not) on a personal and social level.

Examples of such 'musical things' in action include:

– what instruments people can play, and play with others; which are personal or shared, etc.
– the sonic affordances of different instruments and technologies – wired and unwired guitars, drums, microphones & amplifiers, the playability of small percussion instruments, etc.
– supporting materials – music, lyrics, props, paraphenalia, costumes etc.

You will find further sections focus in on this subject as the story unfolds ...

By 2007 we find Gary noting in Book IV of his field-note log:

> Eloise – really going for her cymbal-playing: there is noticeable and genuine development in how she interacts with this instrument in relation to the music and the musicking situations. It mediates her participation. (Gary, Field-note Log, March 22, 2007)

Over the years this cymbal playing develops further: in intensity, rhythmic complexity and sheer uninhibited participation. It is not just Gary and Sarah who notice this development. Other members of the SMART Music group also comment on Eloise's emergent musicality. 'One person I love to see every time is Eloise', says Simon, who has worked as a professional musician – 'because she's so focused, and her timing's marvellous, and you can see here's a person who is extremely ordered in her life. Not a controlled order, but you can see the order in her life, and the pleasure she gets from just doing it, it's great to see that'.

In this way Eloise and her cymbal fuse together in SMART Music – both within a single session, and over time: as image of the 'musical Eloise', but also as carrier of certain personality traits and values – an exemplar of aspects to admire, but also a simple but confident musical voice contributing something key to the whole. This person-instrument identity becomes increasingly faceted over time, as Eloise and her cymbal come to be attached to myriad qualities in ways that afford yet more points for connection with others – through reference to Eloise's past, here-and-now in the collective culture of SMART, and between Eloise and other SMART members. For example:

> Sarah notices her relationship with this instrument, and the Tibetan gown she's wearing today seem to go with this persona. At one point she plays the cymbal with two guys on the drums – 'beautiful, natural if bizarre scenario' says Sarah. (Gary, Field-note Log, March 15, 2007)

***

> Bobby tells Lady Eloise that her new haircut looks good, and she gives him a toothy grin. In the front row they make the most incongruous pair – he a skilled soul drummer; she, with a cymbal & beater, an enthusiastic amateur. Yet there she is making increasingly gleeful sounds during the Blues – what unexpected participation! (Gary, Field-note Log, November 22, 2007)

***

One day Eloise shows Gary with pleasure that the cymbal she's playing was made in Turkey, which leads her to reminisce about her travels there, the music there, the ecstasy of the 'whirling dervishes'. Gary's notes of sessions over the years often note a recurrent moment when, as he plays piano during a musical item he looks over to Eloise on the front row playing this instrument – and catches a look of pure glee on her face. She's caught up in the on-going excitement of the music, but more than this, in her own ecstatic *participation* in this flow, through her vigorous beating of the cymbal – in time, or slightly out of time with the music. Sometimes he sees her trying to inhibit this response, as if it's unseemly! Gary writes in his log that he's seldom seen anyone so transported by music. A photograph shows Eloise at this period caught in full flow, with the metallic brush about to sweep downwards towards the cymbal. This elderly, seemingly sophisticated lady in a headscarf (reminiscent of the Queen at Balmoral) is orientated towards three other players in the ensemble that afternoon, playing a jazz number: a pianist, a singer standing up and also in full flight, and a seated guitarist.

***

For a period of about six weeks in 2012 Eloise is ill. The cymbal is brought out weekly and put in its precise and habitual place, just in front of a chair on the front row of the cafe, just behind the back of the piano. On the cymbal rests the jazz brush. During these weeks the cymbal stands for a particular person's long-term participation in SMART Music, her unvarying place in the cafe, and her unvarying vehicle for participating in the on-going music. It reminds people of her absence, through this strong reminder of her presence.

When Eloise dies shortly afterwards, this cymbal is not brought out again in this way. There is no overt discussion of this; it's simply that her musical voice is no longer there, and for the time being this instrument can't be anyone else's voice. But when an afternoon of SMART Music is dedicated to Eloise a month later, many people mention her cymbal playing, and the vigour of her commitment to being in and amongst the music that this small instrument conveys to everyone. Eloise is remembered fondly in full ecstatic flow as she vigorously beats the small cymbal to the rock 'n roll being played by nearby guitars, piano and drums.

***

Before Gary leaves for a sabbatical during the autumn of 2011 Eloise beckons him over after a SMART Music Session:

> Eloise says she wants me to know before I go 'I've not had mental lapse ... *or a drink* ... for 10 years now, and a major part of that is the benefit of music therapy!'. She is adamant about this, keeping saying 'I really *mean that*, I need you to understand that ... '. Like Jeremy, Mary and some others, I've known Eloise for over 10 years now, and followed her musical pathway from one-to-one in Willow, to the Willow MT group, to SMART Music. Hers has been a rich musical pathway, and one that I've shared too ... (Gary, Field-note Log, 21 July 2011)

On the voice recognition software Gary uses to transcribe the mass of session logs, 'cymbal' comes out as 'symbol'. A little mistake, but it anticipates so much of the story we tell here. For participants in SMART – service users, staff, music therapists, researchers – music both enacts *and* stands for many things: it can mediate identity, offer materials and modes for transformation, transport, transfiguration, transcendence; it can bridge the distance – social, age, illness – between people, and give them experiences and stories to share together. The story of the SMART Music project over 10 years is a tale of how music can be a profound agent of change. How this happens and with what consequences, and how the processes involved are inevitably collective, holistic, *ecological*, is a complex story of musical people, music things and musical situations coming together.

4. SMART the Place, its Values and Resources

SMART's philosophy, as conveyed by its web page

The people at SMART are a democratic bunch so we all sat down together some time ago and decided what our 'core values' would be. These are the things we believe in, that underpin everything we do. In the end we decided to base them on the *Institute For Compassion and Wisdom, 16 Guidelines for a Happy Life:*

We try to think with . . .

- Humility
- Patience
- Contentment
- Delight

We try to act with . . .

- Kindness
- Honesty
- Generosity
- Right Speech

We try to relate to others with . . .

- Respect
- Forgiveness
- Gratitude
- Loyalty

We try to find meaning with . . .

- Aspiration
- Principles
- Service
- Courage

We also believe in good cake with good coffee; flossing our teeth regularly; trying to deal with life's ups and down with good humour; and that listening to/playing music at least once a week is good for your health.

You do not have to share our beliefs but we do ask that you respect them when you visit us.

There are various projects and opportunities for companionship on offer at SMART. IT skills training, floristry work experience, gardening, bridge building (to link to community activities and opportunities), fitness and football training, kitchen and serving skills and of course the cafe ('food is good for mental health'). There are also clubs (including a holiday club). There is a pharmacy help group and a mental health advocacy service. There is also an art group, and of course the three music groups: the original SMART afternoon session, open to anyone, whether SMART member and service user or member of the public, and, for members only, a rock band, *SMART Band,* and a choir, *SMART Singers*.

You have to go down a flight of stairs to get to the SMART basement (or use the stair lift). This is where the music happens.

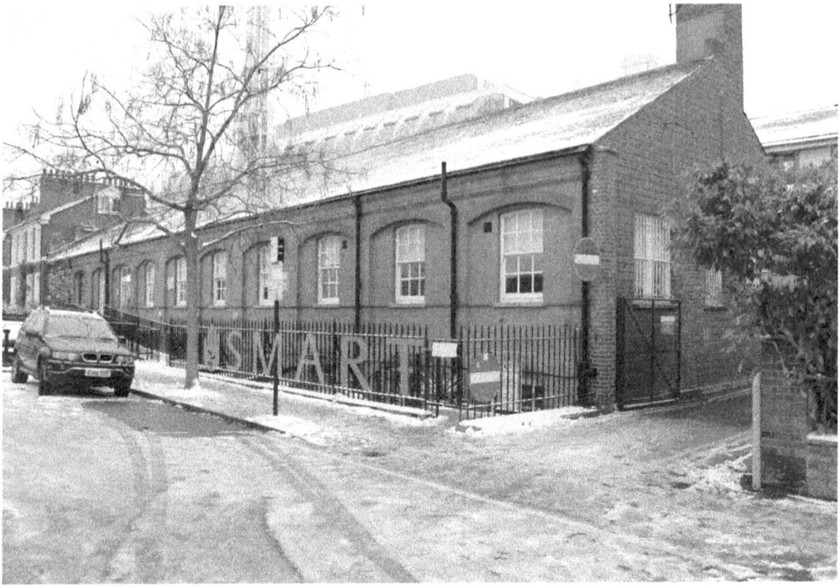

Figure 2 SMART from the outside

Immediately to the right are kitchens and, as you come into the SMART cafe and look directly across, there is a door out to the basement garden, sheltered partly by the walkway to the ground floor entrance to the floors above. Ever since smoking was banned at SMART in 2006, the garden is where to go if you want to smoke (or otherwise be a little distanced from the main cafe area). It's mainly men who hang out here (or in the back of the indoor space, coming and going to the outdoor area). Sometimes they are called in to perform a number or take part in a group performance when SMART Music is going. Sometimes they rebel and initiate their own music group in the smoker's area, the music clashing with the music inside for a few minutes.

At the back of the room is the cafe's serving area, with a SMART member who is on the catering programme behind the counter. There is usually a nice display of cakes and a blackboard to the right announces the day's specials ('Spaghetti Bolognese, with or without meat'). It's common, on a SMART Music day, for members to come early and eat, then set up for the group at 2pm.

Within the main space of SMART, the cafe tables are arranged in rows, three or four to a row, five or six rows. At the front, and pushed toward the wall when not in use, is an upright white piano – which has migrated from a nightclub to the hospital site (where the underfloor heating was cracking it) to here. Off to the

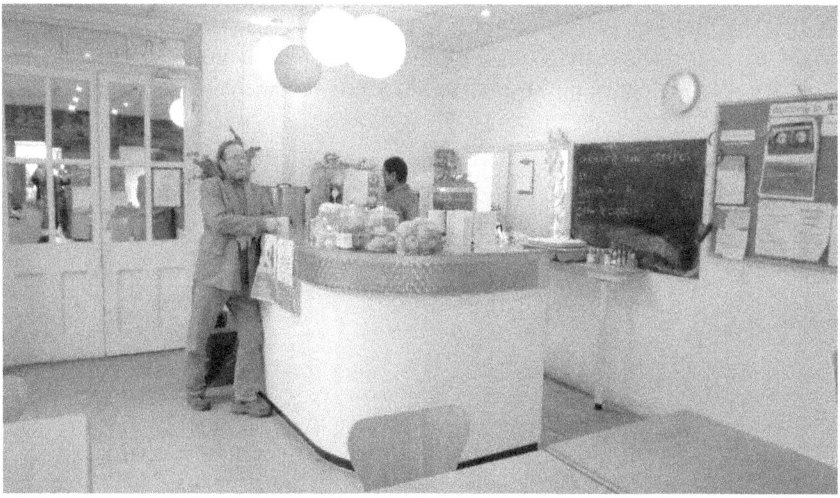

Figure 3 SMART cafe

right of the piano is a small office with a transparent door. This is where Amelia, SMART's Chief Executive works. To the left is a hallway off to the left with more offices and toilet facilities:

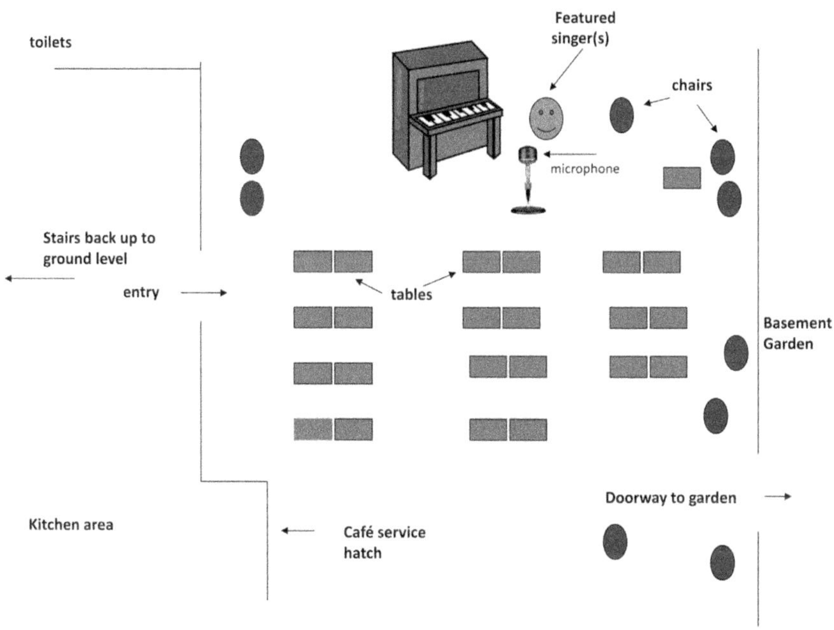

Figure 4 SMART cafe topography for music afternoons

During the first year setting up for a SMART Music Session meant hauling the boxes of instruments, songbooks, electronic equipment and other instruments from the second floor of the hospital to SMART's basement.

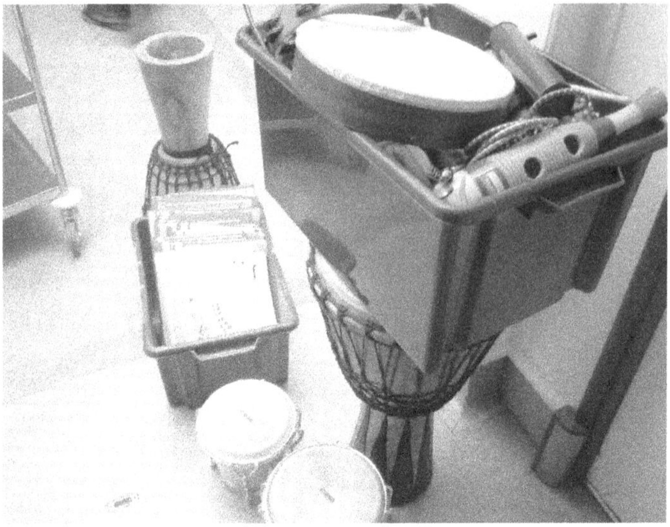

Figure 5 Musical things

In 2007 SMART invested in its own set of instruments, to which participants add their own. The piano is turned to face the group, the mic set up alongside it, and the music books (more about these later), red, yellow and blue, are distributed. Then the tables are set, not for dining but with a good selection of shakers, beaters, rattles and tambourines – ready for people to pick up casually as they sip their tea. An instrument just happens to be there, waiting for a hand to tap or shake it …

5. Barbara's Tambourine

A tambourine sits nicely on a table, alongside a cup of tea and piece of cake; it can be picked up and angled to play with one hand. It's not too loud, nor too soft; it's not too exact, or too vague in its sound. Barbara weekly selects this tambourine to place on a table about three rows back by the window. Next to her Kathleen sits with another small (but more variable) percussion instrument – a shaker usually. Barbara and Kathleen are old school friends now in their 70s, affectionately known as 'the ladies' by other SMART members (and in log notes). They met another elderly member, Peggy, in the next door general hospital, and she invited them down the next Thursday for tea and music. They've all become regulars at SMART, coming every week. None has a diagnosed mental health problem, though their own needs surface as the years go by – isolation, and for Barbara, early onset dementia of a particular kind. They come as 'members of the public' who find their own place and purpose within this unusual musical community.

The ladies will sing the songs they know (though resolutely staying at their table – never coming up to sing at the front). They look mildly disapproving of more modern songs, and will seldom suggest songs to sing. But it would be wrong to say, that they don't much participate. While their participation is 'peripheral' (they sit unobtrusively to the side at their habitual 'station'), Tia notes (from her own even more peripheral position over on the other side of the cafe) that these women have their own way of being active: over the years, that activity takes the form of what might be termed musical micro-gesture which in its way is as important – to the ladies, to the group – as any of the more overt forms of solo singing at SMART. The latency of this micro-musical conduct is developed by Gary and by Sarah. It consists of noticing individuals' musical gestures, contributions and – perhaps – wishes and acknowledging these within-and-through their own playing. So initially, and perhaps generally imperceptible, gestures are amplified by the two music therapists as part of the on-going musical flow. For example, just adjusting to the timing or the timbre of Barbara's tambourine playing for a brief phrase catches the connection between her and the on-going music – which Barbara will notice (perhaps in her hands first?) and look up and smile at Gary. When this happens, Barbara is knitted more explicitly (audio-visually) into the collective musicking. Increasingly she does the same to Gary – she searches out his personal and musical attention – *Hey, Gary, do you notice me, and what I'm playing here?* – and again there's recognition, contact and connection between her part and the musical/social whole.

A film catches this scenario, when Arnold films a SMART Music afternoon when Sarah's *Musical Minds* group visit from the East End. One of the fleeting shots of the 'hinterland' of the musical scene catches Barbara tapping her tambourine in time to the song whilst dreamily looking out of the adjacent window. Where is she then? In the music? In her thoughts and memories? Who is she with then? It's difficult to say, and perhaps the answer is multiple: she's in and out of time; in and out of space ... But she's also very much *in the music* in her own way ...

6. Mary and Her Guitar

Sometimes the tale of an instrument is more about absence than presence. Mary reminds Gary of the interview she did with him when she was an inpatient in the hospital next door, more than a decade ago in 1999. She describes how, in her early days of music therapy, she'd learned guitar as a young woman, but then smashed it during an episode of illness. Music had always been helpful to her, she says, in keeping her stable and happy, but suddenly she found herself cut off from music and its help. Music therapy in the hospital had helped her re-find how music helps her, in sickness and in health. After one stay in hospital when she'd had individual music therapy sessions Gary interviews Mary as part of a research study of what benefits people find from music therapy in an in-patient mental health setting[8]:

> **Interviewer:** Why do you keep coming back to music therapy sessions?
>
> **Mary:** Because I thoroughly enjoy it! I can express myself, I can get up to those high notes ... and I love music ... I used to play the guitar ... but when I was ill I smashed my guitar to pieces ... but you brought out my music again ... playing the percussion instruments, singing ... When I first came in to hospital I'd lost my voice completely, all I could do was whistle ... I love singing with the choir too ...
>
> **Interviewer:** What do you feel after a music therapy session?
>
> **Mary:** It's a good feeling ... a spiritual feeling ... it helps me to concentrate on something, not to hear silly voices in my head that don't belong to me. It also helps relax me, and give me an incentive to come here. It's so enjoyable!

Mary reminds Gary that when they first worked together in the hospital she'd lost her voice. She could only whistle. Gary had suggested they work then on Stephen Sondheim's song *Anyone Can Whistle.* It's not long before her voice comes back again, and she performs this song at a Mayday concert in the hospital – an event that she quotes for the next decade as somehow emblematic of her recovery. For Mary, that difference could then be narrated, laid down in the form of a music-health-illness narrative, a tale of progress through music.

How does music therapy help someone like Mary?

Through respective accounts of *communicative musicality*, Malloch and Trevarthen (2009) and Ansdell (2014) have described our innate and natural psychobiological capacity for responding to music. This response-ability facilitates communication and relationship, allowing for the sense of shared situation. It is also the bedrock of skills-based musicianship, the scaffold of the various forms of social musicking in which we take part. Illness can interfere with this capacity of communicative musicality, but equally it can be 'repaired' through careful music-therapeutic work, and then by access to situations where social musicking brings people back into music, and musical communication again.

Two particular episodes in Mary's music therapy at this time became key examples for an interdisciplinary research project that Gary did with a psychiatrist, music psychologist and two other music therapists – looking at how communicative musicality and affect modulation relate. The following vignettes illustrate how music

[8] Ansdell and Meehan (2010).

within a therapeutic context can promote contact and relationship even within severe illness states, and how it can help to shift away from unwanted states of affect:

Pam [Mary] hits the xylophone hard with the beaters and throws them towards the piano, which they hit, causing the piano strings to vibrate. She shouts 'This fucking life!' and becomes very upset. (The therapist [Gary Ansdell] later finds out that the outburst was caused by her seeing the letter names on the xylophone spelling out abusive messages to her from an internal voice). Immediately after the blow-up the therapist encourages Pam to come to the piano, to sit beside him, and encourages her back into musical engagement again. She begins playing a few notes on the top of the piano, which leads into a short piano duet and then into shared singing with the therapist. Pam takes over the singing herself after a short time (accompanied by the therapist on the piano), becoming involved and expressive. The music seems to take her somewhere else. After the music cadences she sighs and says 'That's better!' The entire episode has lasted just over four minutes.

A week later there's another key episode in Pam's [Mary's] therapy – this time it lasts two minutes and 40 seconds. Pam is 'high' and tells the therapist how uncomfortable and irritable she feels. A sung duet between Pam and the therapist sounds like a speeded-up cabaret item, including a rapid to-and-fro sung dialogue with Blues singing and yodeling. Within the dialogue the therapist nevertheless manages to 'sculpt' the musical interaction such that the duo both go 'up' together, but somehow 'land safely'. In the last phrase Pam's voice softens and relaxes as she cadences – somehow music and person have been modulated together. In clinical presentations of this and other similar examples of music therapy with people in psychotic states, colleagues have generously commented that few other interventions would manage this rapid modulation of such volatile affective episodes, and in a way that is humanly satisfying to the patient. How is music (through music therapy) able to achieve this? What does this tell us about the need for, and the potential of, music therapy within mental health provision – especially for patients experiencing psychotic states of mind? (Ansdell et al. 2010: 4–5)

This research explored music therapy in a traditional one-to-one format, held in a private room. This is something that some patients with severe mental health problems sometimes need at certain stages of their illness. But often they need something more and different from music and music therapy when on a later path to recovery, where the emphasis is on re-finding their place within the community, and then accessing and re-building social and cultural resources to keep them well. The Community Music Therapy movement has tried to broaden the possibilities of music therapy, creating musical opportunities that are more social and closer to everyday musical experiences (Ansdell 2002, 2014; Pavlicevic & Ansdell 2004; Stige & Aarø 2012; Wood 2016). But often these experiences importantly connect to what has gone before, in more intimate music therapy formats:

> Mary sings *Anyone can Whistle* in front of the group today – a symbolic song from her one-to-one music therapy in the hospital, six years ago. She's still able to sing it. I think of the continuity from those sessions into the new context here at SMART. Mary's position in SMART Music is interesting – neither core, nor peripheral – very much of her own choosing. (Gary, Field-note Log, 28 Sept 2005)

Mary's musical activities take her on a pathway from traditional music therapy to the Community Music Therapy model that the Chelsea Project represents. Partly this is also because Mary is increasingly able to locate her own health-promoting musical resources, one of these being attending SMART Music Sessions once they get going in 2006. Mary can be seen during this period as an exemplary 'pathway case study' for the SMART Music project and its associated research arm. Partly because Gary has known her as a music therapist for so long, but also partly because, rather like Eloise (described earlier) the relationship between Mary's musical participation and her wellbeing is so clear. Mary describes her musical participation as the litmus test of her wellbeing. In real time, as we have already described with the emblem of *Anyone Can Whistle*, her musicking provides a platform for mini-narratives about her progress (her, 'that's better', after four minutes of musicking which places a cap on the musical proceedings). These narratives can function as partial scripts, reminders of how and where things are going, definitions of the situation. They are resources by which pathways away from illness are laid down and Mary is one of the people we will describe who help us to define and illustrate the notion of 'musical pathways'. As with Eloise and her drumstick/brush, we find Mary moving from musical moment-to-moment, step-by-step along a musical pathway that involves many small changes that refurnish the spaces and fields of real-time action.

Elsewhere (DeNora 2013b), Tia has described some of the minute shifts that led up to Mary's 'That's better' which we described above. Those shifts include the move from xylophone to keyboard (and all the cultural connotations associated with each of these instruments), a physical repositioning (sitting together at the piano, facing in the same direction, companionably and in a way where both are using the 'same' musical resources). So too, at SMART, as Mary recovers and lives successfully if precariously in the community, she takes part in SMART Music, and the SMART Singers – and when she occasionally gets re-admitted to hospital she re-joins Sarah's music therapy group there. There's a thread of Mary using music to perform both her health and her sickness, but also of her using music, and musical helpers (in the form of music therapists, music therapy groups and other resources) to pave a path between physical locations, and states of illness and health over the years. Where Mary goes, so goes her music. Early on in their project work together, Gary described to Tia how he could predict, from the way that Mary sang, whether she was becoming 'ill' again (an over-elaboration of the melodic line and a pressure in the voice being the musical 'symptoms').

In this on-going work – for musical work it indeed is at times for Mary – she attaches strongly to particular favourite songs, and these become firmly identified with Mary the person, but also Mary the performer – whose fragile performances are signs of ability, resilience, hope and triumph over adversity. *Memory, Annie's Song, Anyone Can Whistle, Any Dream will Do* ... these are dependable musical things that Mary attaches to and makes her own. She transports them to different situations within this network and community, and each time they are both the same and different. Every time they seem to accomplish something for Mary, and are powerful for others, showing how music works 'in circulation' within the present and the past for people at any given time in this musical-social situation. It is not the music 'itself' that does this work for Mary (e.g. the song *Any Dream Will Do* ...) but rather it is the work – emotional work, memory work, social work, embodied work, musical-interpretive work – Mary does with these songs, which is what allows the songs to 'do for' Mary. There is in other words Mary's *investment* in music that empowers it to act 'on' her in ways that are health-giving.

But sometimes, for some people at SMART, this investment comes at too great a cost:

> I say to Peggy 'sometimes music is really ambivalent for people – they love it, but it's also difficult for them because of how powerful it's been in their lives – the memories, and history they have with it'. I say this partly also for Simon to overhear, and I see him tacitly acknowledge this. Peggy talks about how certain songs are very sad for her, especially *Memory* from Cats, 'It reminds me of my old boy – that was our song when he was very ill – we'd dance a bit to that'. She says how it sometimes upsets her when Mary sings this song at SMART – 'but that's all right ... my memories are important too ... '. So again, this emotional ambivalence that music brings – positive sadness etc.
>
> Spookily on cue Mary chooses just this song today, and I see Peggy get up and rush to the back and burst into tears. Sarah comforts her. It's clear that the usual reaction has been exacerbated by the conversation we had earlier. Things are fine five minutes later and Peggy is smiling, dancing, re-engaged, her mood having moved on. So it doesn't seem a negative experience overall, just part of exactly that potent involvement of music, memory, and people.
> (Gary, Field-note Log, 21 July 2011)

***

Gary asks Mary whether he can show a short video of one of her triumphant performances singing at SMART Music at an upcoming mental health conference he's speaking at. 'Will there be psychiatrists there?' she asks. 'In that case, *yes,* you tell 'em that music therapy works!'.

Mary increasingly uses her songs for a variety of purposes: to show people how she is, to achieve something, to dedicate her thoughts to other people who are ill; and then one day to indicate her love for Tim, another SMART member with whom she's started a relationship. Mary and Tim sing a duet to show this to others. Paradoxically, as Mary's mental health gets more stable her physical health declines (perhaps with the impact of 30 years of antipsychotic medication?). She's unable to get to the group for three weeks, but decides to do some music therapy at home for herself and Tim. She gets her guitar out (she's not told us that she's taken this up again), and plays and sings *Greensleeves*. She leaves a message on the hospital answerphone telling Sarah this. It turns out that this is the night she dies. Sarah hears the message a day later. Tim confirms the guitar story.

We would like to say that this tale has something of a mythological resonance for us: Orpheus and his lute – bringing a kind of musical enchantment into the darkest corners. Mary and her guitar, reunited at the end. We know that probably seems over-dramatic, but the facts of the case through the tracing of Mary's pathway show us precisely this trajectory: Mary, who in her darkest hours cast aside music, then re-connects with music, literally embracing it – in the shape of her guitar – in her final weeks of life. *'Now farewell, adieu / To God I pray to prosper thee / For I am still thy lover true / Come once again and love me'* runs the final verse of Mary's last song, *Greensleeves*.

7. Researching Musical Pathways

These three opening stories – Eloise's, Barbara's and Mary's – are key examples of what we're calling 'musical pathways' in this book. These pathways are, we will argue, the main significant outcome of how music helps people in this place, through this project.

People in the SMART community varied in their attitude to our research. We were scrupulous in regard to research ethics: consulting, informing, getting consent and generally reassuring people. But some of the research participants had previous uncomfortable experiences with medical research, and many of the participants experienced variations in their mental conditions. And so, as we described earlier (in 'The ethical moment') there were occasional troubles with informed consent, when some participants sometimes felt unease or suspicion, or simply forgot there was a research project, or what this project was about. On the whole, however, SMART members were only too happy for us to take interest in their passion for music and its helping effects, and they actively wanted us to promote something which most found to be a good thing for SMART and its community as a whole. The rhetoric of the evidence-based movement has filtered down thoroughly now, so people know that without 'the evidence' current services may be vulnerable, and new ones not commissioned.

The occasional person such as Roger had more specific advice to us about what research should be in relation to the music project:

Roger on research

The important thing about research ... When I had a car and I used to work on it myself ... there's the thing about doing everything in a rush ... spark-plugs, points, carburetor ... and then you fix it ... but sometimes you don't know which bit you've fixed! So when you want to replicate ... to learn from failures, when things don't go right ... So the music's important because everybody has an emotional content ... but this needs ideally mixing with the intellectual content and working out why. I think it's a great shame that health, and mental health in particular ... there's a lot of talk about preventative measures, and lots of talk about outcomes, measuring outcomes ... but they *don't* really get measured when you look closely ... But this *does* do a small bit, this project ...
And taking part itself is therapeutic! So there will be roughs and smooths ... Because it would be folly for us to presume that there's knowledge out there, and we can obtain it all ... because there's no such thing as obtaining all knowledge ... life's a *quest* ... to inquire and to fully, intelligently utilise what one's learning *whilst* one's learning it ... and that's not always easy! Life often gets in the way!

Roger, interview (2012)

As Roger says here, a lot of the focus in research on mental health is on objective 'outcomes' and their quantitative assessment (think of RCTs, attitude and depression scales, brain scans, hormone assays). These are generic measures, designed to produce 'generalisable' (read 'scientific') results, to offer statistical power and thus to provide a basis for large-scale healthcare funding and provision. And yet, as Roger observes, outcomes 'don't really get measured when you look closely'. We take this to mean that there is not a good enough 'fit' between what counts as improvement or wellbeing from a 'patient's' point of view and what counts as improvement from the more 'scientific', and more impersonal, point of view as assessed by standardized 'measures'. In company with others, we have discussed these issues in some detail in other writings (Ansdell et al. 2010; Maratos et al. 2011; Ansdell and DeNora 2012; DeNora 2013a; 2013b; DeNora and Ansdell 2014). We will not repeat those arguments here. What is more important now in conveying how we researched this project is the question of how to find 'fitting' ways of describing what 'outcomes' might mean in more indigenous terms, and how to 'bespoke fit' those concepts such that they are (a) intelligible to both SMART members and to academic and health-professional readers and (b) demonstrable through actual happenings and tales about those happenings at SMART – there, then, over time and space. And, lastly, if wellbeing 'outcomes' are robust – beyond SMART – then we want to follow how they carry out, back and into, members' daily lives. And so we present and will use, as a way of gaining purchase on the notion of 'outcomes' the term *musical pathways.* In recent years 'pathways' has become a buzz word in healthcare, where it is used to capture the sense of movement, and different routes away from, the things that are linked with and taken to constitute illness, and toward those things associated with health and/or wellbeing. There's also a small history of talking about *musical* pathways:

Ruth Finnegan on 'musical pathways'

The anthropologist Ruth Finnegan made a pioneering ethnography of the musical life of a modern town, Milton Keynes, in her book *The Hidden Musicians: Music making in an English town* (1989/2007). This is not just a study of music or musicians, but rather explores the larger subject of how people move through an often-complicated range of commitments, activities and territorial spaces of action. Among these are *musical pathways* that, as Finnegan observes, may be far from 'least important':

' ... pathways, then, are one of the ways in which people within an urban environment organise their lives so as to manage, on the one hand, the heterogeneity and multiplicity of relationships characteristic of many aspects of modern society, and, on the other, that sense of both predictable familiarity and personally controlled meaning that is also part of human life. In our culture there are many pathways that people do, and must, follow – within employment, schooling, households, sport, church, child-rearing. Within these many paths, who is to say that the pathways to do with music are the least important, either for their participants or in the infinite mix of crossways that make up an urban locality and, ultimately, our culture?' (Finnegan 2007: 325)

What's commonly lost in research on the 'effects' of music on people (for good or ill) is how making music is usually part of a far broader ecology of action and consequence. We've taken Finnegan's lead (amongst others) in pursuing as full a picture of the social ecology of SMART's musical life as we can – tracing the interweaving pathways and trails of musical people, musical things, and the musical situations and events in and through which they converge, combust and transform.

By its very nature, music emerges from coordinated pathways. Music is made by *moving* (bodies, instruments, the calibration of vocal chords and rhythmic entrainment) and, acoustically speaking, by doing something that moves the air (alternately compressing and expanding air in what we speak of as vibration). Making music is also about *moving through* (from beginning to end of song, phrase, note, passage). Whether fully improvised or guided by pre-composed texts, music is made up of comings-in and goings-out: finding a place and lingering in, then moving on and through (think of improvised jazz and the solo/chorus choreography, or of singing in a choir and knowing when to start, move quickly, slow down, or stop).

Similarly, to hear and participate in music is to hear tones in motion, as the musicologist Victor Zuckerkandl (1956, 1973) so eloquently describes.[9] These

[9] See also Ansdell (2014), Chapter 4.

tones may also seem as if they have character and agency – they may strike us as purposeful, dynamic, self-motivating. The sense we have of music in time is – at its simplest – what is often termed the phenomenology of music. This phenomenological sense is one of the things that distinguishes musical sounds from sounds that just happen as a result of everyday physical events that take place in time and space, that is the sounds that we discount as not 'making musical time' (e.g., the accidental sound of an object falling, but not necessarily the planned sound of a bell or a train). While 'music' is also where we find it, in John Cage's sense, here we have in mind the kind of music that involves mutual coordination in time and in ways that mark out a sense of event, duration and – as also, as we will continue to describe throughout this book, 'musical space'.

Our aim, as will, we hope, become increasingly clear, is to add people and situations to this picture so as to convert a traditional musical phenomenology into an *eco*-phenomenology that can be seen to 'fit' and seen as 'fitting' the ways that people – such as the members of the SMART Music project – account for their experiences of and with music: that it motivates and quickens them; draws them into places and occasions; helps them 'get through' situations; helps them feel they belong somewhere (that they can 'take their part'); softens the passage into a social situation – or, alternatively, repels and redirects them ('the music pounding out of that clothes shop/bar tells me it's not for me'). So music is naturally associated with movement and action, with propulsion and attraction; with finding a way in, through and out of physical, relational and social situations. The point of an eco-phenomenology of musicking is to find a way to 'fit' the 'inside' and 'outside' of music together in ecologically valid ways, that is, in ways that make sense and seem to explain what it is that music does, and thus, how it is that music helps.

Thus the research agenda of this project, and our account of it in this book, is not simply to report 'what happened' during the 10 years, but to try to understand what exactly it is about music-in-action that can so powerfully accompany and sometimes transform difficult lives. To understand it in this way means that we have needed to follow it 'on the ground' and through time; that we have needed to focus in two directions at once: down to the micro-detail of musical-social moments, and then zooming up to see the broader picture developing over the long time-span of 10 years – both for the organisation and place called SMART and its links to the mental health arena, but also for the lives of its members. Helping reconcile between these two foci is a mid-level or *meso-level*, where most everyday social life takes place.

Attending to the *meso-level*

The 'meso' is a term used to describe the middle level of social action. It is offered in contrast to 'micro' (face to face and individual action) and 'macro' (large-scale institutions, trends and patterns). It highlights how social change and social stability happen 'in action' and in ways that involve and draw together groups of people, practices (conventions, operations, activities with histories of use) and things. It permits focus on what sociologists call, 'interaction orders' or local realms of action that produce time-after-time forms of stable, concerted action and experience. The interaction order is the place of mutual and entwined forms of collaboration and the place where identities emerge, firm up, are challenged and change. The meso level is, in the words of sociologist and ethnographer Gary Alan Fine, 'where the action is' (Fine 2010). And thus it is the place where it is possible to see cultural forms (music) getting into action and experience, mediating social relations and creating coordinated pathways of various kinds.

8. Furnishing and Re-furnishing the Musical-Social Space of SMART

An example of thinking about the *meso-level* of the project is our continuing interest in the *space* of SMART. We've already described the basics of the layout in Section 4 above. We'll now go one stage further by describing this context in terms of the metaphor of 'furnishing' and 're-furnishing'. This goes beyond talking about the physical layout in objective terms; rather it looks at how the space becomes configured and reconfigured through collaborative social action.

***

Having committed himself to the experiment of putting a music (therapy) group in the cafe space at SMART Gary's first thought is to disturb the usual everyday life of the cafe as little as possible. On Thursday afternoons between 2–4pm the space will be configured a little differently at one end than usual (the piano turned round, a front row with instruments turned to face the piano, a microphone and amp to the left of the piano, a few more rows of tables furnished with small instruments and songbooks), but no more than this. People who don't want to join in can still sit at the back of the cafe, and around the sides, and look and listen from a distance. This way, there is spatial ambiguity, or rather, it's possible to be both 'in' and 'out' of the musical space, to belong to the space (inhabit it) in different ways – most notably, as a musical participant or cafe patron. The space affords, in other words, different ways of belonging and with these, different levels of musical investment. If music seems to be asking too much, one can 'just sit and drink tea' (it is, after all, still open as a cafe!).

In the early months of the group we experiment with different ways of setting out the space. Some configurations work, some don't; it certainly doesn't work when the music configuration dominates the cafe space too much, converts it *into* a performance space, rather than having a performance *area* within the cafe. There's evidence of participants in the music group also thinking about this dilemma as Rob Szymanek's field-note log describes:

> I see Jeremy. He's got something for me (!). But he's also got a copy for Gary – a diagram with notes attached of his ideas for a new layout for the SMART Music group. He's quite keen on the idea that there should be more of a performance space, with the tables moved out of the way and the chairs arranged into 'stalls.' He suggests that we need to implement his ideas, but I pass the buck … .
> [Rob's Field-note Log, Monday 14 August 2006]

An early entry in Gary's log book (stemming from a debrief between Gary and Rob) shows that thinking about the configuration of the social-musical space in these early weeks was also part of thinking about the potential of the group and the situation, and the beginnings of understanding the relationships between levels of musical participation and musical-social space. For example, the following sketch from Gary's log (week 2, 2005) shows the spatial layout of the cafe in relation to his thinking about the musical participation in the group in layered terms – foreground, middle ground and periphery.

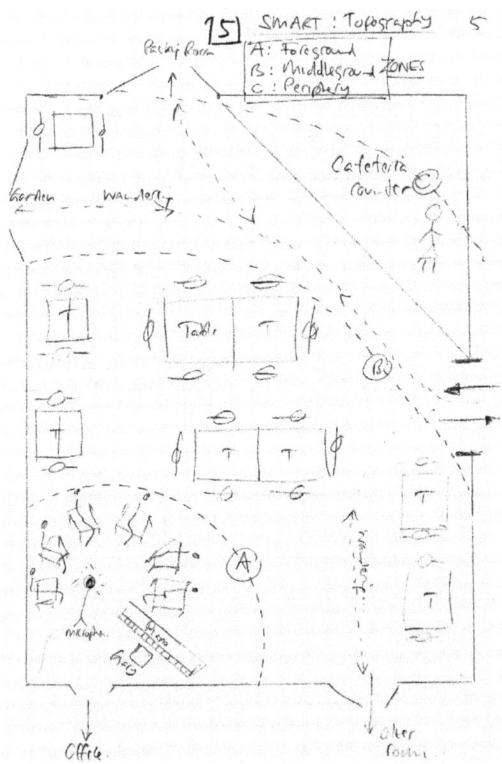

Figure 6 Early sketch of SMART's musical-social space

This theoretical awareness of the uses of space becomes a central theme to our research of this project, and connects to some larger interests that Tia, as a cultural sociologist, has about how, where and when people use music, both for themselves, and for the benefit of others:

DeNora on 'music asylums' and the (re)furnishing of space

In *Music Asylums*, one of the two books that flank this central 'panel' of our book triptych (described earlier), DeNora (2013) introduced the idea of the *musical asylum* (a space of wellbeing, a place or practice that brings relief, respite, or that promotes flourishing). The concept distinguishes between (a) forms of asylum that involve the putting of distance between self and other, self and shared space (*removal*), and (b) those forms of asylum that are created in shared space and through shared practices that modify, tailor, tinker or otherwise refurnish that space in ways that can be understood to *refurnish* space (DeNora 2013a). Refurnishing in this way may involve changes in material space and, connected to material changes, it may involve changes (additions, modifications) to symbolic space. In both cases that space is adapted so as to be made more 'habitable' – to afford security, pleasure, to make it more conducive to the forms of action associated with wellbeing. In this sense, the crafting of space is an inevitably political and ethical matter, since what may be conducive for one or some may be anathema for another or others.

While this theme of the different forms of 'musical asylum' is central to virtually all of what we describe in this book, it can perhaps best be introduced through a discussion of the material details of the SMART physical-social space – in itself, and increasingly in relation to musical activities. In tandem with what people do, with how they make sense of space, material furnishing affords things. That is, it makes some things easier to do, others more difficult. We can trace the differences and similarities between the varieties of these spatial furnishings at SMART through observations Rob made in the weeks he was hanging out in SMART a lot, doing the initial fieldwork and interviews. One day, just sitting there and listening to the normal social life of the cafe, and thinking about the difference when the music group's happening his field notes report:

> I've realised that the special 'geography' of the SMART Music group is something that is part and parcel of the everyday social environment of the cafe: open, free-flow, accepting, dynamic. I speak about this with Dave, the manager. He says it's the fact that the cafe is small, people know each other etc. He also tells me about how in the past, he's noticed how a change in the room's layout for whatever reason can completely change the atmosphere, and then also peoples' responses and behaviours. He mentions the occasions when the tables have been moved into different positions for the Debate nights – pushing the tables together in a square so that people can sit in a round with food and drinks in the middle; the DVD nights – setting up the room with a big

screen, moving the tables out and arranging the seats in rows like a cinema; and the 'three course meal' days – when the tables are set up in rows like a good restaurant. SMART becomes all these different things depending on the layout of the room – a debating arena; a cinema; a restaurant. What about the music group? In a way, it's kind of like a 'hyper' version of the normal cafe situation: interactions, participations, the level of activity; all these aspects are energised slightly when the music group is happening ... Something to think about ... [Rob's field notes, Data Corpus p. 833]

And indeed there is quite a lot of thinking about this aspect in the early weeks and months of SMART Music. Directly after the first ever SMART session, Gary, Rob and SMART staff discuss the space when it is in use for music. They observe what they perceive as 'zones' corresponding to levels of musical involvement (see also Fig. 6):

Without much planning the cafe space organised itself during the afternoon into a topography of three 'zones' radiating from the musical centre: (i) a *foreground area* around the piano and the members up for direct engagement and performance; (ii) a *middleground area*, with people still using the cafe set-up as usual (to drink, chat, hang around) – but orientating towards the musical action – showing interest, smiling, tapping one of the small percussion instruments on a table in front of them, clapping, even occasionally singing a phrase of a song they know; (iii) *peripheral area* – the edges, corners (including Sadie, behind the bar), corridors of the space, where people are peripherally participating, or being peripherally influenced by the music (including potentially to avoid it by walking out). The key point is that this first musical event in the SMART cafe showed multiple levels of participation and influence in/by the music, and that the cafe remained *one space* despite what was happening. The music reached into and influenced this space, as did people reach from their perspectives into the music and influenced it. [Gary's Field-note Log, Thursday 13 January 2005]

This formulation is neat, but perhaps premature, as what the developing narrative on this group shows through the logbooks is how this picture quite quickly shifts. The musical-social space develops, with less differentiation between foreground and background areas, and more sense of a single zone of participation, the whole of the cafe.

***

So far we've discussed 'furnishing' in terms of the relatively large aspects such as physical furniture, areas of action and so forth. There's also another key dimension to furnishing, which seems more modest, but is arguably just as important – the area of objects, decorations, costumes and props, the furnishing that people individually contribute to the overall scene. Here we have cups and cakes, flowers and pictures, and of course specifically musical paraphenalia (either that provided, or personally contributed by members – e.g. Mussei's 'Christian horns' with their farty noise, Roger's range of harmonicas, Jane and Jeremy's sheet-music, and so on …). All of this together musicalises and personalises this material space and creates new forms of furnishing (potential musical spaces; musical asylums) that can be occupied and altered.

This furnishing and refurnishing is both conscious and non-conscious, individual and collective. Our theoretical and methodological strategy is to give equal attention to this dimension as to the 'actual musicking', as these musical things inflect both the musical people and the musical situations through their subtle or major refurnishing of the environment. For example, the introduction of an object (e.g. bringing in a cake, a mouth organ, can provide a means for making other things change, or rather 'adapt' to the new object). So, bringing in one 'little' thing is a pebble in the pond of the material ecology: it might cause some things to suddenly seem more prominent, more important, or more useful/valued and other things more marginal or less valued. We need to attend to the use of things that 'have consequences' and are dynamic and loaded with meaning and implication for the space.

9. The First SMART Music Session: Thursday 13 January 2005

Everyone is a bit apprehensive and self-conscious. Gary has never done music therapy in a cafe before; Rob has never been in a mental health setting; the SMART staff are hoping it won't get too out of hand, be too noisy … and the members, well they haven't got a clue what's going to happen in the next two hours. The staff have simply said there's some kind of music group happening – it turns out that many of the musicians in the SMART community have come along to check it out …

The instruments have been informally set up, Gary is behind the white piano, a small group of members are in the front-row configuration, whilst the usual life of the cafe continues behind them. Twenty or so red folders of song-words which Gary uses in the hospital setting have been put out on the cafe tables …

> Gary: 'How about starting with one we know? *Let it Be?*

> Gary plays the introduction and a surprising number of people immediately start singing. After the song starts a man opens a violin case, takes out the instrument and gradually starts playing – unobtrusively at first, then taking a solo. Rob also joins in with his clarinet, and a few people pick up the small percussion instruments placed on the cafe tables and play along. The song ends, people clap and whoop …

> Bobby: 'Not bad, eh Gary?'

The rest of the cafe has quietened now and orients towards the music, even if most people are still on the periphery:

> Gary: 'What next? Jeremy ... how about you pick one of your favourites?'

Various people call out possibilities, but Gary waits for Jeremy to choose. He flicks slowly through the red folder ...

> Jeremy: How about the Judy Garland one ... ?
> Peggy: *'Over the Rainbow ... ?* I know that one too'
> Jeremy: 'But I don't know the verse ... .'
> Bobby: 'I don't know it at all ... '
> Peggy: 'Oh yes you do! You will when the music starts ... '

On this cue Gary launches into the introduction to this song, and sings the verse (it's true, people don't know this so well, but have a go even if its on the wrong notes ...). There's a surge of singing at the chorus, and the man playing the violin is more confident now, playing a gorgeous counter-melody that floats over the music, enveloping the singing. The performance is as heart-felt as any this song has had in its long and varied life. [Gary's Field-note Log, Thursday 13 January 2005]

SONG 2: *Somewhere Over the Rainbow*

We can make this very detailed account of the second song because there's an audio recording of the session. Recording, listening-back and analysing the details of the musical-personal-social process is key to the Nordoff–Robbins tradition of music therapy, and links well with the ethnographic approach of this study. It forces us to notice details, to test our assumptions about people's participation and their/our narratives about that participation against the traces captured on the tape.

The two columns (which could be further 'thickened' if we had a 360 degree video recording to work from) show how the performance is not just the notes, but the combination of musical elements along with the physical, verbal and situational *paramusical* aspects that pull the musical-social performance together, and push it out into the social space. (We talk about these aspects in some detail later on.)

Musical	**Paramusical / Background**
	background chatter + tinkle of tea-cups... chatting....[conversation about selecting this song]
0:10 - few quiet notes of a violin tuning-up	
0:12 - female voice (Mary?) quickly tries out first phrase *'...over the rainbow...'*, which overlaps with...	Gary scans front-row people... 'front-row' participants look towards Gary for an entry cue...
0:14 - piano plays intro to song strongly, pauses....	
0:20 - Gary sings first line of verse...*When all the world is a hopeless jumble...*	peripheral talking audible, someone calls 'Dave?'
0:24 - other voices join him in a jumbly fashion, with characterful individual voices emerging in the texture (not a blend); slightly out of pitch and timing... Faint violin in background	Gary looks around, gathers as many people as possible through eye-contact and head movement to join the chorus...
1:02 - Chorus: *Somewhere Over*....more voices enter, stronger singing... different registers, but more focused pitch	
1:10 - violin audible in texture, shadowing melody (helping group pitching) + and clarinet providing counter-melody. Overall texture = thick, messy, interesting...	more coughs, chair scraping...
1:56 - C-section: *Someday I'll wish upon a star* - violin helps singers pick up phrase...	'Ooh, Hello there!' (A shouts to B - singer to friend just coming in, timing speech in the pause between two sung phrases)
2:18 - Bit of a strain for all voices at the climax, *...that's where you'll find me...* clarinet covers with a little twiddle at end	Gary looks up to singers, says *'sing up!'*... (they do!)
2:20 - final *Somewhere...* strong singing, with clarinet now confidently doing decorative motifs between songs, helps bind it together as singers flag a bit...	
2:48 - coda section - *If happy little bluebirds fly...* people don't know this so exactly, so it goes a bit messy with pitch and rhythm again. Gary, violin, clarinet to the rescue with emphatic playing...	Bobby makes a face at Gary & others as if to say 'What's this bit?' People looking towards each other to time final note...
2:50 - *...why oh why can't I.....* slows down and leans into the final phrase - full singing + violin and clarinet doing flourishes up and down to embellish the final note...	Clapping, cheers... 'Not bad....' 'Very good Simon, nice...' 'Very good Rob!'

A note on the musical and the paramusical

Traditionally there has been a clear but false division between the 'purely musical' and the 'extra-musical' (that is, non-musical). Seeing music as more fluid and continuous within human experience and practice would rather suggest how *para*-musical phenomena accompany or work beside the musical, whilst not being purely musical themselves. Rather, the musical and the paramusical substantiate and transsubstantiate each other – the 'musicality' of a movement, communication or style of identity shows up for us within musicking. But these aspects are not necessarily separable *from* the music: they are an aspect *of* the musicking and not just a result of it (and as such are *para*musical rather than 'extra-musical'). A paramusical phenomenon is always wrapped up in the immediate ecology and need of a situation, and is never an abstract entity that you could isolate – either during or afterwards. Take away the music, and the paramusical feature can also disappear – even if its echo often remains. This is perhaps no more than saying that overall we must preserve musicking for its own sake, not to achieve something else (even when it often does just this). (Ansdell 2014, p. 99)

In the current text we will make the following non-definitive distinction:

musical means musicalised sounds (not just pitches, but also rhymicised sounds that may have minimal defined pitch) that derive causally from human action, intention and organisation as some level, and that combine and associate to form musical concatenations, follow musical logic (at some level) and form musical effects and experiences.

paramusical means any other 'things' that are caused, initiated, influenced, modulated, or co-occuring with musicalised sounds – things which are shaped-up (spatially, temporally, in terms of their trajectory, intent, or affect) either from / in-relation-to / alongside-with the musical track. Such paramusical things may be: actions (individual or relational), responses (individual or relational), thoughts, associations, emotions, verbal/non-verbal comments and elaborations etc.

The musical and paramusical tracks are often parallel, but ultimately distinguishable (or at the least it's a useful heuristic device for socio-musical studies!).

Returning to the first SMART Music session we see how the song *Somewhere Over the Rainbow* gathers people and instruments into a thick inclusive texture – which is also punctuated and inflected by random environmental aspects such as coughs, moving furniture, tinkling tea-cups, chat and calls. But rather than being just a distraction, this is part of the scene and some of these seemingly peripheral sounds and actions are part of the musical 'whole' (as we described earlier when we spoke about Barbara, her tambourine and micro-participation). The musicking focuses action and the varying voices, but in a particular way, that we might call 'messy', or 'heterophenous' to be technical.[10] That is, the musical togetherness is

[10] See Turino (2008) for accounts of 'participatory music' textures, also Ansdell (2014) pp. 208–11.

not exact (either in rhythm or pitch – it's full of 'participatory discrepancies') but it nonetheless achieves a felt togetherness for the participants. You hear the voices 'together separately' through their individual timbre ('it's Bobby, Peggy!'), but also aligned, focused and going somewhere together. And you know these participants themselves hear, or recognise, this 'togetherness'. For example, they 'know' when to call out to a newcomer ('Ooh, Hello there!') and how to adjust and accommodate to others' musical, and paramusical, requirements, needs and requests (Gary's instruction to 'sing up!', for example, is immediately effected). You hear mutual help, and mutual accommodation *within the music* – piano, violin, clarinet, drums all do musical things to keep the song on track, and to keep togetherness.

In a sense then, and even in this, the first-ever SMART Music Session, the musical and the paramusical are constantly, and in real-time, creating each other and through that process, creating their creators. So, for example, at the end of *Somewhere Over the Rainbow*, when we get clapping and cheers and when the words, 'Not bad' and 'Very good Simon, nice', 'Very good Rob!' are uttered, those words accomplish several things at once. The words, spoken about music, effect a chain of consequences. They:

1. Evaluate the music, what was just produced, and thus the participants who have made the music
2. Produce and enhance the identities of the speakers, who as musicians, are gathered – via music – into a who and who can be what, when and where
3. Evaluate the situation, which is also laying down a marker that this form of activity is good, worth repeating
4. Constitute the speakers' rights to evaluate
5. Constitute those speakers as bone fide members of this community
6. Create new resources for participants (e.g., skill, confidence, claims to certain musical spaces, repertoires, instruments [remember Eloise's cymbal])
7. Furnish the musical/paramusical space with more detail, more opportunities and more possibilities for future action

There is a musically/paramusically fuelled cycle here in which new things are drawn into the vortex and new things are generated from that movement over time. This cycling and re-cycling is the mechanism by which the pathways that interest us are laid down. Through it and as a by-product of it heterophenous voices and heterophenous pathways mutually make each other. This pathway creation at SMART builds upon the basic musical features we have just described – a thick but inclusive musical texture that allows for heterophenous togetherness and that taps, draws in, then plays back out various paramusical matters over time so as to keep the cycle in motion. This is the paradigm of the ensemble numbers in SMART Music; a paradigm of how to approach the goal of creating musical community.

Gary: 'How about something a bit different this time?
Peggy: 'Something a bit jazzy! Get me going' (Peggy, mid-80s, is helping Gary to make something of this first session, she's injecting energy and enthusiasm).
Bobby: '*One-Note Samba?* – here, I'll play the drums ... '

The piano leads, but quickly people and instruments pile in, and there's a more improvisational feel this time, in contrast to the relatively conventional renderings of the first two songs. This time there's a jumble of drums, piano, clarinet and violin, with a tapping and tinkling backdrop of tambourines and an occasional cymbal. At first it's all together, then Gary calls out names – either of people he knows, or of instruments where he doesn't know people – calling for a solo from them for a stretch of the music. People and instruments rise up from ground to figure, but still supported by the on-going lively musical background. This figure/ground interchange allows the group to display itself to itself, its constituent parts and the whole that is greater than, and supportive of, these parts. A few direct voices of encouragement are added – Peggy is heard saying to the violinist 'Come on, Simon!', and Mary improvises singing for a while. The form is of alternating solo/chorus, where people emerge and then settle back – both musically and socially. It ends with a bang!

Someone says to Gary, 'Simon plays the piano too … ', so Gary moves aside for him:

Simon: 'OK, it's request time, folks ... What's it to be?'
Peggy: 'I'd like some tango music please – Argentina!'

Simon plays *Don't Cry for Me, Argentina* – and at the end bows to the clapping, and retreats quickly to the counter at the back. Gary sits back at the piano:

Mary: 'More tango, Gary ... '
Peggy: 'Yes, I want to dance!' (this cues kind laughter from people, looking at this octogenarian lady)

Gary plunges into an improvised tango, and instantly people grab percussion and there's a messy but energetic participation roughly around the tango rhythm. Peggy gets up to dance, tries to grab Jeremy as a partner, he recoils slightly, so Peggy continues on her own, dancing on the spot, playing to the audience. After a few minutes Gary reduces the energy of the music, and segues into *Girl from Ipanema.* This isn't in the song-folder, but Mary sings along with *doo-doo,* Bobby picks up the rhythm neatly on the drum, Rob improvises a counter-melody on clarinet … The room has now been transformed, with the music now the centre, and a definable periphery in which several people are oriented towards the main musical action. Gary notices in the last song that the woman behind the tea-counter is smiling broadly and dancing on the spot as she serves drinks …

> Gary: 'Wonderful! Let's take a tea-break now – twenty minutes … '
> Bobby: 'Well done, Simon, I never knew you played that violin thing … '
> Jeremy: 'Tea, Peggy?'
> Peggy: 'Yes, nice and strong … '
> Rob: 'Mary has a lovely voice … '
> Sadie (the lady behind the tea-counter): ' … and Jeremy too … '

***

Twenty minutes later the music resumes, but by now it seems that everyone knows exactly what's going on. Nerves have gone, people have left who don't like it, and people have stayed and settled to join in who've found something quite interesting is happening …

People at the back of the cafe say they can't hear it when people play solo, so we get out an amp and put a mic on a stand at the side of the piano. Now it looks a bit like an open-mic set up in a pub. Gary asks Mary if she wants to sing a solo. She picks *Where is Love?* and sings confidently, the cafe hushing for her in a particular way. People clap enthusiastically at the end, and Mary looks chuffed. Jeremy follows this up by suggesting he does one of his mother's songs from the 1930s. Gary doesn't know it enough to play a piano accompaniment, so Jeremy sings unaccompanied, standing at the mic, prefacing the song with a short educational introduction telling us who originally sang this song, in which film. As with Mary, he's attended to closely by the audience (it's noticeable how the acoustic of the room seems to change for different people singing). Jeremy, despite a nervous and halting delivery, is given a big clap at the end.

Someone suggests a waltz, so Gary launches into an improvised version of *The Blue Danube*, with violin and clarinet *obbligato* parts, and an energetic *oom-pah-pah* backing on mixed percussion. Peggy's up on her feet, grabs Dave the manager, and they do a few rounds of the periphery (she can dance well, he can't!). After this Simon resumes his place at the piano and does a medley of popular and jazz songs, which people join in with in an informal way. Gary returns after this and picks a simple song, as some of the musical focus has been ebbing away. *Amazing Grace* is sung and hummed, Gary semi-directing people's participation. Focus returns. Then with 10 minutes to go Mary asks for 'more songs from *Oliver*', and there follows a medley, ending up with a high-energy version of *Consider Yourself*. The session ends with *Summertime* with improvised breaks, solos and a high-energy cadence. Everyone's surprised by what's happened …

***

Gary, Rob and the SMART staff have a brief feedback once the instruments have been cleared away and the members have left for the day. 'It worked!' Dave says (with some relief it feels). There's a general agreement that any fears of it being too much, too noisy for people had not been realised. Somehow the cafe had gone on with its everyday work and simply accommodated the musical event (and *vice versa*). Dave commented that the music had 'energised the cafe', and he was amazed what people had done in this first session: 'I've seen a few people in a completely different light – I'd never believed they were so talented!'. People's strengths and talents had emerged, and also their musical generosity, as they supported each other.

As we discussed what had happened in this first session some themes came up that were to lay the ground for much of our serious thinking about this project for years to come:

1. ***Zones of participation*** – without much planning the cafe space seemed to have organised itself during the afternoon into a topography of the three 'zones' discussed previously in Section 8.
2. ***The cafe musicalised*** – at the best moments of the afternoon the dynamic space and atmosphere of the cafe changed according to the musical activity. It energised to a musical buzz in the big moments, then shrank to a hush to listen to Jeremy's unaccompanied solo. The clatter softened as the collective ear followed the trajectory of Simon's beautiful violin melody in *Rainbow* ...
3 ***The individual participants musicalised*** – in the sense that the music 'takes them' into varied levels of energy and intensity, tempo, pitch, style, volume and with it possibilities for paramusical action and experience, for example ...
4. ***Musical performances of self and relationship*** – As Dave commented, amazing voices emerged – people were seen and heard in a different light (by staff and fellow members) via their various musical performances. They were appreciated by others for this, and supported to do so in a group culture of appreciation and encouragement (laced with humour). It was also the performance of relationships – of musical support through accompaniment, or more collaborative versions of musical ensemble – all illustrating Christopher Small's (1998) definition of musicking as the *performance of relationships.* Performances highlighted the web of relationships in the place through how people are seen, heard and appreciated. Ability, personality, health, beauty is performed musically, and heard musically. SMART members became SMART *musicians* ...
5. ***Positive heterogeneity*** – differences of age, taste, class, ethnicity and illness level are immediately obvious in the group. But this first session showed what was possible to negotiate between these aspects within musicking.

The repertoire ranged between jazz, the Blue Danube, show songs, 1930s songs, more recent popular songs. (We were not aware of course at this stage how many people thought 'this is clearly *not* for me' and voted with their feet. Rob's interviews a year later showed that clearly this group was not going to appeal to members with fixed musical tastes for House and Techno! Taste flexibility only goes so far …).

6. ***Who's running the group?*** – Was this a music therapy group? Just a music group? Gary noticed how he used some of his skills as a music therapist to encourage people into the music, to shape and balance the session so that it included as many people as possible, and didn't get stuck; how just occasionally he made an intervention to modulate someone's slightly manic playing that looked like it was disturbing people. But he also commented on a feature that was to become more obvious as the sessions went on: how the 'therapeutic' function of the group was not left just to him, but somehow shared and distributed amongst many of the active members. People collectively helped the session to work, and its contributors to be their best …
7. ***Talking about music's help*** – Rob and Dave mentioned how freely people had said to them how much they loved music, how nice it was to have live music at SMART, and how much it helped. Sadie, the lady who danced behind the food counter said to Rob: 'I was feeling rotten this morning, but I forced myself to come … and after the music I just feel better … '

***

With this first session also came a clear agenda for practical work and theoretical exploration:

- How does music radiate, disperse or modulate within a physical/social space like the SMART cafe (both the positive and negative aspects of this)?
- How do people find a comfortable position in this musical space? How do they move around it, and beyond it?
- How does active participation and performance emerge? How is it configured and re-configured – both spontaneously and strategically by Gary and others?
- How does physical and musical space relate and inter-relate? How does relational spacing and timing work in musicking (for better or worse)?

Several days later Gary listens back to the audio-tape of the event, and another dimension stands out when he's listening back, but not physically in that acoustic. The tape highlights the acoustic ecology of the event; exactly *how* music is within this space, with these people, their ongoing action (relating to its functions and habits as a social space). Music can be heard variously within it: in relation to talk, the phone ringing, the overall ambience – and can be heard to be constantly changing in response to musical events and people.

10. A Musical Ecology at SMART and How to Describe it

The broader research questions were quickly emerging for us – namely, what makes a musical place? and, What makes a musical pathway? A pathway to what?

The very first session shows clearly the simple fact of musical things (the 'template' of the known song – its words, melody, character etc.; available musical instruments), coming into relationship with people's own capacity for making music, there and then. It's a story of musical happenstance, or fortuitous musical-things-coming-together, linking and re-linking in various ways across time and space. We think of this as the construction of a 'musical ecology', an interdependent variety of things and processes that sustain and develop within a particular locality:

An ecological perspective on musicking

Although this concept is more familiar today in relation to the natural world, it makes a lot of sense to think of human social and cultural life as ecological too. The origin of *ecology* combines the Greek *oikos* – the household – with *logos* – word, or in a more philosophical sense the order, principle or 'logic' of something. Thinking ecologically means exploring how people manage to live together more or less successfully within both their natural and their social environment. Recent movements such as 'community psychology', 'health psychology' and branches of sociology have increasingly used an ecological metaphor to explore how people thrive and sicken, adapt and develop in relation to their ever-changing physical, social and cultural environment.

Certain key principles are common to both natural and human ecologies. The most important of these is that everything in an ecology is connected and interdependent. As with a spider's web, a change in one part of an ecology is registered, and may have important effects, somewhere else in the web. A second key principle is that ecologies work through a subtle interdependence and exchange between living and non-living things and processes. Whilst each entity normally keeps its own boundary and identity, it is also porous and in continual interaction and transaction with other things around it. Processes of communicating, collaborating, improvising and recycling are key to keeping an ecosystem flexible, resilient and sustainable.

A meso-level of analysis helps us to see these ecological principles in action within musical situations. It means attending closely to how music is part of a complex process of interdependent interactions between people, practices and things within a particular place. We could see a 'musical ecology' in terms of the original Greek sense of household management – as one of the sub-systems that helps to make and keep our broader social world habitable. (Ansdell 2014: 27)

In the accounts of the early days of a musical community being developed at SMART we have seen how people in musical action linked and were linked to myriad musical things that make up the ecology of SMART, and that also permeate their everyday lives: instruments, songs, genres and the paramusical things like word-sheets, food and drink items, CDs and other paraphenalia such as dress and comportment relating to musical occasions.

In the human sciences and the humanities, a recent welcome trend has been the encouragement to treat the things we research more 'flatly', without too many pre-decisions about what will work, how it will work (don't, for example, assume that music, or some forms of music necessarily have the power to cause certain things to happen, e.g., listening to Mozart and spatial reasoning, or listening to lullabies and feeling sleepy). We agree, as we have described in the two books that accompany this text (DeNora 2013a; Ansdell 2014a), that it is not a good idea to assume that some things are 'bigger' or more important than others (e.g., the socio-economic determinants of health and illness versus what happens in a single moment of action). To the contrary, sometimes the so-called 'littlest' things loom large. Instead, here, we are looking at how people and things act together, such that unique and characterful trajectories of joint action can happen. This perspective is directed toward the *gatherings* and *concatenations*[11] of things, and the progressive tinkering and negotiating with them that allow patterns and capacities to accumulate and develop.

We see how collaborative and mutual forms of musical action produce outcomes that no one individual (healthcare client, medical professional, etc.) could achieve, for herself or for another. So how is music, then, something to lean on, to build upon? This question provides the central plot line for the stories we are telling here.

And to tell this story, we too are 'leaning' on a few further narrative devices. People, events, 'theories', materials, spaces, performances, songs are 'followed' across space and time within the particular evolving musical community of SMART. The musical stories around musical things, people, events and outcomes are the basic building blocks of our narrative pathway and they are the basic building blocks of SMART members' journeys in, through and out from the SMART Music space. How are these blocks hewn, arranged, contended and consolidated? How, for example, a 'musical person' or a 'musical thing' (such as a song, or a tambourine) is rendered into being, attached to, how it takes on definition over an interval of time (a minute, a year) and what is mobilised to make this so: this is the crucial story here.

---

[11] Concatenation (from Latin *concatēnāre*, to link, string or chain together) is the logical corollary of a 'flat ontology' – that doesn't try to reduce or force things into a neat vertical hierarchy of relative (and often abstracted) importance in order to explain what's 'really' mattering, acting etc. It assumes rather that *every-thing* is potentially significant in some way within the whole – the network of actors swirling within a given situation.

Telling this story relies on the 'longhand discipline' of following, noting and noticing (out of the corner of the eye and the ear), mapping, charting, trailing, sketching … trying to keep our attention on the 'person+'; that is, the person *with* and alongside all the things that allow them to become musical, to remain musical (as individuals and together), and to 'change musically' (and paramusically). Every time a link is added the whole chain changes – just as it does when (within the internal world of music) you add a tone, and the harmony changes, and the meaning of the musical past, present and future is transfigured.

In this way we are attempting to follow a 'musical person' or a 'musical grouping' – and their pathway and 'career' over minutes, weeks or years, and to substantiate how all the various musical things concatenate along, around and with them (chosen instruments, songs, styles, clothes, narratives, performances, etc.). But, in the interests of symmetry, it's also possible to follow one of the 'musical things' as if *it too* had a line of development of its own, a life of its own within the field of play: following a song, for example – how it is established, appropriated, re-appropriated, changed, given a new owner and a new meaning, taken from place to place, used to inspire, to mean something (different to different people), translated between immediacy and history. Equally, a more physical thing like a tambourine, bell or guitar – how does it travel, attach to a person and a meaning, settle and travel again? What role does it take in the emerging collective story being played out and told?

In light of this strategy one point to emphasise here is how when we 'zoom in' with our analysis – to an individual person, to a particular song, to a few seconds of musical interaction – we are resolutely not implying that you can reduce the overall complexity to its constituent elements, and then add up these individual elements to explain the overall effects. Rather, any focus on individual elements is always to take the 'flattening strategy' of looking 'sideways' from them, and towards them, as part of the whole picture of the musical ecology – and to see how the linkages, gatherings and concatenations function to construct outcomes for both individuals and the situation as a whole.

11. 'The Man on the Violin'

One of the participants of the first SMART Music session referred to 'the man on the violin' who unexpectedly emerged to play. This was Simon. At the time, the people in the room are clearly conscious of the beautiful sound Simon made, but they also accept it as something quite natural. 'I thought I'd give it an airing,' says Simon later. 'I thought it was a sawn-off shotgun you'd got in there' says Roger. ('Truth is, the latter would be more likely in this place than a classical violin,' Gary thinks to himself.)

After this initial 'airing' the violin goes back in the case and does not reappear for several years though Simon himself appears most weeks, hanging around the back of the cafe, usually chatting to Sadie at the drinks counter. They talk about music (Sadie having been a regular at Soho jazz haunts in their 1960s and 1970s prime). Gary is puzzled that Simon doesn't repeat his performance of that first session, but doesn't ask as the overall policy is to let people decide how they want to participate in SMART Music – it's their choice. Simon and Gary often talk about music and musicians during the tea-break, and when Rob does his first round of interviews in the summer of 2006, Simon agrees to talk to him. More of Simon's musical life story comes out in this – a difficult account of his fundamental ambivalence to music, and in particular to performing music. Simon gives Rob what Gary recognises as a classic 'music-health-illness narrative':

Music-health-illness narratives

Music therapists have long noted how willingly and spontaneously people (in clinical settings and not) tell stories about themselves, music, and illness – with music as a character in their story very like another person. There's a long history of health/illness narratives in the sociology of health/illness (Frank 2004, Charon 2008, Charmaz 1997), but adding 'music' as a character perhaps illuminates something particular and important about how music helps. The psychiatrist John Meehan and music therapist Gary Ansdell (2010) suggested the term 'music-health-illness narratives'. In the study Ansdell and Meehan found that when patients talked about music therapy, they often told a story that interleaved an account of their general relationship with music with aspects of both their illness and their health, as if these three strands naturally belonged together. They called such accounts 'music–health–illness narratives' and suggested that they typically had a three-part structure of: (i) an identified pre-illness relationship to music, and its usually positive role in their life, leading to (ii) how illness has disrupted their relationship with music and their use of it as a helping resource, ending with (iii) how music therapy has started to re-establish their relationship to music, such that it can be helpful again. Both the form and the content of these narratives confirmed that music therapy was often experienced as 'continuous' with their previous and on-going relationship with music in their everyday life.

At the point when Simon came along to that first SMART Music Session in January 2005 he'd not played for years, and had experienced the same ambivalence that had driven him out of his career as a professional musician – and away from music as a whole in many ways. It seems that for people like Simon, music is simply *too* powerful. Where it helps many people, for Simon it feels like there's always the risk that it will singe him badly. Another analogy Simon uses (especially in a second interview he gives to Gary in 2009) is with drugs – quite simply, with music it's easy to overdose! So keeping the violin in its case is a way of restricting 'use' for Simon – he can tolerate being on the periphery of music and musicking, but needs to be careful of his own direct involvement.

The following years between 2006–13 are a story of Simon's conscious and perhaps less conscious attempts to regulate and titrate his musical participation in SMART Music. Concretely this means his moving backwards and forwards physically in the space over months and years, depending on how he feels in himself (in relation to his illness), but also how he feels able to join in, and often to create, musical occasions through playing violin or (increasingly) piano.

The violin becomes an *obbligato* instrument (decorative, enriching, supportive of the main musical line), increasingly functioning as another musical voice supporting the other 'acts' during the music afternoons. Simon and violin stand to the right of the piano, and he spontaneously improvises lines that complement Gary's piano accompaniments to singers, or else Simon and Gary join together to give more character to an improvisation based on an idiom such as Spanish or Middle Eastern elements. The violin really enhances the musical experience for everyone, and Simon gets many comments about his 'beautiful playing'. At first people are surprised at the sheer quality of his musicianship, having previously known him only as the nice man who hangs around the place certain days. In a sense this revelation of him as a skilled musician is quite shocking to all – members and staff alike. When he plays Simon looks transported – eyes closed, swaying with the music, fluent and elegant. When Gary asks him about this in the interview he says that he closes his eyes merely so as not to see that audience, since his major ambivalence is about performing to please people.

Daniel increasingly asks Simon to play piano for him when he sings classic jazz songs. Simon can usually be persuaded. Gary is happy with this, as Simon's repertoire and ability in this style is far above his. Simon and Daniel often need to negotiate the speed and style of a performance, and are more or less successful in this negotiation over the years. But it's the violin that somehow carries Simon's musical persona at SMART. For one week only it's substituted for a viola. Then back to the violin. There are renewed long periods where the violin disappears, even if Simon himself doesn't disappear. He merges back into the background of the cafe, and the ongoing music. When he and Gary catch up with each other in later years of the project, they lapse quickly into musicians' conversation – the latest performers in the spotlight, the composers they enjoy. The underlying feeling Gary has is often a sadness for Simon that he's far away from most of that now, but happy to be so; that he's happy to be around SMART and SMART Music, but is being cautious.

Then at the Christmas event in 2012 when Gary visits (having left the project) Simon tells Gary that he's playing violin seriously again – classical repertoire, with an elderly pianist who has started coming to SMART Music. Both of them practice, both enjoy playing together. Simon is also happy that he's been able to help another SMART member who's a competent accordion player into a good West End restaurant job. Simon still has his connections.

Simon also still has his absolute, unwavering love of music. But there are still risks, still the need for caution and regulation. Is music healing for Simon? It's a difficult question. Perhaps, like the homeopathic theory, there is a potential hidden poison in the remedy. Dose is crucial.

The following extended extract from an interview Gary did with Simon highlights music's double-edged character and serves as a cautionary tale for anyone who thinks that music can do 'only' good:

> **Simon:** I do tend to limit it, because it is ... It's a dangerous drug to me ... it's something that needs to be controlled.
>
> **Gary:** I'm a bit, I'm not quite getting that, so ...
>
> **S:** Well, I mean you have to, you can go and look at the lives of certain artists, composers, like Beethoven, Schumann, Tchaikovsky ... writers like Ernest Hemmingway, Van Gogh ... You know, it's something that can take over completely. And I'm certainly not saying that I'm a great artist like any of those, but the effect is the same you know. It can take you to extremes very easily. Some sort of, I don't know, escape valve I think, shutting off from pain or discomfort. So it's a question of trying to face up to reality more ...
>
> **G:** Mmm. So for you ... music, it takes you out of life, rather than the other way round?
>
> **S:** It does, yeah. It goes to extremes ...
>
> **G:** Is that when you do music on your own, or with other people? Or just any kind of music?
>
> **S:** Both, anything ... It's like the chicken and the egg. If you're becoming unwell, you can start to want to use that or actually, I think possibly, using it in itself can lead to the illness, you know. So I do try and limit it.
>
> **G:** Do you have any idea how it leads to illness?
>
> **S:** I dunno how, I mean it's obviously done by whatever the cause of the condition in the first place is. It's like anything, it's to do with a lack of balance somewhere you know, like anything. You might think 'I'll have a couple of drinks, and oh well it's not having the same effect, I'll just have one more', and your saturation level needs more and more and more to achieve what you feel you want. So I do tend to sort of detach myself. And also in my case, I think behind it all there's a sort of [sigh] in many ways an obligation to please people, and to do the right thing. And at the same time as I do that, I'm not happy. I never have been happy having any recognition for it. So [laughs] it's not the best use of any skill really.
>
> **G:** So it's very complicated for you, isn't it?

S: I mean, because I was in a position where I was right at the front of everything as a professional and people would clap quite loudly, and whatever and say 'that's lovely music blah blah blah, and thank you' I learnt how to do it … whereas before I couldn't do it at all. I'd just run off, you know, if somebody thought I was good at something.

G: As a professional you learnt the tricks of the trade. To kind of …

S: Yeah it's like acting really. I mean it's the same as you know, how many comedians who are largely of the same mindset, not any different. They do suddenly get tremendous acclaim and then the second they stop and go off they're completely and utterly miserable. And depressed, you know. It's extremes of mood in a very short space of time.

G: That's quite a different story from many people who use music here.

S: Oh absolutely, yes.

G: Because in a sense for them it's very often a very health-promoting thing. It's the thing that's the opposite side from their problems. But with you it's a much more subtle story, isn't it? A much more complicated story. The relationship between music and your health and your illness and you know, your hopes and stuff. [pause]

S: And yet, it could be the same. If you look at when D—plays with the other base guitarists and B--. If you gave them free reign they would go on and on and on, and get louder, and to me, more miserable, singing blues and stuff. Which they enjoy doing and they're very good at. But it is, you know, they push themselves further and further and further and they'd be up until six o'clock in the morning if they were able to. And they're sort of overdosing on the emotions and feelings they get from it and the way they express themselves.

Whereas for most people, it's a very simple format and it's something they know that cheers them up and that … not just the music in itself but that there's a focus for them. People, someone can come round, someone can sit at the back [pause]

G: And that's how it's designed I suppose. It's this kind of chance for people to be recognized. To do something, to be appreciated, but at their level. But it is different for pros isn't it? Maybe you and D. It's the same, slightly the same story. There's a real ambivalence. It's 'I've got this talent, I can do this, but it's also, there's another side to it, there's a different side to it as well … ' It's reconciling that with …

***

G: Simon, this is a bit of a blunt question … .but you know me now! We're talking today about these two years 2006–2008 … .and I think you know I get your story about music and your involvement in SMART Music. I understand the complexities of that on all levels, but there's one thing that's quite obvious to me observing. Which is that you have participated more and more over these two years …

When I first started this afternoon in 2005 I remember you standing at the back of the room, and now you contribute, so much that you stand at the *front* of the room mostly now. Mainly with your violin, but you do other things, you play the piano sometimes, you play what needs to be played to help the music along and you give a lot. You help me and you give a lot to people. There's a real change it seems to me … and it doesn't quite square with the story you're telling me, do you know?

S: That comes from the feeling of an obligation to please people more than anything. And to be seen to be useful and [pause] it seems to be my role in life, and most of my family. My sister's a nurse, and she's a total martyr and a slave to everybody all her life. And my dad the same, dad was pretty much the same and his mother was the same [laughs].

G: Yeah, it's a family trait, is that right? So do you feel pressured to do it? I mean, have I exerted pressure to …

S: No, no, not at all … [pause]. I'd had quite a bad patch … . I was depressed for a very long time; six months I think it was … and you probably noticed around that time that I had played the piano a bit, which is, there's somebody else there when you play the piano and its, the piano's there and everything else's there.

The violin, it's a bit, I always had, especially when it was put out in bands, and leading dance bands and going around tables and stuff. There's this thing sticking out in people's faces, you know, it's very confrontational, and it's precarious and if you seem to go wrong you know about it straight away. Plus I'd hardly played the violin for hardly 10 years or more, hardly at all. I'd hardly touched it for years so it took a little while to come back … .generally recovering slowly …

G: So kind of feeling you could somewhere? You suddenly felt, people gently encouraged you to get up there and …

S: Yeah. But then this is the situation that I need to be very careful. You've said 'do a few things, do this do that'. And it's a sort of partly feeling 'well I don't want to let them down, I don't want to refuse'. Well, it wouldn't be half bad for me to try something. But then have I think 'is this the right thing for the music and will it be a problem?'

Like yesterday when D said 'can you play something?', I thought OK fine … and there was B sitting there and the first thing I should have said is 'no drums

> please' ... which is common sense, whatever it was, I don't need it. But I thought 'oh no' you know, don't make a fuss, don't upset anyone, it's a party.
>
> **G:** Yes it's difficult, isn't it?
>
> **S:** But those sort of situations can be very stressful and dangerous for me really. So the 'Arts' a dangerous thing' I think. From someone who's balanced like you ... I mean obviously you've got your own problems in life and everything ... . but you're using it as a balancing thing for people, music, to help them. But it's obviously difficult for you to see the other extremes of anything to do with the Arts. One can tip the balance quite easily.

So, for Simon music is both the best and the worst of things. It is dangerous in that it can tip the balance into illness. It can bring with it too many obligations – to perform, to please, to conform, to entertain, to play a pre-defined, and sometimes non-negotiable role. And it can be taken in too great a dose. At the same time it is an escape valve, a source of identity and a validation of identity and a means for feeling emotion and for connecting to others. In short, music is no mere panacea but a complex substance that has good and bad effects – for different people, at different times ...

12. Finding a Place and a Path in Music

> 'Who and what exactly makes, transports and transfigures this particular kind of musical place and space?' [Gary's log, 4 Feb 2010]

Simon's story highlights the intricacies of musical participation – the business of finding a place, part or role as a musical person within a musical community, and the variety of ways of finding a pathway within such a space by way of entrances and exits, passages and degrees of proximity and distance to the musical action. For other people at SMART it's perhaps less complex, but the 'mechanisms' of such finding of place and pathway are equally crucial, and help us understand more of the benefits and risks of musicking in sensitive environments.

Coming back to our idea of an eco-phenomenology of music we see how music is naturally about moving and moving through; coming in and going out; travelling towards and living through; finding a place and taking a part for a while, then moving on. To be in/with music is to be in movement, in passage, on a pathway, seemingly going *somewhere*. This happens both 'within' the life of the music itself, and simultaneously in the paramusical social life that happens when people are in the process of musicking.

We wrote earlier about how music draws people into places and occasions; helps them 'get through' situations; helps them feel they belong somewhere (that they can 'take their part'); softens the passage into a social situation – or, alternatively, repels and redirects them.

These 'musical movements' can be seen 'externally' and heard 'internally' within the unique processes that music affords. For example, to sing a particular voice in a musical texture (low/high – top/bottom – soprano/bass) is to find a place and a part within musical space. Then thinking of the dimension of time, musical process gives you hints about when there's a time to come in, to make one's entrance and exit within the musical texture (a rhythmic judgement of time and thus a sense of propriety, musically conceived). Different idioms, different cultural traditions of music construct these processes in different ways – that both reflect and continue to build musical-social reality. There are some particular and important characteristics of what we might think of as 'participatory music':

Thomas Turino and Christopher Small on 'participatory music'

Thomas Turino (2008) describes the aesthetic and practical differences between 'presentational musics' – where control, relative perfection and presentation *to* people is the norm, and 'participatory music' where the priority is to involve everyone in a given social situation, where process trumps product. In another book in this Triptych DeNora (2013) suggests that the dichotomy may not be so clear since the criteria by which 'perfection' are registered are both numerous and, at times, self-contradictory. As Pierre Bourdieu (1984) has put it, there is no autonomous way of judging art; judgement is always linked to some people, times, situations and values. That said, we have a feeling of what Turino means. Music that is 'participatory' often makes use of various techniques (musical and paramusical) to cover up or otherwise make sense of the 'messy' ways that people come in, go out and play around within the music. (Tia's field notes from her first-ever session in 2006 say, 'Note: people drift in/out, like attending Catholic church'.)

So 'open forms', which allow for what Turino calls 'feathering', accommodate messy musical beginnings and endings, lulls and extended transitions where people negotiate and experiment with what comes next, with whom and how. Texture and timbre are often loud and dense (heterophonic) for similar reasons in order to provide a 'cloaking function' to reassure and support less able participants. Roles and responsibilities of players change and mutate as people move in, out, forward or back in the musical configuration, or in the texture, finding their place and function with the broad musical relationships – but also being together in the dynamic intensity of the forms of vitality. Something of these features can be found in African and other ethnic musics, jazz, folk and other popular music traditions.

Christopher Small's (1998) *musicking* model offers another way of representing the complex relationships between the physical performance space and the people and tone relationships that interact within it, one that connects well with our discussion so far of musical/paramusical features. The following diagram shows Ansdell's (2014) visual/summary interpretation of the musicking concept, showing the reciprocal relationships musicking sets up between: (1) tone relationships, [includes tones and their sounding materials/instruments etc.] (2) people relationships, (3) situational relationships. Small's point is that these basic levels all inter-penetrate and add further complexity through second-order and third-order relationships ad infinitum. But what's conceptually complex is *not* complex in our experience within musicking. Rather, that's what it's all about, and that's why it's satisfying to us. There's a natural connection between how tones and people and places and occasions go together to make something that is far more than the sum of its parts.

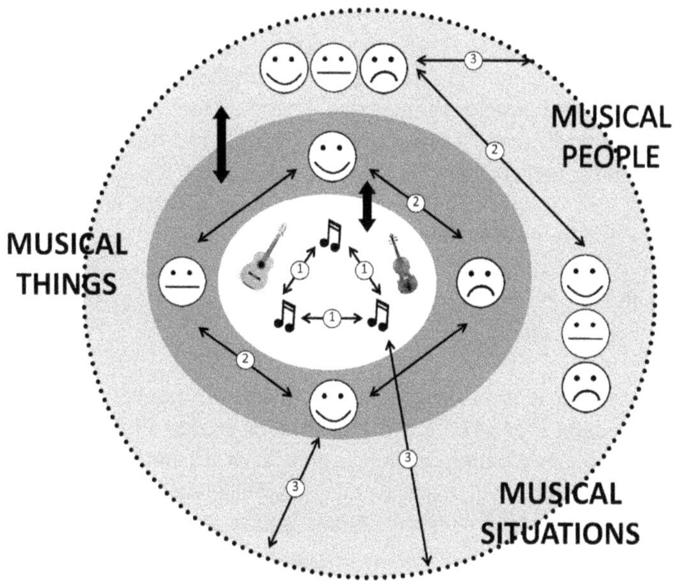

Figure 7 The ecology of relationships in musicking

Add to this picture of 'how music works' in social life the situation of the people who attend SMART and SMART Music and a further complexity appears, but one that takes its logic from what music affords in terms of movement, appearance, passage and placing. This varies over a wide variety of parameters that we were able to witness, track and try to understand because we were there over a 10-year period:

- ***Long timespan*** – the open space of the cafe, and open choice of participation at SMART Music – whether to come or not; when to stay away, come back, find a place again (despite having been ill / in hospital etc. for six months or not). SMART Music is still there.
- ***Short timespan*** – within a particular afternoon/event: finding your time to arrive, be there, depart.

- ***Immediate timespan:*** Finding a time within the flow of the afternoon to make a musical appearance, to be noticed, to fade out, to go away.
- ***Exact timespan:*** Finding an exact point in a given musical item to come in to the musical process, be there, go away, fade out, do something else …

The data we collected has a wide variety of examples of these categories, all of which of course interpenetrate both with themselves and with the other dimensions of tone relationships and people relationships. So, for example, there is one long-term member who 'engineers' a variety of long-span and short-span entrances and exits which afford him recognition, drama, continuity, characterisation, respite and reprise, but also long-term development within this socio-musical frame. With other people we see something less linear, something more like phases or cycles linked to the ups and downs of illness that determine their pattern of participation over time. But underneath these surface variations, the structure of the various SMART Music projects facilitates a patterned way of engaging musically that is supportive and accommodating and that enables diverse ways of appearing, disappearing and generally belonging.

Parallel to such 'timespan' aspects is an equivalent 'space-span' aspect, based on the way that the physical space of the SMART cafe (and related spaces) afford and disallow aspects for members' musicking:

- ***Wide space-span*** – the physical layout of the cafe and its special arrangement for SMART Music and other groups allows different spaces for being, participating, hiding, coming forward and backward, retreating, positioning for social, musical and relational advantage etc. It also relates to the acoustics of the physical settings, and the spatial relationship between main-space and sub-spaces (e.g. garden, back-room, kitchen, offices, street …).
- ***Narrow space-span*** – more precise musical-social configurations that afford particular modes of playing, performing, acting with, coordinating and occasional negative aspects such as acting against, subverting etc. This level links to the 'internal spacing' within musicking – how registers, accompaniment/soloist, ensemble, texture, timbre and 'orchestration' are managed (consciously and non-consciously).

These two meta-dimensions (time/timing in musicking; space/spacing in musicking) enabled the dynamic movements of musical occasions (and their progressive patterning over the years): the movements *through* - the passages, pathways, entrances and exits that form the structural grid by which people and their music, and the collective music takes on a narrative and dramatic shape. They also enable the parts, and roles that people come to take on, develop, try-on, reject and move on from …

We also noted two other kinds of pathways: 'spiral pathways' where directions of movement work in more than one plane (up *and* down, in *and* out), and secondly, 'paving the way' through music. Here there's a sense of how people in collaboration with others, can pave the way to expanded and changed identities and associated health states, paving block by paving block, as it were, where some of these paving stones are musical performances and musical encounters.

***

Talk of 'pathways' inevitably suggests a now long-running concept in modern healthcare theory of 'care pathways'. Whilst not unrelated to this, our research in SMART has helped perhaps to return the concept of 'pathways' in recovery to a more distinct meaning, rather than the rather formulaic and generic idea it's become. (We'll have more to say about this bespoke understanding of the pathway concept later on when we return to the subject of how to assess 'outcomes' in music therapy.) An incident at SMART illustrates this, when Gary reported some of the project informally to the manager, Amelia:

> Talking to Amelia (she's currently bidding for the new Borough tender for daycare services), leads to a discussion of the service needs for ensuring pathways for people. I mention what we've learned about this recovery concept through the music project: that a 'musical pathway' can be from that chair (I point to the back of the cafe) to the microphone to sing a first ever song in public – where the pathway is about 4 metres, but over a timespan of 6 months!). But it's very valuable and significant within the 'personal scaling' of *that person* and their history and situation. Whereas the general talk of 'pathways' in mental healthcare is often generic, formulaic, one size fits all ... theoretical ... Or, I say, there's the other type of momentous musical pathways between here at SMART and the main hospital atrium for a public performance .... [Gary's log – June 2011]

13. Everyday Ritual, Everyday Performance

It doesn't take long for SMART Music to become a regular, ritualised event in the SMART weekly timetable. Because of its beginnings (in 2005 SMART had few plans or formal expectations of it) Gary could experiment not only with the musical situation, but also with the frame of the event as a whole. Was this a music therapy group? Not exactly, but on the other hand it was an event that was regular, sustained, safe and reliable (in key ways it has always conformed to at least some of the classic therapeutic boundaries of space, time and person – though this statement we know would be puzzling to a psychodynamic therapist who automatically understands the therapeutic frame only as private, confidential and closed once business begins). SMART Music inevitably took some of its shape from the working practices and attitudes of the music therapists who ran it. At first

Gary just called it 'SMART MUSIC', partly not to frighten people away, but also to not over-define or constrain it. It could be what it needed to be. They reverted to the basic philosophy of Community Music Therapy: *follow where people and music lead ... whilst retaining your expertise and skills as a therapist.*

The characteristic routine and shape of Thursday afternoons established itself relatively quickly, involving the following key stages and priorities:

1. Setting-up the 'musical-social space' together with the members. Physically this space was co-extensive with the everyday social space of SMART – the cafe itself – on purpose, *not* creating a separated out 'therapeutic space' in the back room.
2. Starting the musicking as soon as possible, but with full allowance of people drifting in, drifting through etc. In this sense some of the basic 'rules' of traditional therapeutic boundaries were being breached from the beginning.
3. Having an interval/ tea-break about half way through – for chat, mingling and for the music therapists to find out how people are, and how the afternoon is going for them.
4. Having a 'second half', often with enhanced participation, culminating in
5. A 'finale' of sorts – culminating in a 'last song', usually being a gathering of forces and enhanced togetherness at best, incorporating goodbyes and mutual appreciation.
6. 'Breaking' the stage together, and returning the cafe to its normal configuration, putting the paraphernalia back into storage for next time …

This outline description highlights how this everyday event shares its form, shape, 'rules', features and perhaps purpose with many other social and ritual formats: in the relationship between the characteristics of the space itself (before/during/after); the transformation of the space and people's behaviour/experience within it by re-configuring the space, adding aspects (both material – things, foods etc. – and quasi-material – music being a fluid addition [as we outlined in the previous section]); configuring and shaping time within 'special' boundaries; having a contrast between within/without in terms of time, space, activity, feel, specialness etc.[12]

The connection between the musical occasion and ritual process is strong here, and it's no surprise that aspects of ritual theory have been increasingly used within Community Music Therapy literature to describe and understand the situations, conditions, behaviours and affordances of socio-musical transformation at work in events like SMART Music.[13]

---

[12] Victor Turner (1982) *From Ritual to Theatre*, p. 1: 'The word *entertain*, incidentally, is derived from OF *entretenir*, to 'hold apart', that is, create a limial or liminoid space in which performances may take place'.

[13] See Ansdell (2014), pp. 31–236, 239–40, 243; Stige, Ansdell, Elefant and Pavlicevic (2010); Aigen (2014).

Ritual performances/performance rituals

Rituals and performances often mirror each other, both ceremonies of belonging. Rituals incorporate everyday things and behaviours and make them special by artifying and musicalising them through formalisation, repetition, exaggeration and elaboration. Reciprocally, on returning from a ritual, the everyday can seem special again, even sacred. Many people today would say the same of art. But because in the West now we tend to separate out the various art forms and concentrate on their unique features, we are apt to miss just how many aspects of ritual still remain in our ways of approaching and using the arts overall. For the key aspect of any ritual is that it affords not just display or repetition, but also potentials for individual and communal transformation.

In his book *Musicking* (1988), Christopher Small sets out to highlight the ritual aspects of musical performance by explicitly choosing an event – a conventional symphony concert – whose very familiarity masks its ritual for many readers. Small nevertheless shows how, just like any other form of musicking around the world, a classical concert functions ritually 'as an act of affirmation of community ('This is who we are'), as an act of exploration (to try on identities to see who we think we are), and as an act of celebration (to rejoice in the knowledge of an identity not only possessed but also shared with others)' (1998, p. 5). But whilst ritual is the grand frame of musicking for Small, a specific musical ritual need not be grand itself. Rituals range from the relatively mundane and small scale through to the sacred and spectacular. Ritualisation can be as simple as the framing or re-framing of small gestures of everyday interaction, whilst in other situations its grand displays are designed to stoke utopian dreams. What all levels of ritual seem to share, however, is a way of gathering people together to catalyse and then to support *transitions* between roles, experiential states and situations – either individual or collective. This is perhaps why rituals and ceremonies become crucial at times of crisis, uncertainty, or where a new personal or communal identity is actively being sought. Ritual helps us to come together, and then to move together towards something different.

Some key features that all rituals involve to a greater or lesser extent:

- a cross-sensory blend of action, music, symbolic speech, stylised movement, costumes, fragrance, lighting, staging – synthesising verbal and non-verbal forms of communication;
- participation and immersion in a shared scene and narrative structure that either derives from a collective history or is in the process of creating a new tradition;
- intense psychophysical states of anticipation, excitement, anxiety and ecstasy, bringing about transitions and transformations in feeling and thinking, both individual and collective;
- reconciling differences between individuals and sub-groups within the larger frame of the whole event.

The connections between these features and the stagecraft and emotional characteristics of the performance arts are obvious. A ritual relies on an infrastructure that organises and mobilises the staging, props and witnessing/participating audience that are necessary for its transformative purpose. There's also a characteristic structure of most rituals that the first generation of anthropologists identified and codified from their comparative studies of many cultures. Most ritual processes have a simple three-part process: separation, liminality (or between-ness) and return to normality. At whatever level of complexity or importance, we are taken out of everyday life and its structures and rules, and out of quotidian time and its usual demands. We then experience a period where things are in flux and possibility, then we return again to 'real life' – but somehow transformed, either in social status or in a more individual and existential sense. This pattern could stand true for an adolescents' initiation ceremony in a traditional society, for a contemporary Western transition to marriage or to a new job, or for the experience of living through a concert or religious service.

Music therapist Brynjulf Stige (2010) has used anthropologist Randall Collins's theory of *interaction rituals* to study the process of a music therapy group with adults with learning disabilities. Stige observed closely just how naturally the therapist and clients assembled together a small-scale everyday ritual situation within their group, picking up and elaborating everyday communicative interactions in a creative and musical way to build something that was more than the sum of its parts – and that had an overall transformative effect on the whole group.

An 'interaction rituals' perspective suggests, and as ethnographic work on music production has documented (Atkinson 2006; 2010), that a performance situation of any type has its 'staging', repeated format and 'props' that function to support and focus social interaction and meaning between people in ways that would not necessarily happen otherwise. The performance frame may be very modest, spontaneous and informal, but it will typically involve the following key features:

- *Bodily co-presence* describes how people involved are physically orientated towards one another as much as possible, heightening their mutual focus. When physical gestures are 'musicalised', they become more noticed and significant to the group, pulling people further into face-to-face interactions.
- *Mutual focus of attention* describes how an individual's musical responses and interactions become increasingly 'circulated' and shared amongst the group as a whole. The music helps the group to find a mutual focus of attention and interest that can lead into joint action.
- *Shared mood*: the 'feel' of the songs and spontaneous interactions is both subjectively experienced by individuals and intersubjectively shared, with the highlights creating unexpected releases of musical and interpersonal emotion. Everyone experiences a similar progression through the charged time and 'musical shape' of the session. Randall Collins suggests that the key to interaction rituals is that they are 'emotion transformers' for the group as a whole.

In many social and therapeutic contexts, these ritual features are repeated weekly, and they gradually shape and reinforce feelings of belonging and solidarity. Music therapy groups take time and careful repetition to bring out the potential for greater social interaction, and for the group members the regularity of the weekly session is often itself a helpful ritual. Brynjulf Stige suggests that what he calls 'ritual outcomes' can be viewed as therapeutic outcomes too. Social space is opened up and energised, and a sense of group mutuality and solidarity prepares for transformation – both individual and communal. [adapted from Ansdell 2014, pp. 31–236]

Sarah and I discuss how SMART Music creates a special event weekly, but is also a very normal, everyday event as well – a weekly ritual of specialness for people. Psychiatric culture tends to leave out this need, but if we look at everyday musical culture it's always an evocation of some kind of *specialness* – when people perform, witness, support, achieve, risk, experience some peak moment, share conviviality, etc. [Gary's log, 7 June 2007]

14. Emerging Outcomes

By the end of 2005 the Thursday afternoon group – SMART Music – is established and successful for the people who now participate in it, and support its development. Many of the themes we've written about above are beginning to shape our thinking about what is happening in this nascent musical community, and what's important about this in relation to people's health and wellbeing.

The staff of SMART emphasise the musical 'flourishing' of individuals, but also what's quite apparent is the musical flourishing of the community more generally. This shows up in particular in events where either appreciation or trouble is concerned. Here we begin to see how music helps in more precise ways. Early examples of this are celebrations and 'bad days'; unexpected appearances of music; realisations of everyday happenings that are qualitative outcomes of the project and of people's collective work on musicking together. Here are five vignettes, occurring between March and October 2005. These are not 'high-points', just everyday events recorded in Gary's log:

- There are more people today, more instruments being brought along, it's raucous at points – full participation. We sing happy birthday to Eloise for today, and then to Sadie whose birthday was yesterday. Music as a vehicle for celebration, ritual, here in this community. Bobby has brought along friend who's an ambulance driver to witness him playing drums and singing. Feeling that SMART Music is a social achievement for many people now, they've carved out their place here. [Gary's log, 10 Feb 2005]
- SMART staff give some feedback: Anita: 'I get so emotional here on Thursday afternoons – we sit here blubbing'. They talk of surprising events for them – people doing what they thought they couldn't do, how music makes people feel powerful. 'They all have their own music, it connects to their past, they feel powerful when they do it in front of others. The music changes this place on Thursdays.' [Gary's log, 26 October 2005]
- I suddenly hear someone playing claves from within the office during an improvisation. It's Dave, the manager – he says he wasn't aware he was doing it really. But we orientate the improvisation to him, giving him a little rhythmic figure to play within the music even though we

can't see him, and he can't see us – it's fun, but also an example of how musicking stitches up the physical and social space here. [Gary's log, 26 October 2005]

- Rather low-key group on a dark wet afternoon. But also comfortable and gentle, which enables some nice things to happen. For example, Kerry has been building up her confidence for a few months, and had a breakthrough today – coming to the mic and singing two songs and a duet with Viv. People found this very moving – a good example of this group as a vehicle for personal development over fairly long scale (from 'I want to do this' to 'I can' to 'I did'). We have seen this progression of participation from the communal singing to individual performance, communally witnessed. Because it's a stable community of people, they know how much of a step that is for Kerry, and appreciate the significance. Later the staff said that they listened from their offices, and found it so moving. [Gary's log, 16 November 2005]
- Dave tells me a nice story afterwards. He is having a difficult discussion with Will in his office during the music group, about the challenges of taking SMART and the staff along with a new plan. At this moment what comes through the wall is a rousing *Climb Every Mountain*. 'I don't believe this' I said to Will – 'it's a sign'. Great example of the music and its message permeating and influencing the whole place. [Gary's log, 26 October 2005]
- 'I was feeling rotten this morning, but I forced myself to come. After the music I just felt better' [Sadie, volunteer behind drinks counter, July 2005]

From these early days of the project it's clear that for many people music helps – though it is not always an unmitigated 'good thing', as we've seen in the ambivalence certain people have to music and musical participation. The pattern is more complicated, and it involves fluctuations, both in the life of individuals, and of the SMART community as a whole – good days, bad days. And yet, it is also possible to speak of outcomes that are overall 'for the better' – though if there is one thing we have learned it is that such more complex outcomes could not be captured by any simple measurement device, in ways that suit experimental formats. The problem we find with the artificial structure implied by a Randomised Controlled Trial is that it implies a unitary 'before' and 'after' and that people are somehow (often mysteriously) affected by a musical 'intervention' (see DeNora & Ansdell 2014). Experiments have time frames that are not necessarily aligned with the lived time of musical engagement as it occurs in real-time social interaction where, in Roger's terms (quoted earlier), you get an admixture of 'the rough with the smooth'. Second, the changes 'for the better' that we have seen, have experienced in ourselves as well, and are able to document are at once more subtle than those that could be measured by, say, an attitudes survey, and more imbued with meaning than could be captured by any physiological or brain-imagery techniques.

Third, they are – frankly – simpler. The evidence is often literally under our noses, directly accessible through observation, experience or report from others.

By the end of 2005 our research observations (greatly helped by Rob's interviews and the co-research that many of the SMART members are giving us by generously sharing their experiences, evaluations and insights) are that we can see qualitative outcomes of the music project in terms of:

1. Music affording individuals shifts of mood, participation, engagement, vitality, motivation, hope.
2. Musical activity and participation in the group affording positive appraisal of self and others through performance, and an opportunity to characterise the self through music choices (songs, styles, occasions, renderings).
3. Performances and participations affording staff an alternative (and mostly more complete and positive) way of understanding and appreciating members.
4. Music in the space and place of SMART affording ambience, energy, atmosphere, community and mutual appreciation and celebration.
5. The musical events affording topics of conversation (on music, on musical achievements), on-going preparation and focus for in-between session musical work.
6. A positive event to look forward to, to structure the week.
7. There's something organic and self-generating about how music is emerging in this community.

15. Interlude

By the end of 2005 the Thursday group, SMART Music, had become an established feature on the SMART weekly routine. It regularly attracted up to 20 people who came specifically for the music group. A further group of people would simply be there because of the cafe and would experience the group by default, and would often join in peripherally in some way. Of the people who came to sing and play it seemed to satisfy them, more or less. The unique nature of the group – blending age groups, social and ethnic groups, musical tastes and aesthetics – partly followed SMART's inclusive attitude (people were primarily there because they were coping with a mental health challenge). But as the music group matured during 2006 it was also clear that it couldn't cater for everyone's needs all the time. As news of the group went around the local community it also attracted 'ex'-musicians who had lost touch with music and wanted/needed to play again. The aesthetic mix became more complex.

Rob's fieldwork in these early years included hanging around the cafe/ organisation for a prolonged period every day for a month in the summer of 2006. During this period he did a series of 29 interviews with anyone who was prepared to talk to him about music, whether or not they had anything to do with the new music project. Two interesting and useful things came out of these interviews: firstly, ample evidence for our research hunch that there's a powerful connection between music and mental wellbeing for many if not most of the members of the SMART community (and that sometimes this involves a very personal and private relationship to music). Secondly, whilst many people were very satisfied with the new music project, and had found it transformational for them, others felt that whilst it was a good start, more and different forms of musical participation were needed at SMART. They gave suggestions, and we listened ...

During 2006 Gary continued to facilitate SMART Music on Thursday afternoons, whilst continuing to work with Sarah in the adjacent hospital site to bridge patients between there and SMART (building on the strong informal relationship between the two organisations that'd existed for years). Alongside this practical work, the project gradually concentrated more on the idea of 'musical bridging' – and how this helped people transition between the physical sites of care, but also bridging experienced states of mental illness/health in a smoother and more positive way.

Finally, by the end of 2006 arrangements were made for Sarah also to work on the music project at SMART for a full day from 2007, working with Gary on Thursday afternoons, but also initiating some complementary music groups on a second day, Wednesday. Music between the hospital and SMART sites would now be more formally bridged and coordinated ...

At a research level, we were amassing more evidence at exactly the fine-grained level we were looking for: seeing just how, when, and why people's detailed engagement with music and musicking in this community seemed to help – both with their immediate experience, and with movements towards long-term recovery. Patterns were emerging of how exactly individuals used music, how they collaborated together to mobilise music within SMART, and how the combined musical work of the members, Sarah and Gary increasingly 'rippled out' through the immediate and wider community.

16. Occupying and Navigating Musical Space

Six months into the project, a sense of musical space (or terrain) has developed in the Thursday afternoon SMART Music session, such that individuals and groups can now be identified by their musical tendencies, by the places that they tend to dwell within when musicking. Daniel, for example, becomes known primarily for his jazz standards and for his participation on electric guitar, Jeremy for the songs his mother taught him, and Simon for his exquisite obbligato playing on violin. We started to think about the SMART musical space graphically according to three dimensions: scale (what are the more and less frequented musical forms, genres, works, instruments in general terms? – as indicated by the different font sizes in Figure 8), depth of involvement (how frequently and with what levels of intensity do they occupy these parts of the space? – the weight of each line below), and individual levels of attachment (how much does this member of SMART take part in this form of musicking and to what extent? – through what do the lines in the diagram pass and linger on?).

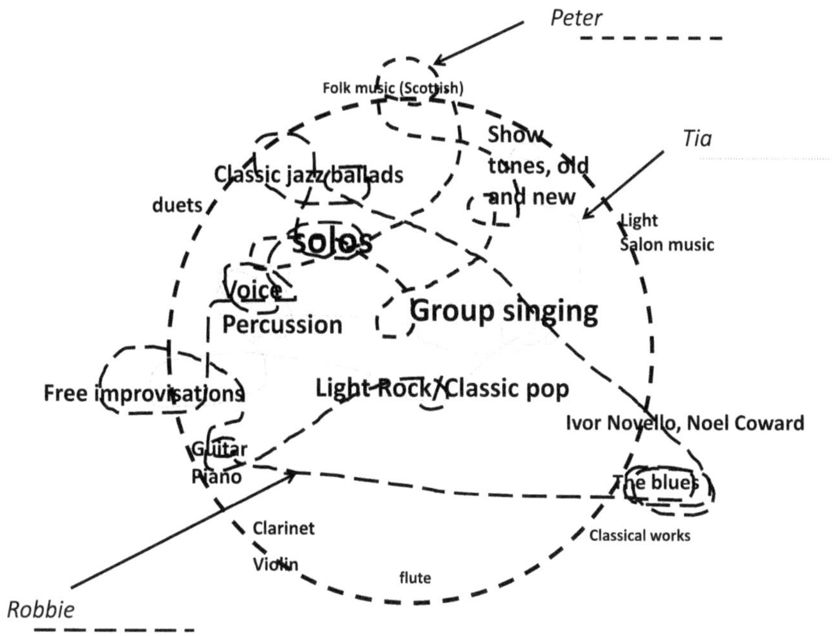

Figure 8 Three individuals' 'musical trails' in SMART Music space

Thinking about the musical 'furnishings' of the SMART space in this manner can be useful because it helps us to map the main and more marginal places in the SMART space and consider how that space, musically, changes over time (thus allowing us to consider the question of cultural change from season to season, year to year). Second, it allows us to understand the dynamics of that change – the who, where, what, when and how it changed, as new musical and paramusical materials are adopted and drawn into the space, as other materials are pushed to the margins of that space and allowed to lapse. Along with this second question, thinking about SMART's music spatially also lets us consider individuals in terms of where they are situated musically, how that situation overlaps with other members, drawing them into closer alliance with some members and distancing them from others. Simultaneously, it allows us to think about how individual musical practices may expand or contract, drawing them into the musical orbits of others and through this making links, forging socio-musical capital between individuals. This forging of links in turn is the mechanism by which the overall musical culture at SMART comes to be developed and expanded, how the musical space not only develops as it comes to be increasingly diversely furnished, but how that diversity of musical furnishing also offers opportunities for action, and change, within the space.

One of the most basic processes by which the space is furnished is through individuals' 'signature' tunes where social relations are interleaved through the sharing, or partitioning, of these tunes. Such tunes become 'places' for occupation in several senses. First, they offer forms of musical occupation (forms and styles of musicianhood). They configure musicians who, to perform them, need to align their own bodily-musical features with what it takes to produce *that* song as opposed to *this* one. Second, they produce identities, demonstrate musical affiliation and attachment through the ways that, over repeat performances, they demonstrate which part of the musical space a performer occupies and/or may claim to occupy. Widening one's repertoire thus means access to varied ways of musically presenting one's self, which means an openness to varied forms of musical connection. Such openness in turn offers a musical, or as Simon Procter (2013) has spoken of it, proto-social form of musical capital, – the basis, in other words for growing social capital understood as relations and meaningful links with other people. But singing someone else's song, or venturing onto their musical terrain can achieve varied results. On the one hand, it may be a tribute. On the other hand, it may be read as a takeover bid. Third, signature tunes offer place holders for occupational wellbeing and health; they endure through the vicissitudes of illness/health and their performance can be read as a demonstration of 'wellness within the illness': even during 'bad times' the songs remain – sometimes as an actual support. If they can be sung, however tentatively, then that aspect of self is demonstrable 'well' and thus a resource for further improvement. Finally, fourth, the repeated performance of signature tunes can demonstrate both up and down turns in health/illness situation and as such, the ways a singer comes to occupy the same song on different occasions can offer diagnostic methods for gauging the singer's health/illness state (how strained is the voice, how halting the melody, does the voice sound congested, is the melody so over-ornamented that it becomes unrecognisable, how entrained is the singer to the song and to the accompanying musicians?).

The other aspect of musical space is how certain 'formats' of musicking develop at SMART Music; that is, the configurations and social-spatial dispositions of people and musical instruments that follow from certain styles, choices and set-ups. You will recall that Session 1 of SMART Music began straight away with a group number. The aim was to involve singers and a variety of instrumentalists who happen to be there waiting. The format is at once some kind of *ensemble* – everyone playing together, using everything. But there's also within this first session a few solo songs, one unaccompanied, one with piano and other instruments accompanying; there are some improvisatory versions of known songs and an improvisation using just a musical idiom (tango). As with SMART Music as a whole, little is planned, so such juxtaposition of musical format has musical-social significance at some level just by virtue of it happening this way. In many ways the first session set the tone and agenda for formats for the following years, but we should still keep an eye on the evolving significance and affordance of the appearance and balance of solo, duet, ensemble, improvisation, song performance, idiomatic group jam, etc. All of these create and inflect musical-social space. Gary sometimes intervenes with the (therapeutic) strategic aim of balancing individuals' needs against those of the group, or with the intention of breaking up something that is dominating or 'too much' (for example, too many solos in a row, too much group, too much noise from amplified instruments etc.). But there's also a more natural and spontaneous mix and flux of the overall musical shape – an ebb and flow that is perhaps musical in itself. That is, there's a shaping of the intensity, pace and 'narrative form' of the session that is partly managed through changes in format. This variation also attends to some of the precise musical-social needs of the participants: to be heard and witnessed (as individual performers); but also to make musical relationships and collaborations, to forge musical community and bring together the cafe as a whole.

***

The following sections will present aspects of what we gradually began to understand by the second year of following the project in terms of this occupation and traversing of physical and musical space through trails, tracks and pathways. We will look at individual and collective repertoire, and how this developed over time. Also how singers and songs communicated subtle non-verbal understandings within this space, and how all of this together helped to establish and strengthen this musical community.

17. Jeremy's Songs

Jeremy tells Gary how he threw a lot of his mother's sheet music out of the window when he was ill some years ago. He retrieved enough of it, however, to keep selecting songs from this repertoire for the last 10 years of SMART Music Sessions. In one sense these songs formed something of a time capsule for Jeremy: a time when he was with his musically-talented mother (a pianist and singer) in South Africa in the 1940s. The songs come from his mother's era (the 1920s and 1930s). His long-term psychiatrist, Dr M, makes the mistake of criticising these songs at one point – pointing out that Jeremy's attachment to them and what they represent is a millstone around his neck that prevents Jeremy from moving on in his life. Jeremy is outraged at this attack on the songs (it seems very much this, not an attack on Jeremy, but his songs …), and he goes around the SMART community telling people of this outrage. 'These songs' he tells anyone who will listen, 'saved my life'.

This ambivalence as to whether Jeremy's songs help or hinder his life revolves perhaps not around the 'fact' of the songs but rather the songs-in-action. When Dr M describes them as 'millstones' he's thinking of how they perhaps trap Jeremy both in a past era, and in a past relationship (with his deceased mother). Certainly *one* aspect of how the songs help (from Jeremy's point of view) is that they are 'comforting', as they represent a tangible connection to a significant intimate relationship in his life, and a relatively stable and happy time in his life (South Africa, as a child). In this psychological sense the songs evoke (and perhaps more directly, *invoke*) a person and a place. The problem with this aspect is that it seems to have been unchanging during Dr M's 30-year support of Jeremy. Are these songs helping or hindering Jeremy's life?

Crucially, in Jeremy's first interview with Rob, he describes how he likes SMART Music because it gives him a chance to 'air' his songs. Jeremy quickly develops a routine on Thursday afternoons of bringing the crumbling sheet-music to the sessions, and singing two songs (with or without accompaniment). These are prefaced by an elaborate and often witty prologue that introduces the song, and who the original singer was (often a singer-cum-film star of the 1930s/1940s such as Jesse Mathews). Jeremy then explains the connection between a song, his mother and himself – and then sings it. This routine becomes known as 'Jeremy's spot', and it's usually received with appreciation (which includes appreciation for Jeremy as a person – a valued daily figure in the SMART community), but also a measure of wry puzzlement at the sheer out-of-time character of these musical items. They are not just one but two generations back, and seriously outside of any current popular musical repertoire. Occasionally, a few of the older members (in their seventies) will recognise one of the songs and partly sing along with Jeremy. Some songs become known by other people through sheer repetition by Jeremy over the years at SMART.

But the key aspect of Jeremy's songs within the SMART musical space is the *performative* dimension; how Jeremy 'airs' them – the songs-in-action, within a real social setting where immediate musical-social relationships are being forged and developed. The first performative aspect is how Jeremy (with the musical help of Sarah, Gary and later other musicians) manages to get a lot better at singing his songs, and singing them with others. Through performance the songs are let out of their time capsule, and become a way of being musically with others, whilst keeping their personal value to Jeremy. He airs both the songs and the relationships that they symbolise. The past becomes the musical present.

A second variety of performance is to *use* the songs to fit purpose here-and-now. Tracing the various special occasions of the SMART community over the years shows how Jeremy cunningly and wittily adapts the old songs to fit new situations. Goodbye and anniversary/appreciation for SMART members come up many times. More touchingly, at points of illness, stress or confusion, Jeremy uses the songs in a coded way to express what he can't always say more directly.

Then there's a very gradual change in how other people interact with Jeremy and his songs. He joins the newly formed SMART Singers in 2007, a group who choose their own song repertoire to work on (often with some of the same agenda as Jeremy with his private songs – that is, to say through sound and words what can't always be expressed easily otherwise). But of course there's a mis-match between the song repertoire that Jeremy favours and defends (his!), and the more up-to-date repertoire that the other singers are both familiar with, and want to work on. There's some conflict at times, charted through Sarah's notes – how Jeremy feels that others don't respect or accept his songs, and how he can't identify with their songs. Some more history comes out from this: that Jeremy left the UK in his thirties for a culturally insulated South Africa, and therefore missed out on pop music developments in this country for the next 20 years. He cites Dusty Springfield's *Only Want to Be With You* as the last pop song he heard. Sarah's careful musical and therapeutic work in the Singers gradually shows Jeremy that he's wrong in his assumption that nobody is interested in his songs, or wants to sing them – they do. But they also expect their acceptance and interest to be reciprocated – that Jeremy actively try to sing their repertoire. And, bit by bit he does just this – in the weekly rehearsals, and in the occasional internal and external concerts. Jeremy never looks entirely comfortable singing rock ballads, but he gamely tries …

Soon there's a revolution in repertoire for Jeremy, which feels as symbolic as with his own traditional favourites. He declares to the people at SMART Music that he's bought a *Take That* CD, but also a CD player, is shopping for classical music at HMV, and enjoying listening to a wider range of music, which keeps him from getting lonely at home.

This is not to say that the pile of songs is deserted! 'Jeremy's spot' still happens at SMART Music, and usually the song(s) come from the old pile. But his 'musical pile' has also been aerated, infiltrated by others songs, genres, eras … We believe him when he says that those old songs have saved his life. The point is that the new songs are helping forge a path forwards, not just backwards, and Jeremy's musical branching out makes more points of contact with others and their songs. Here music, and musical broadening can be seen to pave the way to deeper and more relationships. It offers, as Simon Procter terms it (2011), 'proto-social capital' …

18. How a Musical Repertoire Emerged and Developed

One origin of the more general shared repertoire of SMART Music in the first year or two is the 'Red Book' that travelled across from the hospital site to SMART for that first session (along with the percussion instruments and other equipment on the trolley). Gary had been using these red folders of photocopied word-sheets for the previous five years in his work in the hospital. It was built up, and gradually varied as songs patients said they wanted to sing were added and then sung in individual sessions, groups or (from January 2000), the 'Willow Choir' that grew out of a carol-singing group the previous month. The red book consisted of a slowly evolving repertoire of middle of the road popular songs that the wide social and age constituency in the hospital could relate to in some ways. As such, the repertoire was a musical reference point for people to join together singing and playing.

Much the same logic informed why Gary brought this book and its repertoire over that first day to SMART. Copies were put out on the cafe tables and as a 'safe starter' Gary suggested for a first song that people find something in the 'red book' to sing together. As we saw earlier, *Let It Be* emerged as the first choice, and *Somewhere Over the Rainbow* the second (chosen by Jeremy). Quickly, however, in that first session the repertoire of music expanded beyond the red book's possibilities, as people offered their own music, or as spontaneous choices (*One Note Samba, Girl from Ipanema)* came up. Right from the beginning, the musical repertoire of the group was a fluid combination of accessible choices (through songbooks) and personal offerings that stood for very personal taste choices and repertoires that the wide variety of participants contributed.

The red book served passably for a while, but represented a limited choice, and tended to encourage people to only sing what they could see in the book, getting into a habit. When Rob was appointed as a research assistant to the project four months over the summer of 2006 he had two tasks: to conduct a wide variety of interviews with SMART members about themselves and music, and secondly to help Sarah (now in the hospital site) to compile some new books, both for her use and for SMART Music, enlarging the repertoire of available songs for people. We talked about how to do this and consciously decided to involve members in this process: partly for the straightforward reason that we wanted the books to represent the taste range of the users, but also as a research tool to elicit the process of selecting and negotiating a repertoire. What would this tell us about the relationship between these people and music?

Rob's writes a very illuminating diary entry into his field notes on just this subject on Monday 31 July 2006, one that reminds us about the mutuality of 'care' in SMART, and the power of split-second interactions to make things right, normal and easy:

> Just after 12 Tim shows up in the cafe. By now I've piled music books onto a central table in the cafe, and sat down with a newspaper and a tea. We get chatting about the new song books, and I suggest that he looks through all the music books, to choose five songs he'd really like to include. Over the next 10 minutes, the meeting turns into a very insightful experience for me. I give Tim a piece of blank paper to write down the songs of his choice. His handwriting speed is quite slow, and he writes long sentences with particular attention to detail, making sure all the information is there on the page: 'Five Songs for the New SMART Songbooks, as chosen by Tim. Monday 31st July 2006'. It turns out to be a strange moment for me; I don't really know Tim all that well, and so in the silence caused by his concentration, I start off feeling a little awkward. But then I realise something: Bingo! One of those moments when the world seems to light up. Something is made clear to you. Here it's the fact that actually there's no need to be awkward with Tim. He's relaxed. And then suddenly I think, well, that actually there's no need for awkwardness with anyone in any walk of life. Suddenly it's all clear: another moment when my experiences at SMART force me to rethink my approach to people in everyday encounters. Getting to know individuals *here* is revealing about how people

interact in general. People are very *human* here, I think. Very *direct*, reacting to situations with what seems to be a gut instinct. People really show their emotions clearly in their body language, on their faces, in their expressions. With Tim, he's relaxed; at ease. He's feeling no awkwardness, so why should I?

To make things about a million times better, Tim then starts singing almost every song in one of the books he's looking at. Just reading through the contents page, he reels off the whole of each song down the list. He looks up from the book as he sings, singing to the room, to me, looking me right in the eye. Again a moment of awkwardness. But then it's ok again: he's fine with it, and actually, I'm fine with it also. He sings songs I know and I join in with him. The cafe continues around us. I'm not sure if people are really listening. It doesn't seem like anyone is watching us, or paying us any special attention. [Rob's Field notes, Data Corpus p. 30]

This is such a rich event, and goes to illustrate how some forms of knowledge, attachment and taste really need to be demonstrated and *enacted,* rather than just told. And how this is often a relatively slow process of witnessing and working alongside people, until the research epiphany comes. Rob organises a 'songbook committee' and people take their choosing very seriously. The outcome of this process is a set of three songbooks – henceforth known as the Red, Yellow and Blue books (each of which also accumulates and loses songs over the following years). A Green book comes out each year with Christmas songs. This core repertoire somehow anchors the SMART Music Sessions for many years. There's a ritual of putting them out and collecting them back (Eloise does this for a few years, counting them meticulously when a few start to be 'borrowed').

Other aspects of the development of the musical repertoire includes:

- Using published collections of songs that members bring along. Jane at one point starts spending her money on collections of 1970s and 1980s songs, or of favourite artists (Abba, Bert Bacharach etc.), and bringing these along to SMART Music and SMART Singers, for use by her and others.
- As downloading sheet music becomes possible, certain SMART Music members begin to do this themselves: finding a song, practising it during the week at home, and then bringing the music along to the sessions (which Sarah and Gary are expected to sight read without problem or error!). Daniel does this in particular.
- Borrowing music from the library: Nick does this regularly, pursuing particular 'taste trails' (e.g. French popular songs, then Germans songs …) often in a kind of private conversation with other SMART members – Eloise with the French songs, Anton with the German, etc.).

The subsequent history of repertoire development is a cross pollination between the three emerging groups at SMART during 2007 onwards. Dependent on the stage of this process, certain musicians become part of the different, but often overlapping music groups, to which they bring a song(s), which then goes into the mangle and is transmogrified by the immediate musicking of that group. For example, a song may begin in the SMART Singers group, and then someone will bring this song back to SMART Music on Thursday afternoon for a more open performance – where it gets a different treatment because the 'backing boys' put electric guitar and drums with it. Increasingly, people bring *their* music as well as relying on the core repertoire. They are confident of a basically receptive and appreciative reaction whatever the style, and however unusual and surreal the juxtapositions are within the two hours: a mish-mash of Mussei's reggae, Noel Coward, full-on Blues, wistful 1970s, a little light classical …

In *Musical Asylums* (DeNora 2013a: 117) Tia takes this theme one stage further by attempting to map the, as it were, differentiation of SMART Music space by genre, style, person, physical space and frequency of association between these things. As researchers we began to realise that SMART offered an interesting case for the sociology of musical taste and musical affiliation. As in the classic work of Pierre Bourdieu (2004) we could see that people and types of music tended to cluster, and that not all people at SMART participated in the makings of all the forms of music there or, when they did, they did so less frequently and/or from the physical periphery of the SMART Music space. So, as we just saw with the case of Jeremy, branching out from the songs his mother taught him to embrace a wider repertoire and thus occupy a greater portion of available musical space, members of SMART Music dwell and migrate over time from musical place to place, overlapping, sometimes conflicting in their views of how such space 'ought' to be occupied (as Tia describes in *Music Asylums*, one afternoon Gary got caught in a stylistic altercation over how to sing a jazz ballad) and sometimes bonding over shared musical commitments.

But whereas classical perspectives in music sociology might direct us to potential hierarchies and rankings of performers (preferred renditions, abilities, training, connections, experience), genres and styles ('high' versus 'popular'), there is something very unusual about the aesthetic democracy (or perhaps anarchy) of these SMART Music events. We are suggesting that the social-therapeutic process of cultivating a community that can and does tolerate difference is part of what allows music at SMART to 'help'. Through musical participation people find new aesthetic experiences as they try out each other's repertoires, and through this engagement find new relational and social experiences, and new opportunities.

19. People and Songs: Charting Song Attachment and Migration

Who sings what, and why? Does a song change owner, and does an owner change song? And, then, as we witness the singing of songs over many years at SMART, how do people keep singing their songs, and how do their performances change?

These kinds of questions became more fascinating as we accumulated enough longitudinal data to begin to answer them:

Studying songs empirically

The project logbooks over the period 2005–11 regularly record the songs people sing within SMART Music, Singers, Band, as well as in special events and occasions. Four hundred and twenty-six songs are specified in this data, though obviously thousands more were actually sung during this time. Those recorded in the logs usually comment on particular aspects of the people/song relationship: e.g. a person singing a song for the first time, or making an unusual choice. The logs provide a good longitudinal record of:

- someone singing the *same* song over a long period (or periodically), such that it becomes identified with them, or expressive of them in a particular way.
- someone requesting a song, or that another member sings it – for a particular personal or contextual reason often.
- when a song becomes symbolic of something (a person, event, etc.).
- how a song develops a 'career' of its own – changing 'owner', venue, format, performance style etc.

In order to look at this dimension we listed all of the songs in the summary data files (A–G), along with their singers/groups, and then looked for patterns within this.[1] This was worth doing, as to an extent it both confirmed and made a more subtle expression of a 'hypothesis' that we'd developed during the project fieldwork about how songs and singers related/developed over time (as in a–e above).

As a result of this exercise songs/singers could be accommodated into the following schema:

Ubiquitous Songs [16%] – usually 'old favourites' in the songbooks that could be relied upon to start off a session, or to revert to as 'something everyone will know', for more nervous singers to be sure they knew if trying out a solo; as a reassuring small repertoire of songs, such as (these are just the best examples each time):

Beatles (*Let it Be, Yesterday, When I'm 64, Hey Jude)*
Spirituals (*Swing Low, Amazing Grace)*
Summertime
Moon River
Danny Boy
Girl from Ipanema
I am Sailing
Somewhere Over the Rainbow
Annie's Song
Blue Moon

---

[1] Specifically: (i) we looked at all specific references to songs/singers in the summary files; (ii) coded these experimentally for the first file, then settling on a simple four-category system (see main text), (iii) coding the remainder of the files according to this; (iv) producing percentages for each category. There are of course drawbacks to this analysis: the logs don't represent *all* songs sung over the 250+ sessions, and are probably biased towards what is noteworthy to the researchers. But it does nevertheless present corroboration of patterns we perceived more informally.

'Tethered' Songs [40%] – where there's a close identification or 'tethering' of song to a singer over time (both part of the person's musical presentation, but also an acknowledgement by others of this being 'their song'):

Memory, Where is Love? Send In The Clowns, Anyone Can Whistle – Mary
Raindrops Keep Falling On My Head – Jonathan
What a Difference a Day Makes – Daniel
Dancing on the Ceiling, These Foolish Things ... – Jeremy
Won't Sleep Tonight [one-off] – Peter
Ol' Man River, Somewhere – Tim
Leaving On a Jetplane, My Baby Just Cares For Me – Ella
Cabaret – Gemma
Streets of London – Roger

'Migrating Songs' [37%] – which may start off with a particular person, then 'migrate' to other singers within/over time; between the Thursday group and Singers, Band, from/to regular and special musical events etc. As they migrate they may take on different interpretations, instrumentations, combinations etc. It might be interesting to think more about what it is about these particular songs that afford such migration. Sometimes it's only a few people who 'share' the songs, sometimes they are widely shared in various formats of musicking ...

Autumn Leaves
Cry me a river
Whiter shade of pale
Sway
Strangers in the night
Daydream believer
Nightingale sang in Berkeley Square
Smoke gets in your eyes
When I fall in love
Annie's Song
Lady is a Tramp
Fly me to the moon

'Novelty Songs' [7%] – being unusual, not in the normal repertoire, seasonal, or cued by current events or anniversaries:

In the bleak midwinter (Henrietta)
Pachelbel Canon (Tony)
Schubert Impromptu, Blue Danube, violin solos (Simon)
We'll Gather Lilacs, Cliffs of Dover (suggested by Eloise relating to historical anniversaries)
Congratulations (birthdays etc.)

There are further sub-categories that could be pulled out, such as links between ubiquitous songs and tethered (people gradually appropriating common songs); between ubiquitous and tethered songs that migrate to other music groups; collaborative treatment (*Whiter Shade of Pale, Blue Moon, Fly Me To The Moon*); songs that seem to slide over most of the categories (*Nightingale Sang in Berkeley Square, Danny Boy, Autumn Leaves*). But in general, the emerging picture is of a relatively small repertoire of 'common songs', but with an important balance between songs that almost only tether themselves to one (or sometimes a few) people, and those which migrate between and amongst the broader group.

We explored the relationships between people and songs a little further, and more closely, through a few small case studies of 'people/song careers': both (i) starting from *people* and following 'their song' longitudinally within different contexts and appearances, but also (ii) starting with *key songs* and tracing their 'career' over the data. To do this we re-examined the long list of songs made in order to code for the previous section, and looked at the 'ubiquitous songs' category, listing these separately. We then searched the log files (A–G) for each of these songs for frequency and detail of mention. *Summertime* came up as the most useful song for the purpose, appearing in a variety of formats, ensembles, solos etc., and appearing throughout the data set. For a 'tethered' song we chose Mary and two songs that we already knew were key to her: *Memory* and *Where is Love?* We again searched the log data for mention of these two songs in connection with Mary.

Interestingly, this more 'empirical' approach did not quite yield exactly what we'd expected. We'd expected more drift between songs and singers, whereas it actually seems that people and songs remain more static. Fewer songs actually have migrating careers. SMART musicians, however, certainly have careers with songs though – and perhaps this is the more accurate story, in that they are remarkably faithful to their songs, and their favoured styles. What happens, though, in terms of performances and reception over the years?

Two songs which emerged in the very first SMART Music Session continued to have a particular significance in the SMART musical community. One is a 'tethered' song that we see re-occurring over the remainder of the data – Mary singing *Where is Love?* The other is the classic jazz standard *Summertime*, from the 'ubiquitous' song category. The following sections will trace the 'career' or pathway of these two songs (plus a third, *Memory*, also strongly associated with Mary) across the data set to the end of 2012. Several interesting things come out of looking longitudinally in this way: how songs develop, change, don't change etc. in relation to people, situations and their own psycho-social and life changes.

20. The Songs Mary Sings

When Gary has worked with Mary before in the hospital setting she's sung *Where is Love?* both in individual and group music therapy sessions. So Gary is not too surprised when Mary suggests this song in the very first session of SMART Music on 13 January 2005. He writes in his notes: 'Mary sings *Where is Love?* confidently'. It's one of her 'signature tunes'. The next mention in the log is on 9 March, when Gary notes that Mary sings the same song, takes a while to get going but is quietly listened to by others, and appreciated.

In Session 55 on 20 July 2006 Bobby wants to sing something, but doesn't know what. We suggest picking something from the songbook, and Peggy suggests *Where is Love*. Someone says 'Let's dedicate this song to Mary, she's still in hospital, and she loves that song'. But it becomes apparent that Bobby doesn't really know the song at all. Gary ask him 'do you know it?' and he says

'I don't have to know it, I just sing it!'. And he does just this – he makes up his own version, with Gary providing jazz chords in the background. Bobby improvises the song using the words and serenades Peggy directly (who graciously and humorously accepts the honour!). It's a good counterexample of someone entirely ignoring the performance history of a song, and doing their own thing. It's also a good example of a song still being 'tethered' to a singer even when they are not physically there performing it.

By September 2006 and the first session after the summer break Mary is out of hospital, and has returned to SMART Music after four months away. She negotiates her re-entry into the group by singing this signature songs, *Where is Love.* Then later, at a session in November that year a member newly attending the group innocently picks *Where is Love,* and there's clearly some feeling that this is Mary's song, but of course this lady doesn't know that. But Mary is fine singing *Memories*, another one of her signature tunes. Songs, its clear, are associated with people, but not owned.

Mary ends up back in hospital the next spring and is actively missed by people in the SMART community. During a session in March 2007 Sadie suggests 'Mary' song, *Where is Love'* and Tim gets up to sing this, dedicating it to Mary. By April Mary is back again, and on 5 April (in Session 78) asks again to sing *Where is Love*. She is so pleased afterwards, saying 'I can still sing'. Sarah says afterwards that earlier in the week Mary had told her that she thought she'd never be able to sing again.

***

A parallel 'signature tune' for Mary was *Memory* from *Cats.* The emotional content is similar to *Where is Love?* – a combination of wistful sadness, vulnerability and hope. The way Mary sings these songs somehow mirrors these qualities. Again, *Memory* is a song that accompanies Mary across different care and social settings over more than 10 years.

She first sings *Memory* in the fourth session of SMART Music. People listen carefully and applaud; perhaps surprised by the accuracy and commitment Mary brings to her performance. The next mention in the logs of this song in relation to Mary is during one of her phases of hospitalisation (June 2006), when she comes over to SMART Music during a few hours leave from the ward. Sadie and others come over to support her, sit by her. Mary sings *Memory* in rather uncontrolled gusts. It's clear that she's still ill – but despite this she somehow rises to this performance. By September she's better, though still vulnerable and lacking confidence. When she sings this song in Session 58 it's noticeable how much others help her musically, gently singing alongside, making sure that she gets through the performance.

We might say that Mary was musically 'escorted' here in Session 58 with the others gently singing alongside, but there are other times where we can see her pathway as it became extended, times in fact when we can actually watch Mary (in concert with others) doing the (simultaneous) work of laying down a bit more pathway and moving along that new extension. In 2007, for example, when Mary joins *SMART Singers*, she also continues to attend a performance group that Sarah runs in the hospital site. So, in Session 93 of SMART Music in September 2007, Mary announces that she'll sing *Memory* – 'I'm practising for the concert in the hospital, 18th of October, and it needs to be good!'. She goes on to sing with a well-focused voice, good tuning and breath control – amazing given her recent serious period of physical illness over the last three months. She's focused and determined here. She's also ably accompanied by Eloise on cymbal.

Memory and Mary feature in the periphery of the recorded soundscape of SMART Music on a BBC Radio 3 feature in February 2008. The following week at SMART Music Mary selects *Memory*, and announces 'This is the song I sang on Radio Three'.

On 2 October 2008 Gary writes in the log for Session 139:

> I found myself very moved by Mary today – I uncharacteristically well up at one point when accompanying her on the piano as she's singing *Memory*. I haven't seen her for ages, she is one of the people who fade and suddenly pop up again. She just says 'sorry, I've been ill'. I know from Sarah that she and Tim were briefly engaged, but then broke this off. But there they sit together today, two vulnerable, lovely people. When Mary gets up to sing *Memory* her voice is strained and forced at first (I'm scared that this is what happens when she's getting ill), but then it settles, and is controlled and beautiful at moments. Simon plays a beautiful obbligato part on the violin, and it's magical. Perhaps I'm so moved because songs like this are like a precious continuous thread in her harrowed, inconstant life. It's the way this music accompanies her across the difficult voyage of her life that moves me.

One of the thoughts that the music therapists, Gary and Sarah, have over this period is whether people like Mary get 'trapped' by the same songs within these groups. Mary and *Memory* is an example of this. But we're ambivalent: is this the right interpretation, or is it rather a case that the songs afford a sense of confidence and skill when performing, and are reinforcing a precious if precarious musical identity? And, in everyday life, as Tia knows from her research (DeNora 2000), many people describe how music – the same music, over and over again – becomes a 'rock' or point of stability in the face of otherwise turbulent times. It's a companion and a comfort and provides the sense of continuity and hope that the good times will come again.

When Mary dies at the end of 2010, members of the SMART community plan a memorial for her, held in the chapel of the main hospital. Sarah and the SMART musicians are central to this event – a musical celebration of a musical person. There are a few hymns, and then a group of musicians from SMART have prepared a few of Mary's favourites, including *Memory* and *Where is Love?* It was amazing how much these songs were felt to be Mary's songs.

21. Picking a Song

Why do people pick the songs they do? Sometimes, as we've suggested, it's because of historical reasons, or because they see a song they know on the index page of the Red, Blue or Yellow books. Sometimes they pick it for someone else, and sometimes when they can't think of anything they just take pot-luck. But sometimes it's also more conscious, or perhaps sometimes an unconscious selection that projects a message outwards to others, or backwards to the singer themselves about how they are, and what they can't say directly at that time. In her interview Henrietta talks about this:

> **Henrietta:** So even choosing songs ... it reflects in certain ways how people are ... I mean you'll have one day when you sing *Summertime* because you're feeling quite good ... and another day you'll sing *Streets of London* because you're *not* feeling good. And even that's a subconscious way of letting out of your head what's going on ... through music and through the words. And you don't even realise you're doing it! Sarah'll say 'Pick a song' and whatever mood you're in ... it'll kind of suss it out in a way ... from the lyrics, and you know the songs ...
>
> **Gary:** And it's a safe way, isn't it? Because sometimes you just don't want to *say* how you are, do you?
>
> **H:** No, so you just find a song which seems to sum up where you're at ... even if nobody else realises you're doing that ... which is *more* safe! You just happen to have picked a song ... that for you that is cathartic ... and *clearing* in that way ... which is great. There's probably lots of times that after the event I've realised and thought 'Oh ... ' or somebody's said 'Why did you choose *that* song?' and I say 'I don't *know* ... ' but inside my head I kind of knew but I just didn't want to say ... because the whole point of choosing a song was that you don't *want* to say how you feel straight out ... So using the music you can get out how you're feeling for yourself, without it being so ... it's keeping a certain level of protection for yourself ... . but not letting people in too much ... which can be quite frightening ... but still letting the world know ... whether they know it or not ... actually how you feel. And I think a lot of people have a problem communicating how they feel ... and that causes a lot of problems ... so that's a way of ... . whether you're belting out *Rhapsody in Blue* or *Twinkle Twinkle Little Star* ... or whatever ... it doesn't matter because it's meaning something to you on some level.

22. *Summertime* – the career of a song

A buzz of amiable chat ... a burst of laughing ... clinking of knives and forks ... a few stray beats on a djembe ... the rattle of a shaker ... SMART cafe's ambient background sound on a Thursday afternoon at 2.55pm ...

Gary shouts out 'Summertime' ... . 'Porgy and Bess?' asks Jeremy; 'page 6' says Bobby; 'Yes, bottom of page 6 says Peggy ... ' ... Bobby says jokingly to Sally, 'You'll need a microphone for this ... .' and she laughs him off, retreating backwards quickly through the cafe with a cup of coffee, saved from the microphone. Bobby laughs, calls 'You're too shy-shy ... '. Meanwhile Gary plays a jazzy introduction on the piano, waiting for people to find page 6, and giving time for a few other musicians to gather ... Roger takes out a harmonica from his pocket, tries out a few long in-out notes, and Bobby taps out a few helpful rhythms on the djembe ... We're musically treading water for a bit, waiting for just the right time to start the song ... And then suddenly a clarinet joins the texture too ... .then a few more bars of improv with all the instrumentalists ... Gary calls ... 'Here we go ... ***Summertime ... '***

Gary starts singing, backed up by Clare and others: ***'Summertime ... and the living is easy ... '****. Other musical lines on piano, harmonica, clarinet and drum weave around the main melody, supporting it and making it our unique version – here, now, with these people, and infused with their musical voices ...*

' ... .Oh your daddy's rich, and your mama's good looking ... ' *... a tambourine enters in the middle of the soundscape, playing on the off-beat. Other sounds – some small musical instruments, some the scrapes of coffee-cups and cutlery – join the texture too. Any sound is welcome ...*

' ... .So Hush little baby, don't ... you cry ... .'*, the end of the first verse leads into a free improvised section, whilst a few people discuss who should sing a solo during the next verse ... . Roger takes advantage of the space and launches into a harmonica solo – waa, waaaaaa ... sculpting the arcs of melody through this tiny instrument that's just popped out of his pocket ...*

Then it's the second verse ... ***'One of these mornings ... ' ... .*** *Everyone's joining-in now; the music has flow and fullness ... Is that metallic sound we hear someone playing on the spoons?* ***'Then You'll spread your wings and take the sky ... '****, and some collective spirit spreads our musical wings, raises the energy, and gives the music a more rhythmic character, with a tambourine beat, and a clarinet melody that glides up and down the musical space ...*

'With Daddy and Mammy Standing By ... ' *... Another improvised break, and this time Bobby suggests a rhythm –* ***da-daa*** *– which the players here and instantly* *echo back to him for a few musical exchanges ... developing a light-hearted musical conversation between drum, piano, clarinet, and harmonica ... which then speeds up ... It's a musical game now ... this is really* ***playing*** *music – it's always play, even when it's serious ... . The speeding up comes to a point we can't go beyond so Gary pulls it back to a shaking pause, when all join in at a moment when we know it's just about to lead back into ...*

Summertime ... and the living is easy ... *Everyone together, loudly this time, for this final reprise, giving it all they've got ... then slowing up together for the final line ...* ***So hush little baby ... Don't ... You ... ... CRY ... ...*** *the climax – which involves maximum shaking, banging, then a glissando down the piano, and a final drum bang from Bobby. Clapping and whooping.*

Summertime*, never sung and played like this before ... or ever again ...*

***

This song emerges, perhaps inevitably, in the very first session of SMART Music. It's a ubiquitous jazz standard, a standby that almost anyone will recognise and be able to sing or busk along with. It has qualities that permit multiple interpretations in terms of ways of singing/playing, of speed, ensemble and style of performance. Gary writes in his notes on the first SMART Music Session how *Summertime* shows up the social and collaborative side of musicking, how the song adapts to the people and situation; how the people step into the song and find themselves together differently as it sails on …

The next mention of *Summertime* in the log is in September 2006 (Session 57). It's probably been sung many times before, but the log tends to note changes or unusual aspects. Ella's mother had died the previous week and she said that she wanted to sing a few songs for her mother as a tribute: 'This song is for my mother, who passed away a week ago today – and if I know mum, she's sitting right in this room now … So were doing it for you, mum'. She tells us that her mother had run a record shop and knew many musicians, and how her childhood had revolved around her mother's favourite music. She manages to sing *Summertime*, although she understandably stumbles over the line 'with mama & papa standing by'.

In February 2007 Tim sings *Summertime* in his extraordinary double-bass voice. But as Gary accompanies him on the piano there's something strange in their musical interaction: Tim can't quite find the groove of the song, and Gary can't quite find out how to help him. He keeps waiting for the next line, and then coming in artificially late. The real problem is that he's aware of this, and says later 'I couldn't get in sync with you today'. Gary wonders what makes the difference with Tim between when he can and can't get it together in this way? This is the downside of this flexible song, that can be stretched and shaped to suit any number of different singers … but for someone who's struggling with their timing (both internally and relationally), it perhaps gives too little temporal definition.

Tim has another go at this song in a different SMART Music format a few months later, this time within the *SMART Singers* group. The previous week they'd successfully performed a set of songs in the elderly patients' ward in the hospital, and Tim wants to reprise the songs that went down well there. Today he and Henrietta do some work on singing *Summertime* in a variety of different ways, partly seeing what would work best if they performed this with the SMART Band – a possibility for a forthcoming summer gig. Sarah writes in her notes how *Summertime* is useful as a musical frame for encouraging singers to be a bit more free in their singing, to dare a bit of improvisation …

In November 2007 (Session 99) Ella takes the song up again, and it's clear that she's been experimenting with her interpretation of it, probably a cross-fertilisation between the Singers group and the Thursday SMART Music Sessions. This experimental feel to her performance is helped by how various instrumentalists in the session (we've now come to the stage of development in this session where there's almost a 'support band' on the side – guitars, violin, accordian etc.) join Ella and between them they sculpt a way of making the song work, here and now.

The cross-fertilisation continues, with this song as one of the foci during the next six months as the music groups plan to collaborate on various events, pick shared repertoire and then perform together. A highlight is in July 2008 when SMART Singers and Band provide the music for the retirement party of Richard, a well-liked and respected services manager. After various specifically chosen songs, *Summertime* emerges for a more spontaneous jam between the various elements: Daniel and Henrietta take turns singing solo verses, then various invitations and combinations are semi-directed by Daniel: Simon (violin), then Bobby (drums). The downside of this spontaneity is that there's something of a struggle to establish exactly *how* to play this number: on the beat, or a little behind the beat, or a lot behind the beat (Daniel) … This needs negotiation in the music, but it just about hangs together …

Claire sings freely from the fourth 'row' back of the cafe, but in all the years of SMART Music she has declined to come up to sing a solo. One day Claire has been singing earlier with SMART Singers in a lunchtime concert in the Atrium of the main hospital. It's gone well, and her confidence is higher. Later in the afternoon music session Claire does her usual scat/jazz singing, starting from the back of the room. But then she's suddenly there, at the mic – and sings *Summertime*.

In November 2010 another joint event between Band and Singers involves a laid-back version of *Summertime*, with Jim singing and the Band supporting. Jim manages to temper his sometimes over-exuberant expression, and there are also instrumental breaks for guitar and harmonica. People around the cafe are humming, tapping feet …

Summertime is itself a musical space – to be in comfortably, or challengingly; a musical object to change and re-shape according to mood (or according to whose version you may have been listening to most recently); to inflect according to who you're playing it with; to expand into a flexible structure that can incorporate both pathways out (solos, elaborations), and then pathways back to the safe ground of the chorus. It's always the same, and different; always Gershwin's, but always our very own – here and now.

23. The Grain of the Voice: Song Performance at SMART

This account of a single song takes us on to the next aspect of the evolving song repertoire at SMART – the *performative* dimension. It's not only *that* somebody sings a particular song that is interesting or significant, but exactly *how* they do so …

> I move across and sit with Tim and Mary again, and we start talking about the music group. Mary calls Tim the 'double bass', and Tim responds by singing really low with his voice. I say, yeah, but he can also sing quite high, and Tim again sings a really high note. Mary mentions she's looking forward to singing again, and sings a few notes of *Memory* from *Cats*, the musical. I talk to them both about the singing lessons I've been having, and how my teacher has been training me to be able to stretch my lungs open. For the next 10 minutes both Mary and Tim are trying to do it, too! I have to warn them that they must continue to breathe at the same time (I don't want them conking out on me!). It's all fun and games. A few minutes go by and Mary is just staring at me. I ask her if she's feeling alright, but she's just trying to stretch her lungs apart with her muscles again. Tim and her then practice singing and stretching the rib cage open at the same time, the result being a string of sustained pitches. It's nice to see both of them responding to each other musically, one changing their pitch in relation to the other. I'm pleased, because it seems to cheer Mary up a great deal. [Rob's Field notes, 22 August 2006]

Not just songs, *singers!* This is a crucial aspect to what music and musicking in SMART is. People, individually and collectively, love certain songs and styles of songs, but they also come along to hear each other sing them – it's the *person*-in-the-music that matters. And it's clear that people characterise themselves in such vivid ways that have a profound influence behind *how* people hear them, respond to them, understand them. As Rob's vignette above illustrates, these musical characterisations also become part of the activity and performance of musicking – *working* on how the sounds of music are made with and through the body; taking pleasure in each other's musical characterisation, and how these develop.

Musical performance and personalism

A long history of social theory has explored this idea of self and identity as a performance rather than an essence. Erving Goffman's famous book *The Presentation of Self in Everyday Life* (1959) showed how social life requires us to strike a balance between making an expression of ourselves whilst managing a favourable impression on others. This balancing is often a precarious social and cultural performance. Our 'social skills' and knowledge help most of us keep the performance going for most of the time. But stressful circumstances or illness can quickly undermine this competence, and show up the whole game. At the least, it seriously questions what it could mean to 'just be yourself'.

However, there's another angle to the theme of self-performance [...]. A 'heightened performance' on a real or metaphorical stage can sometimes be the making of us. It can represent a breakthrough into broader social competence, and towards a fuller reflexive sense of the self. [...]

Recent theory from both music studies and therapeutic theory has been moving towards similar conclusions. A 'turn to performance' promoted by Christopher Small (1998), Nicholas Cook (1998, 2003) and others is rebalancing the almost-exclusive attention to abstract musical texts with a new interest in performance processes. Cook (2003) summarises this as a move from a concept of 'music *and* performance' to 'music *as* performance'. In an analysis of this shift, Stan Godlovitch (1998) outlines a stance he calls *personalism*. Why do we attend musical performances? Godlovitch suggests it's not just to hear the structure of musical works being reproduced, but to hear real people performing them live. We witness something at stake for these performers, something humanly vital happening:

> Personalism reminds us that performance is a way of communicating, not especially a work or a composer's notions, but a person, the performer, through the music. Personalism intimates that a proper understanding of performance must ... appreciate ritual forms of communication, action and its significance, human benefit and reciprocity, and a good many other concerns belonging naturally to social conduct. (Godlovitch 1998, p. 145)

Another useful suggestion comes from the anthropologist Victor Turner (1982), who was particularly interested in the connections between ritual and performance. He suggests that our assumption that the word and concept 'performance' means projecting a work 'through the form' is only one possible etymological interpretation. Instead,

> *Performance* ... is derived from the Middle English *parfourmen*, which is itself from the Old French, *parfournir* – *par* ('thoroughly'), + *fournir* ('to furnish') – hence performance does not necessarily have the structuralist implications of manifesting form, but rather the processual sense of 'bringing to completion', or 'accomplishing'. To perform is thus to complete a more or less involved process rather than to do a single deed or act. (Turner 1982, p. 91)

This sense of performance as completion of a process assumes then that something *needs* completing, both in the cultural form that is the performance vehicle, and in personal and social life. It suggests that in the creative 'carrying out' of performance something is transformed, personally and socially. In this sense, performance events are closer to ritual events in being both heightened social events and potentially reflexive ones – showing back to people something about themselves and the society they belong to. Turner became especially interested in the rehearsal or preparation process for performance. He commented on how an actor moves from taking up a role (= 'not me') to assimilating this in performance as 'not not me'. The aim, says Turner, is '*poiesis*, rather than *mimesis*: making, not faking'. He sums up his concept of performance: 'A performance, then, is the proper finale of an experience' (1982, p. 13).

There's a tendency today to think of performance as 'showing off' to an audience. But we might also usefully think of other performance-based activities and contexts, such as when a sportsman's performance is a case of 'bringing it off' rather than 'showing off'. This accomplishment might only be possible when witnessed and spurred on by an audience. Thinking of the self as performed in this way reinforces the understanding that, as an ongoing psychosocial process, identity needs appropriate props, a stage and an audience. As Goffman famously said, 'All the world is not, of course, a stage, but the crucial ways in which it isn't are not easy to specify' (1959/1990, p. 78).

Given these positive affordances of performance, it is perhaps no surprise that therapeutic theory is now belatedly acknowledging this truth. A good example of this is the work of the radical 'social therapist' Fred Newman, who makes the wonderful definition of performance as 'being who you aren't, doing what you can't' (1999, p. 100). He maintains that human development is an 'unnatural act'; that we become who we 'are' by continuously 'being who we are not'. Newman's critique of traditional therapy is inspired by Vygotsky, the pioneering Russian developmental psychologist. Vygotsky (1978, p. 102) suggested how a child can find herself 'a head taller' in ability and confidence when inducted into what he calls a cultural 'zone of proximal development' based on talking and doing things with more developed others. In this zone, adults literally perform above the child's current developmental level, but whilst in that cultural performance space the child then finds herself performing 'beyond herself' – raised a level. A similar process could happen to any of us.

This idea links in turn with Victor Turner's (1982) definition of performance as something 'completed' along with others. Newman's work takes a performative stance on therapy itself – where he encourages people to learn to perform themselves differently in ensemble with others. The aim is to transform the whole 'zone' of relational experience such that people experience themselves differently together. Newman writes that people in his therapy group 'were learning to perform beyond themselves ... they were breaking out of the habit of simply being themselves to discovering not who they were but who they were not' (1999, p. 129). [Adapted from Ansdell 2014, pp. 130–33]

This way of thinking naturally links performance to wellbeing, and suggests how this link will show up clearest in the *how* of performance: in what Roland Barthes (1991) called 'the grain of the voice', that reflection of who we are at a particular point of performing – in terms of our body, mind, personal and social relationships. As the music therapy theorist David Aldridge (2004) has written, what we hear in music therapy are 'health performances'.

We will stay for a while with Mary and Tim in following this theme. The following descriptions come from a commentary that Rob made of selected musical excerpts from the first year of SMART Music that he was compiling onto a CD for research purposes:

Mary sings 'Memory'

I will always remember Mary's voice. The Sufis believe that a person's soul is heard through the voice, that the voice tells you about the past, present, and future of that person. Mary's voice is on the one hand so full and round and harmless, and then on the other so broken. She can really *carry* a tune and sing it well, but then it seems like there are markers of something sad underneath – something to do with the tuning, the various breaks in the voice. With Mary's voice you can feel overwhelmed with an incredible positive warmth – here is someone giving it their all, trying hard, enjoying the moment. But other side of her voice is almost traumatic to listen to because for me it's like there's an almost innocent quality, but one that's been hurt along the way. I don't know if I have the authority to say that. 'Memory' is a song which characterises this duality in Mary's voice very well – a lovely tune, something we can all sway along to and enjoy; but a tune sung to words that paint pictures of isolation and sadness. But then this wonderful thing at the end: hope. I can't help but cry massively whenever I hear it now. I'm also interested here in the support offered on different percussion instruments – and it feels like support rather than 'joining in'. It's just there in the background, like a big hug you can sink into; it's not meant to take the song anywhere else; it's just there to carry Mary, a little extra sparkle that highlights her performance, shows some appreciation while not taking over the moment.

Mary sings 'Somewhere Over the Rainbow'

Another song sung by Mary with that voice of competence, bravery, enthusiasm, innocence, hurt, and hope, and the words match the sentiments of the voice.

Mary sings 'Where Is Love?'

There are a string of songs that Mary sings (*Memory, Send in the Clowns, Strangers in the Night*, and *Where Is Love*) that all share a similar degree of this duality I have talked about above.

Tim sings 'Somewhere'

This is all about Tim's voice. Tim's voice is this great big double bass thing and that people really appreciate it. It acts as a focus for the group, and there's much discussion about it from many people afterwards.

So what is Rob picking up here? Although a sensitive and eloquent commentator, we take his perceptions to stand for what most of the rest of us are 'picking up' and understanding somehow in terms of these people and their situations through the medium of their musical performances. Rob hears a dimension of the person 'within' / 'behind' / 'in front of' the voice – (its difficult to know which metaphor is more accurate here).

Rob intuitively says a lot, but also doubts that he has the authority to say what he is picking up. He finds complexity through the vocal channel of these two people: the 'duality' of Mary's voice, which is brave and broken; Tim's unique timbre and tessitura, which entirely characterises him in this musical community as someone 'big' and a talking point. The voice 'carries' another dimension of the person – one you'd not necessarily know by looking at them, hearing them speak. And it's somehow a key dimension to knowing about them fully (their 'soul').

How exactly is this information 'carried'? Through the tuning, the breaks, the *qualities* of the voice, writes Rob. This dimension is probably something that most people intuitively 'pick up' as a non-verbal communication that informs you about someone's physical and psychological state and intentions. It's information that we need socially in order to know how to respond, and in order to protect ourselves sometimes. It's important, however, to note that it's probably not just a case of a direct and simple communication of emotional state via immediate physical parameters that we hear in some SMART solo performances (and that Rob's comments describe). There's also the important linkage between what the *song* conveys and what the *singer* conveys in /with the song. It's the singer/song combination that's so potent – and so 'revealing'. It's very clear that Mary's songs have an overall theme (whether she's conscious of this or not): *Memory, Rainbow, Send in the Clowns, Where is Love?* A song sequence of words, melody and harmony that convey a complex amalgam of tragedy, sadness, hope, courage … As Rob writes:

> Mary with that voice of competence, bravery, enthusiasm, innocence, hurt, and hope, and the words match the sentiments of the voice.

Roland Barthes writes of the *grain* of the voice as a way of discussing these complexities of personality, persona and performance in relation to songs. He's primarily talking about classical music in his famous essays on this subject, on what you pick up as a listener about the difference between the singers Fischer-Dieskau and Panzera from the grain of their voices. But he suggests that it's just the same with popular music and singers. It's sometimes simplified that this just means the *timbre* of the voice, but Barthes says no: it's rather something that is about the *relationship* between the language of a song and the embodied performance of the singer – an amalgam of text and texture.

Roland Barthes on the grain of the voice

The 'grain' is the body in the singing voice, in the writing hand, in the performing limb. [...] since I am determined to listen to my relation to the body of someone who is singing or playing and since that relation is an erotic one, but not at all 'subjective' (it is not the psychological 'subject' in me who listens ...) [1991: 276]

Barthes is critiquing old-style musical analysis that bypasses the body. He's also showing how music and musicking takes us beyond the binary of usual meaning making: the signifier and the signified. Art, and music in particular, lead us rather towards to an 'extra meaning' which goes beyond this binary, but only by amalgamating the activity of making and conveying human meaning in a particular time and circumstance ('musical signifying' according to Barthes). That is, the body is needed to complete and convey the meaning – which is a meaning to do with soul (desire, erotics, needs, compulsions, etc.): 'my body puts itself into a state of speech ... ' (306).

In this hostelry of the signifier where the subject can be heard, the principal body movement is the one that voice originates from. The voice, in relation to silence, is like writing (in the graphic sense) on blank paper. Listening to the voice inaugurates the relation to the Other: the voice by which we recognize others (like writing on an envelope) indicates to us their ways of being, their joy or their pain, their condition; it bears an image of their body and, beyond, a whole psychology (as when we speak of a warm voice, a white voice, etc.).

[...] The singing voice, that very specific space in which a tongue encounters a voice and permits those who know how to listen to it to hear what we call its 'grain' – the singing voice is not the breath but indeed that materiality of the body emerging from the throat, a site where the phonic metal hardens and takes shape. [1991: 254–5]

Barthes talks of an 'obvious meaning' that we naturally pick up, and which takes us forward without much need of reflection, and then of this 'extra' (or 'third') meaning that he calls the obtuse meaning: ' ... the one that appears 'in excess', as a supplement my intellection cannot quite absorb, a meaning both persistent and fugitive, apparent and evasive ... ' (1991, p. 44). It opens up the field of meaning ...

In the examples of Mary singing above the *outcome* of what people pick up from such an 'obtuse meaning' is their (complex) response to her. Rob describes (quoted above) how what you hear in the *Memory* track is the swelling of audience support for Mary as she goes on singing:

> I'm also interested here in the support offered on different percussion instruments – and it feels like support rather than 'joining in'. It's just there in the background, like a big hug you can sink into; it's not meant to take the song anywhere else; it's just there to carry Mary, a little extra sparkle that highlights her performance, shows some appreciation while not taking over the moment.

Is it that Mary's performance creates both a sense of how she is, and also what she *needs* in this immediate situation from others? We could see Mary's musicking as a 'health performance' that marshals resources for her own support through the processes of identification and empathy.

We're familiar with how we can hear illness in a person in some ways: their voice changes in timbre if they have a cold; if they 'sound depressed' it may be that we pick up a lack of usual dynamic range and flexibility in their 'forms of vitality' (Stern, 2010). We use our 'core musicality' to instinctively read conditions of health and illness (in ourselves and others). We might call this listening to the 'grain' of illness and health. From our experience of SMART over the years we suspect that people are continually reading each other for signs of illness (partly out of empathy, partly as a warning system for the day). This is apparent in music too, but we wonder whether it has a more subtle 'display' within this medium. Again Mary is a good example of this. Throughout the data are examples where Gary makes comments about Mary's mental state in relation to his 'musical hearing' of 'how she is'. Perhaps the sense gained from music is an early warning. This aspect of hearing the 'grain' is different (though related) to the dimension Rob comments on. Gary's comments are less about the 'static' quality of the 'grain of the voice' but the 'dynamic' ones which show up especially in interactive musicking: how there is sometimes an additional quality of 'pressure' behind the singing that distorts the pitching (in ways not related to Mary's natural musicianship); there are exaggerations and distortions of musical timing. These are apparent when trying to accompany someone and in trying to modulate the worst of their 'excess' in order to keep the musical show on the road – successfully for them and the listeners. Other bodies of knowledge (such as communicative musicality – Malloch & Trevarthen 2009; Stern 2010) suggest that illness is often accompanied by problems with self-synchrony and interactional synchrony. The consequence of the problem with these is a problem with everyday social interaction and judgement. All of this can be 'diagnostically' heard.

The 'grain of health' is perhaps simply the opposite of this: a comprehensive and flexible access to the full range of vitality, and flexible self- and interactive synchrony; a comfort within the self, and between self and others. It's perhaps a 'musical' condition or state.

24. The Grain of a Song

A final aspect of the performative theme is how songs themselves have a 'grain' that influences the mood and qualities of musical-social action within SMART. There often seems to be a reciprocal characterisation of singer and song. The singer sounds unique in their delivery (as described in the previous section), but also the song itself gets variously inflected by the singer – the song takes on a 'grain' of individuality, and a further level of meaning is added to it by its immediate performance and reception (rather than 'just' being an internal set of structural relationships between tones and words). Something is immediately conveyed to the audience 'between' singer and song.

A few SMART musicians come with their own songs (Peter, Roger, Steven), which reinforce this singer/song identity in perhaps the closest way. In the second session of SMART Music Peter arrives with guitar and two new songs of his own:

> I wrote these songs while I was on the streets ... It's from the soul ... I don't know whether it's from the Holy Ghost ...

He's an edgy character, and instantly there's a hush in the audience as people hedge their bets and listen quietly. His performance is unpredictable, surging with intensity on certain violent images the words convey in a first song; but his playing and singing is also competent technically. The performance conveys a complex mix of vulnerability and threat, which is in words, music and delivery simultaneously in his second song:

> *It's cold outside / It's dark and cold*
> *My muscles ache / and I'm feeling old*
> *I won't sleep tonight / I'm on the streets*
> *Been through the bins / To get my eats ...*
> *I've got too much fear / I'm all alone*
> *I need a friend ...*

Rob comments about the audience reaction to this song; how it's somehow an emotional education for people like him, to gauge how to react and how to interpret what's being communicated. The point is perhaps that a message is given/sent that is both situational (through the performance here-and-now by this particular man), but also within the 'grain of the song'. It's directed as a kind of challenge to the audience – even if its message is ambiguous – not exactly 'pity me', because it's also challenging, perhaps provocative.

As an opposite scenario to this take Leslie and his bi-weekly appearances at SMART Music. Certainly not on the streets, or consciously attempting to convey a message about his psycho-social state to others, Leslie nevertheless conveys a lot 'in between' the singer and the song. His first song at SMART Music is *Some Enchanted Evening.* He takes the 'performer's place' to the left of the piano, deposits the music for Gary, sweeps aside the microphone (acoustic only for him!) and launches into a confident, charismatic performance. His voice has a trained classical quality, but also elements of musical theatre. All this shows up in his comportment, breathing, facial sets, use of larynx, facial resonance etc. Now nearing eighty we later learn that, at age seventy Leslie had taken up weekly singing lessons with an opera singer, and this is the result! It's a polished, very prepared performance, one *to* rather than *with* the audience at this point. His voice is loud and full of resonance; it judges all the high points of the musical score with accuracy and emotional effect, and he and Gary together pull off a rather splendid performance of this song. A few jaws drop in the audience, people stop chatting and are riveted by this spectacle. Or, one might also add, that they politely recognise that this is a spectacle, which calls for a certain form of attention which they offer, with characteristic hospitality. As Stephanie Pitts (2004, p. 158) once put it, not only does shared music making keep the sense of community alive, so too, shared listening, (and styles of listening, ways of bestowing praise) reinforce identity and belonging. Right on cue, when Leslie finishes, the group claps ecstatically.

All kinds of things are conveyed by this performance apart from Leslie's musicianship, located again somewhere between singer and song: a *standard* of performance (based on practice, preparation and respect for the audience); an authenticity to the original song-context on stage (a now-dated era that resonates with some of the SMART members); a certain attitude that he is with but not exactly *of* this particular group – he's come to entertain (albeit in a very genuine and generous way just as the group show their appreciation in an equally generous way). Does Leslie express his personal 'idiom' through this song and his performance? Yes and no; the ambiguity is telling, and crucial.

Daniel's fine performances are another example of such complexity and subtlety. He sings beautifully stylish versions of jazz standards (styled on Dinah Washington, whose records were a fixture of his childhood home). Before one song he actually says the words, 'I am Dinah Washington' in a way that calls forth a kind of identity claim and holding structure for his delivery style. And indeed, Daniel's Washington-like micro-pauses and rhythmic subtlety allow him to assume a cool, almost quizzical attitude during these songs, a kind of jazz-hauteur that simultaneously allows him, ever so slightly, to 'stand apart'. There is, in other words, an elective affinity between Daniel and 'his' songs, his channeling of Washington, his mastery of the idiom. Daniel also sings raw Blues numbers, with an almost-perfect authentic voice. But again this is cultivated: Daniel is a first-rate musician and spent a period in the States learning Blues from the masters. So his performances are both quintessentially Daniel (anyone would recognise him singing at street level before coming down to the SMART cafe), but also these are performances of the *grain of the song* too.

This is perhaps only to say that any decent musical performance is a *double-performance*, and this is a chief positive affordance. *It's me ... and not me ...* a song performance conveying personality, but also persona; being a direct message, but also a generic message. A song's grain (or that of an idiom such as Blues/tango etc.) is also a 'collective grain' – a *cultural voice,* a dual identity that relates to particular musical qualities, history, cultural niche. Because of this, songs and singers can be directly authentic to their immediate performances, but also ciphers of collective emotions, lifeworlds, situations; spokespersons for collective sorrow and struggle (Blues), or brokenness (Mary and the heritage of Judy Garland).

Lastly, in relation to this theme, the performances at SMART illustrate something common to the musical artworld in general: the flexibility of a song to tolerate a wide range of different interpretations that inflect the personal idiom of the singers without losing the identity of the song. The song becomes, as scholars in Science and Technology Studies have used the term, a boundary object or a mutable immutable object: it can always be the same and yet from rendition to rendition, appropriation to appropriation, be widely divergent or 'not' the same. So having 'a' song to play with – to vary and yet to treat 'as if' it is always 'that' song, is to allow a musical container, or forum, for the performance of differences that themselves can be contained. The song's flexible accommodation performs community: we are all singing, in other words, from the same hymn book, even when in fact we are not and it is this ecumenicalism of 'the' song that binds us together. We 'share' the same songs even when their similarities may be smaller than their differences. The song becomes then a kind of holding form, a way of being able to know that we have these musical things in common. So across the data we have variable renditions of classic songs – *Let it Be, Blue Moon, Somewhere Over The Rainbow, Amazing Grace, Autumn Leaves* – with their pace, rhythmic style, vocal delivery etc. inflected according to the immediate mood and stylistic intentions of the performer. A song is always the singer's, as is a singer always a performance of a song at some level …

The idea of 'double performance' not only applied to the duality of me/not me. It also applies to 'the song'/ 'not the song', to the ways that some renditions of songs so modify the song to fit the singer's vocal grain, or the singer's musical skills and capacities, that it is possible to see the places where the song doesn't 'fit' the singer, or where the singer's musical rendering stretches or reforms the song, making it over into something aesthetically unusual, innovative, unconventional (in ways we think that John Cage would have loved). Rob's comments above on Mary's voice offers a good example of how 'different' voices can enrich the ways we define 'good music'. On these occasions it is possible to catch glimpses of how, in inserting ourselves into a song, we are 'trying on' a persona. Singing is always potentially a chance to play the game of 'could I be like this?' and it is a chance to channel, impersonate, pretend to be, that other, musically conceived (recall Daniel's 'I am Dinah Washington').

There's of course also a long cultural heritage that stands behind each song, and singers at SMART play creatively with the links between the heritage of the song they're singing and their own, sometimes aspirational, performance style. Gemma, in one session, for example does a spirited and characterful performance of *Cabaret* – smartly, even theatrically dressed up in black taffeta. She says 'I *am* Liza', and indeed she is for those minutes. There is give and take involved in finding what will work, will seem plausible, will suit the vocal grain in ways that pull off the attempt to appropriate the song and its various associated meanings and stances. This is by no means only a musical skill. It is rather a life skill, asking 'what cultural artefacts and categories might I lay claim to?', or like trying on a dress ('does this fit me?') it is about ownership, which is, ultimately, about finding ways to make things work or at least be 'passable' ('yes, it wasn't designed with you in mind but on you that dress takes on new depths and connotations – wear it!' or 'well I think you just about get away with that'). This attempt to inhabit songs, to 'wear' them is, we think, nothing less than the activity of joining in with public life, playing with, playing on, stock materials (boundary objects) in ways that further elaborate the realm of publicly comprehended possibilities for, and of, action. And, as in public life – interaction – 'successful' performance depends upon the kindness, and deftness, of others in how they support and accompany it.

25. Musical Accompanying

This account of SMART song performance has concentrated mostly on the individual aspects so far. But what is most characteristic and interesting about SMART performances is rather how they are collectively and collaboratively assembled. Song performances are in one way or another *supported performances.*

This dimension is especially important given the fluctuating needs of many members of this community for support of one kind or another. The project has given us the chance to explore in some detail the nature and potential of *musical* support, which, in a sense is an entirely natural and everyday dimension of any musicking – as when a pianist supports a singer by accompanying her, or how in a band there's a mutually supportive relationship between the hierachical but interdependent roles of drum, bass and lead. Within a music therapy frame such patterns have a further resonance in that musical and personal support are combined within a mutual but asymmetrical relationship between therapist and client(s). The root of the modern 'therapist' role is the Greek role of the *therapeutes*, who accompanied or walked beside someone through a challenging episode of life.

As with many of these familiar themes from music therapy, the SMART Music project (following the broader Community Music Therapy agenda) adds further nuances and questions. This section will look at how people in the various SMART Music groups are supported to make a personal performance through what we'll call *musical companionship.*

Musical Companionship

This concept comes from pioneer music therapists Nordoff and Robbins, who found that the isolated and challenging children with whom they were working often seemed to make a relationship first with music itself, and how a music therapist could then invite the child gradually into a more inter*personal* contact through the musicking. They write of one boy, 'as he projected himself into a new intensity of human relationship, the boy experienced musical companionship' (1971, p. 67). 'Companionship' is perhaps the best way of describing what follows musical contact and connection, where a journeying together in music can begin. The etymological origin of 'companionship' – breaking bread together – conveys the qualities of mutuality and solidarity through something being shared. For musicians, there's also the related sense of *accompanying*, the supportive travelling together through the music that one musician offers another.

We can do this because we share an underlying capacity of *communicative musicality*. The developmental psychologist Daniel Stern (2010), a pioneer in the study of intersubjective communication, further suggests that at least three key types of music-like interaction underlie developing relationship:

> *Attuning* – perceiving the vitality forms of another person and responding sympathetically with your own actions. This calls not for a slavish mirroring, but rather incorporating someone's timing, intensity and shaping in a response that presents your own vital signature too.
>
> *Dialoguing* – creating and developing forms of reciprocal action, ranging from simple turn taking to more complex forms that interleave actions. This involves some degree of shared understanding of the meaning and direction of the communication. Co-action generates something *between* the partners, moving the relationship forward through the mutual contributions.
>
> *Regulating* – making micro-judgements that 'titrate' *how* the dialogue moves forward, and the level of arousal it evokes. This needs a mutual sensitivity to how much, or how quickly, change can happen, such that surprise is balanced with tolerance. This mutual shaping and regulating of an interaction ensures that the relationship stays on track.

Human communication in general (as well as some human–animal communication) rests on the mostly non-conscious working of these 'mechanisms' described by communicative musicality and forms of vitality. But music therapists often make more conscious and strategic use of them when working with their clients. Their skill, shared with the skill of their clients, can allow working on maintaining and sometimes repairing breaches in musical companionship.
[Adapted from Ansdell 2014a, pp. 48–150]

Both on-going weekly work, and specific incidents, within the SMART Music project have given us the chance to see and further explore the various processes that are involved in establishing and maintaining musical companionship, defined as the supportive travelling together through the music that one (or more) musician(s) offers another. This variously involves:

- The basic level of musical accompanying – when Gary and Sarah, or other SMART members, accompany someone doing a solo.

- The 'choreographing' and crafting of a musical moment – with either a positive or negative result – where the music either comes together successfully or 'misses' …
- The process of 'repairing' – when it all goes horribly wrong, and reparation is needed.

A typical scenario in SMART Music is when Gary or Sarah accompanies on the piano a member singing a song. The songs are seldom complicated in themselves, but sometimes the way that people actually sing them is not straightforward. The performances are individualised renditions – either by choice or by 'accident'. The accompanist's job is therefore to 'keep the musical show on the road', to help, or mentor, an optimal if sometimes individual and idiosyncratic performance to feel successful and satisfactory for all.

> Jeremy tells me that he only knows the chorus of *These Foolish Things*, not the verse. I start playing the music from the dog-eared sheet-music as he talks over the music to the audience, explaining a few historical details. I count Jeremy in, and he sings the first phrase 'A cigarette that bears a lipstick's traces', but then cuts the usual pause between 1st and 2nd lines, creating a small uncertainty in our shared timing within the song. I'm used to Jeremy doing this, half-expect it in fact, and compensate in my piano accompaniment by also jumping a few beats to catch-up as he sings 'An airline ticket to romantic places … '. At this point Jeremy decides it would be nicer to invite people to sing along, momentary leaves the song and its internal timing to say 'join in, please!', then jumps back into the song again, the harmony and melody of which I've kept going underneath. We just about coincide on the 're-entry point' at 'places' … All goes well then until Jeremy again ignores the gap between verse one and two, and there's a bump as he sings 'A tinkling piano … ' and I have to cut out three chords that bridge the verses. Again we just about land together and keep the smooth on-going progress of the song, partly as I now emphasise with my piano touch the melody of the song in the right hand, acting rather like a tracking-device. When I listen back to this song again writing this, I also notice that at certain key structural points of this performance – ends and beginnings of phrases – other voices and a stabilising pulse on a tambourine swell up around Jeremy, perhaps intuitively recognising where he tends to 'go off the rails' and needs musical help? [Gary's analysis of recorded excerpt from 2006]

***

A similar form of musical help happens several times when Jane sings solo songs:

> Jane has chosen *Stuck on You* and is in front of the microphone, but spending a long time fiddling with her sheet-music, glasses, the height of stand … during which other members begin to chat and attention is dissipating. I play the piano

introduction, attempting to put real musical focus into the music so that it propels forward and gathers attention back to the song. Jane needs cueing into the first line of the lyrics as it's not really clear when this comes because of the flowing accompaniment ... *Stuck on you /I've got this feeling down deep in my soul that I just can't lose ...* we sing this together, but then this creates another problem, as Jane's a soprano and I'm a baritone (and Lionel Richie was a high tenor!). The tessitura of the song doesn't really suit either of us, and Jane has to switch from one octave to another to sing each phrase. During this I try to anchor the performance with a confident piano, balancing keeping Jane in the musical foreground whilst keeping musical momentum and presence going ...

In his commentary on this song performance, Rob writes 'Gary gives a helping hand to Jane with confidence to sing the melody. He's like a climbing frame, or a piece of solid scaffolding for Jane to walk over. But he manages to make it 'Jane's moment' by not completely taking over, and specifically not singing whenever it seems like Jane has got a hold of the song'. This at least is what I was trying to do – and internally it means that I 'track' the ideal song in my head whilst listening to Jane singing it, then intervene with my voice or piano when I hear the second-by-second need – which is musical *and* personal at the same time. Again, listening back to this now, I hear other subtle forms of musical help seeping in at crucial moments: a guitar strum which helps fill the texture out; Rob's clarinet weaving a counter-melody that somehow glues-together the musical space – which is always a risky area, given that Jane's voice fades in and out according to her comfort with a given phrase, or the ebbing and waning of her confidence ...

Jane finds her confidence at the beginning of the middle-eight ... *Oh, I'm leaving on that midnight train tomorrow/And I know just where I'm going ...* and indeed it's as if she *does* know where she's going now! The other musicians respond by leaving their careful supportive roles and embarking on more daring musical journeys themselves – a beautiful arc of melody coming from a picked guitar, crossing the phrases ... [Gary's analysis of recorded excerpt from 2007]

There's a moving subtext to Jane's performances. Following a difficult incident in SMART Music where Jane had a conflict with Daniel over the 'right to sing', Jane told Gary the following:

This is not an excuse, it's an explanation ... Of why I get like I do when someone I feel is doing too much. I get frustrated ... because *I* want to do lots as well. I know I can't have more than my fair share too, and I know it's difficult for you when people like me get difficult ... But I need you to understand why I need to do more. It's because I *need* to sing, to sing to other people. I think it's because I need to communicate. And I didn't communicate with anyone at all for years ... And now I *can*, and I *need to* ... And I don't have many years left now ... I need

> to communicate, and music is the most direct way of doing this, isn't it? It's the easiest way and the best way. So that's why I need to do this, and I want you to understand why … . [Gary's log, March 2007]

***

In these two examples there's the ongoing musical companionship between singer and accompanist in which both work to maintain the song and the musical relationship that keeps the song on track. There's also evidence of the therapist's strategy to keep the interpersonal–musical relationship 'on track' through the processes of attuning, dialoguing, and regulating. There's also evidence of the therapist intervening musically to make ongoing 'repairs' to the musical-personal fabric such that the performance remains optimal.

One more surprising aspect that came out of the ongoing analysis of the nature of musical support in the project is how there are also often cases where other SMART member/musicians step into a situation in an overt way to both foster musical companionship, and to offer varieties of 'support and repair' to potentially perilous moments:

> It's early days in Ella's musical pathway between hospital music therapy groups and SMART Music, and today she's brought a book of songs to SMART Music. She selects *My Sweet Lord,* but as I play the opening lilting chords on the piano Ella's suddenly not sure how to get going. She sings in a very small, quavery voice, coming in on *Oh my lord,* trying to stabilise the pitch and rhythm for herself … . I'm trying not to be too obtrusive with my accompaniment but it's clearly not enough of a guide at this point … 'You'll have to start me off' she says. I cue her in with my voice, and she's away, a bit like someone having trouble balancing on a bike, then they're off. But I'm not quite getting the balance right between subtle support and guidance such that the performance stabilises … But then we arrive at the famous call-and-response section of the song: … *but it takes so long my Lord* … and suddenly there's Daniel singing *My Sweet Lord,* perfectly placing this echo phrase in a way that almost instantly stabilises both Ella and the song. Other singers follow, and a few percussion instruments emphasise a subtle beat … Ella gathers confidence and her voice swells on *I really want to show you Lord … I really want to go with you* … Throughout the rest of the song Ella remains absolutely in the solo space, but she clearly feels the musical support around her now – keeping her more securely in musical time and space. On the final phrase she and Daniel look at each other and time their singing together – *My … Sweet … Lord.* It's been a collective process of musical support, stabilisation and repair. [Gary's analysis of recorded excerpt from 2007]

In this and other occasions we found how the principles and craft of musical companionship becomes further 'distributed' amongst the other musicians involved.

It's not just the music therapist who does this – the search for, and achievement of successfully being together in music is often a *shared achievement* of musicking, and 'reparative musicking' when necessary. And yet, for craft to be distributed and for achievement to be fostered, the music therapist does employ a great deal of specialist craft.

An outsider's view of the music therapist's craft

It's May 2006 and Gary and Tia are sitting on the top of a London bus on their way to SMART. Tia has started to think about Gary's 'craft' – does he always know what he's doing, or does he just do it. How is the knowledge produced, and how cognitive is it? And how is it different from what 'any' professionally trained musician might be able to do?

Gary explains to Tia that his training was all about acute listening – to the client's musical utterances and acts, yes, but also to the situation of musicking. This training came from the Nordoff Robbins practice of 'listening back' to the taped sessions and – as we've seen so many times so far in this book – 'indexing' on paper the micro-detail of the interaction between the musical and paramusical. So what does Gary listen for and how does he respond? Tia thinks that this listening happens on multiple planes simultaneously. The first of these is Gary's ear for individual musicking practices, iterative, continuous and changing, developing and, sometimes, disintegrating.

For example, Gary tells her something intriguing about one of the participants, Mary. He says he thinks he can tell when she is becoming ill again from the way she over-ornaments the melody lines of 'her' songs. In this sense, how a person musicks is a kind of diagnostic tool, and part of preventative, or at least proactive, healthcare.

If listening is 'diagnostic', and if musicking exhibits symptoms of becoming or being unwell, then to what extent can strategically structured musicking counteract symptoms, Tia wonders, all the while knowing that this question is too simple, too mechanistic. And yet, it would seem that for Mary, and even in context of her conflicted relationship with music at different times in her life, music was a way of redressing the things that otherwise caused distress. It was, in Tia's sense (Book One, *Music Asylums,* in this Triptych) a kind of asylum. And so, fixing-up music was like fixing-up (furnishing) a space for being well. And the musical furnishing of that space did two things simultaneously: it gave Mary a form of shelter and it filled the space that was Mary, which is to say that music was a medium for experience – relationships, self and daily life. Music occupied the space that otherwise other things (confusion, anxiety, depression, loss of focus) might have filled. In this sense, music did not 'cure' anything, but it did eclipse other, more negative, things. Those other things co-existed with Mary's musical state, but they also rubbed up against that state in ways that inflected her musicking and in ways that could eclipse her ability to be socially musical, to be attuned both to the music (its times, requirements and styles) and through that music, to others, similarly attuned.

So, Tia asks Gary, how is what you do different from what most community musicians do? What is different about what you do for Mary and what someone without music therapy training might be able to do? Gary replies that he is like the pilot of a commercial aircraft. Most of the time he's just doing routine work, watching out, attending closely to all the data and double checking that the plane stays on course and isn't going to bump in to anything. But if troubles arise Gary will leap into action so as to safely 'land the plane'. In addition to what Gary did for Mary, Tia witnessed quite a few examples of how Gary managed this task.

For example, as we mentioned earlier (and as Tia has described in some detail in *Music Asylums*) in 2006 there was a tussle between two members over how to perform a jazz ballad. The singing duo were vying with each other (swing style versus ballad style). Each considered the song in question to be 'their' property (as one began to sing, the other quickly joined the performance saying 'this is my song'). Both singers were trying to render the song 'their' way, which meant contradictory tempos, melodic inflections and sensibilities. This sort of musical conflict didn't happen often at SMART. It felt like musical tug-of-rope, with Gary as the 'rope'. It was, to mix metaphors, an opportunity for Tia to see precisely what it took for Gary to 'land the plane'. He hammered out the melody and chords, he sang along, he used his body to chart a middle way through the conflict zone and he sang at the top of his lungs to find a middle way.

Within the musical spaces of SMART, musical territory is an important resource. The songs that members love, that they may be deeply attached to, are salutogenic spaces, that is symbolic places of nurturing, comfort, pleasure, security and thus places for flourishing. This musical ownership is anything but trivial as it becomes a way of both finding and securing self-identity and pathway outward from illness to other places in the 'room' and as a way of negotiating presence, relation to other and current status in the group. So, when Mary returns from the hospital to SMART, after four months of being very ill, her re-entry into musical space is 'announced' by her singing one of her signature songs, *Where is Love*. And when, as we saw, Eloise is ill, her cymbal is prominently positioned in the front of the room, in her spot, as always, and the fact it is mute is both a testament to the fact that it awaits her return and that she remains an important figure in the collective musical ground.

Being able to stake a place in that ground is part of what it means to build a musical pathway. And the skill to be able to foster that claims-making, without seeming to be doing anything more than furnishing 'accompaniment' is a great part of the music therapist's craft. Both Gary and Sarah routinely engage in what Tia came to think of as musical shepherding, joining in a solo song if they perceive that the singer isn't going to manage on his or her own, singing sotto voce or hammering out the melody so as to offer musical scaffolding, modulating up or down to match a singer's pitch, prolonging an intro until the singer is reading to jump in, skipping whole swathes of a verse if the singer makes an unannounced digression, or calling in the rest of us to act as chorus if the soloist seems like they need a breather.

So too Gary and (as we will see, Sarah from 2007 when she joined the project) know how to call on the chorus if a voice needs drowning out, as once happened when a participant came up to the mic and began to improvise overly enthusiastically, ribald lyrics to a song that he used as a serenade for a visiting therapist.

The ability to keep things 'up in the air' under duress, and to effect soft landings, is, in short a big chunk of the community music therapist's craft. But it is by no means all there is to it. As much as being a music therapist might be like being an airline pilot, so too is it like being an airline steward, albeit perhaps in the first class passenger section where the job includes both being charming and playing the host, facilitating the feeling of being at ease and thus able to enjoy the flight, but also ensuring that no one passenger becomes unruly or disruptive and that personal space, adherence to safety regulations, and general cordiality are maintained. But unlike either of these airline jobs, what Gary and Sarah do as music therapists is linked to their great familiarity with their, as it were, flying partners.

Both Gary and Sarah have worked in the adjacent mental health facility and they know the SMART members well, in musical terms, they know these people intimately and they know how each member possesses a unique musical fingerprint. Gary and Sarah know the contours of these prints, their whorls, loops and arches, which they can mimic, blend, support and complement easily. Each member has 'their' songs and 'types' of songs and part of the craft of the community music therapist is to know how to work with members to develop their musicianship (and through it their tastes and sensibilities over time) in ways that bring them closer to their songs and musical aspirations, and that lead them into new and fertile musical terrain. So both Gary and Sarah know how to suggest plausible, useful and pleasurable songs, how to combine one person's songs with another's, and how to use those combinations so as to flatter everyone, and everyone's tastes and skills. They know how to use their bodies and forms of eye contact to cue the timings of things, when to call out instructions for solo spots (e.g., calling out names or instruments), and when, occasionally, just to be silly. They know that the ceremonial features of what they do and what happens is vital and thus when it is important to engage in a doing of heightened, 'this is what we are doing' behaviour, as would any celebrant in any ritual. They also know when to insert a collective number, an improvisation, for all, for some, when to encourage someone to come up to the mic and when not and when to break for tea. They know how and when to just let things happen and when to intervene. They know how to model songs and musical attitudes so as to show how things could be, musically. And they know how to talk about music and encourage talk about music that is, simultaneously, the constitution of narrative about recovery, skill, interrelationship and new (musicalised) identity, something we have seen so far in Gary's interview-dialogues with SMART musicians. Talk, in other words, contextualises, and empowers, what it is that music seems to 'do'.

The skills that Sarah and Gary use are not skills that transfer easily to more casual musical events of a one-off basis or with continually shifting personnel. Gary and Sarah are part of this setting. They are, in other words, institutional musicians who work in SMART and in its adjacent hospital. They are, sometimes almost literally, part of the furniture. Here, and through their roles as musical conductors (think of conductor in the sense of being a mediating conduit) they facilitate and make musical intimacy. They do this in ways that offer participants opportunities for action, respite, asylum and development. It is the attempt to build in structured ways musical relationship over time in ways that are conducive to wellbeing. It is achieved through hundreds of micro and often invisible practices, time-after-time. And in community music therapy it is directed to supporting the joint work of building pathways to wellbeing together. In these regards, the study of music therapy can be understood to contribute to the growing body of studies of craftwork in the social sciences (Atkinson 2013; Zembylas 2014; Delamont and Stephens 2008), including other studies of music therapeutic 'craftwork' itself (Procter 2013)

26. Distributed Sensitivity, Action, and Appreciation at SMART

> … using the verb [musicking] emphasizes that not only is music an activity, but it's also a form of human encounter in which everyone who is present is taking part, and for whom success or failure as an event everybody who is present has some responsibility. It is not just a matter of active performers doing something for, or to, passive listeners. Whatever it is that's being done, we are all doing it together. (Small 2010)

At SMART Music soloists and audience are often interchangeable, as in other traditions of participatory music, but very unlike most other situations Westerners are used to at musical events. In the SMART cafe on Thursday afternoons singers and players come out of the audience, and then return back to it to support others. As the music session develops over the years there's also an intermediate group of 'supporting players' (guitars, drums, accordianists, violin, clarinet, harmonica) who provide musical support for many of the on-going items. But overall there's the sense of people being 'all in it together', and taking collective responsibility for this fact, as Christopher Small suggests. Because of the particularity of SMART as a mental health community, there's also another dimension to such participatory support.

Rob first comments on this when he comes into this situation as an unprepared outsider, and sees how people react to different situations as the 'audience'. He first comments on the performances by Peter, during which the audience is unusually quiet and attentive (somewhat because Peter has shooshed them in an uncompromising way). The song performance and content is unusual by SMART Music standards – the singer's own songs about living on the streets (see Section 24 above). His performance is edgy and slightly disturbing. Rob writes:

> It seems that after Peter finishes singing other people in the room find ways of dealing with the content and expression of the songs. They make comments about the songs being 'good', but there are no cheers, the applause matches the solemnity of the music – people are finding appropriate means of

> supporting Peter without patronising him with some over enthusiastic happy-clappy adjectives. Dealing with other peoples' strong emotions is difficult for most people, not merely those with mental health problems but everyone in general. We don't usually have to cope with these situations in our everyday lives. Peter's moment in front of people could therefore be seen as a positive experience in that it provides an opportunity for people, the music group as a whole, and the SMART community to manage these expressions effectively, like a self-training: How do I deal with this? What is the appropriate thing to say? What do other people do? Is it effective? What is the right thing to do? These were all questions I had to ask myself when Peter played. I learnt a lot in that moment about how to support someone without being condescending. Just by watching other people. I'm sure it was an opportunity for many other people to do the same. [Rob, CD commentary, p. 37]

Jeremy mounts a quite different style of performance, and the audience respond with an equally different style, but similarly with a collective and collaborative support that is somehow part of the performance. Again Rob describes a performance of *Sleepy Lagoon* by Jeremy:

> 'Silence please! Silence' says Jeremy to a room of chattering people, and he introduces another of his solo numbers with a little history of the song and context from which it came. He's bringing the attention of people to what he's doing. In his interview and on other occasions he has told me of how the music group is an opportunity to educate people, and here he seems to parody the manner of a teacher or public speaker. [... .] As Jeremy talks about his song, Roger pipes up with a joke: 'He's like an inexhaustible supply of gramophone reels' and several people laugh heartily. Someone else calls Jeremy a 'stylus', and Bobby jokes further that Jeremy's more like a loudspeaker. Jeremy finishes his introduction; someone [I think it's Gary] shushes the group, and Bobby shouts 'Pray Silence! Silence in court.' You can then hear Jeremy and other people laugh. For me this 'mocking'[14] of Jeremy by other members of the group, something initiated by Jeremy's own self-mockery at the start, is another way in which people support the person performing – by mirroring their behaviour. Jeremy doesn't seem to want his ego to dominate and so makes jokes about himself. The group somehow recognises this, perhaps, and meets Jeremy in the middle by adding their own mockery. In other instances, where someone is quite solemn for example, the group supports that person by mirroring this solemnity. When Jeremy starts singing, the mockery continues with various musical jokes – playing instruments that drown Jeremy out [people laugh];

14 We're not sure Rob has got the right word here. He means perhaps 'teasing' as it's clear that the banter is playful and not upsetting to Jeremy – more a shared joke. This is how Tia and Gary experienced such moments.

> singing in a very over the top manner. The atmosphere is very light and jovial. But it seems as though this is somewhat initiated by Jeremy. This is why I think Jeremy is so very generous in his performances – it's much, much more than just about singing into a microphone; it's creating an event for everyone to enjoy. Jeremy let's people enjoy themselves and add their own enjoyment to the mix. He allows for collectivity. He is the catalyst for collectivity. [Rob, CD commentary]

Rob's key comment for the subject we're discussing is how the audience mirrors the needs/wishes of the immediate situation (either a person, a type of performance etc.). This is similar to how a therapist typically does this – being sensitive and attentive to just how a person is, to how they are doing something, and then 'matching' or 'mirroring' this to establish an intersubjective contact, to support and demonstrate empathy and understanding. This can happen on micro or more general levels. The interesting thing in SMART Music that Rob picks up on here is how this basic 'therapeutic response' (support, understanding, appropriate reaction) is somehow 'distributed' across the 'audience', is a *collective* understanding and response.

Listening back to the excerpts, when you hear both performer and audience 'in action' it's clear how the 'audience' tunes-in, and provides appropriate atmosphere and musical and listening support to different moments, different people. The audience is almost acting like a single organism itself. What, then, is the need in this particular situation, this particular community, that somehow collectively and naturally emerges? Rob makes a suggestion in his notes apropos a comment about Ella:

> The music group – the space provided, the safety assured, the support offered – is an arena in which people can just practice doing music, practice being in front of people. It's an environment that allows people to get better by being themselves – that's what music does as well. Jane mentioned to me in her interview that singing was like a big sigh, like 'the long letting go'. Music is an opportunity to release yourself from everyday constrictions – to behave as a human being: moving, singing, dancing, expressing, feeling. I know that for Ella the SMART group has provided the necessary space and experience to practice being herself in music and getting better at it. And being herself in music is the same thing as being herself out of music'. [Rob's music notes].

The audience response to Mary's singing is fairly constant over the many years she performs the same three or four songs in SMART Music. Mary is well known and well loved in the SMART community, and as such is always a welcome performer, and she is encouraged to sing. But there's more to it than this. As we've noted before, there's a 'duality' in Mary's voice that seems to be automatically heard and understood by anyone listening: the 'two faces' of her and her voice – beauty, courage, strength … twinned with vulnerability, hurt, precariousness. A natural response to Mary is simultaneously to encourage and to protect. In this sense the audience supports her both morally, but also very practically through how they play instruments, and sing along. As Rob comments:

> I'm also interested here in the support offered on different percussion instruments – and it feels like support rather than 'joining in'. It's just there in the background, like a big hug you can sink into; it's not meant to take the song anywhere else; it's just there to carry Mary, a little extra sparkle that highlights her performance, shows some appreciation while not taking over the moment. [Rob's music notes]

'Carrying' is perhaps the best metaphor for what we're talking about here; there's a dynamism and movement in the support, which comes from how the audience are also inside the musical time and space of the performance, not just passive observers. They are also active *participators* in the event – where (as Small states) we're all doing it together, we all have a response-ability to what's happening, and what *could happen next* ... for good or ill.

A last example: an occasion where *Strangers in the Night* is being performed. Gary plays the introduction and the singing is immediately more cohesive than usual, and with no percussion playing along. The atmosphere has a quiet, hushed calm that matches the song, but clearly also the achieved state of the group that day. After the first verse sung by all, there's a period where Gary vamps on the piano asking who'll sing a solo verse: Sadie? No? Roger? Finally a voice arrives at the microphone, which Gary doesn't recognise. Most of the audience probably don't recognise her either. She sings with a small voice in a focused, clear but quiet way. The audience sing behind her, in an equally quiet and focused way, modulating their way of singing closely to the quality and the support needs of the unknown soloist. Rob writes:

> The soloist starts and is very quiet. You can hear the very quiet singing of people in the room. They seem like they don't want to sing over the soloist. It really feels like they're supporting her with a quiet ebbing undercurrent of the melody as a safety net. When Gary asks for everybody to join in again for the last verse, the group singing is markedly quieter than the singing at the beginning. Could it be that people are conscious that loud singing at this point could overshadow the soloist's preceding attempts, especially considering the very quiet nature of the soloist's singing? Is this quiet group singing a way of collectively respecting the soloist? It sounds almost humble. No one voice is heard above any other, as if the group is sending a message to the soloist that 'we are a group, we sing together – and in singing as one we recognise your solo effort.' [Rob's music notes]

***

There are, of course, more overt and conventional forms of response in SMART Music – clapping, whooping and other sounds of appreciation. But again, there's a subtle dimension to this that only emerges as we experience and compare these responses over time. How soon do people applaud or comment? How loud? How sincerely? It becomes clear to us that the 'clapometer' is related to many things apart from obvious aesthetic parameters – sound of voice, style of performance, objective 'bringing off' of the performance. Rather it's often a subtle response to the relationship between the present moment (how the performance has gone) and what the audience know of the performer's history, current state, effort and aspirations. Appreciation and recognition at SMART Music is a complex and subtle situated interpretative process on behalf of the 'audience' that relates to how Christopher Small (2010) has written about the 'misunderstanding and reunderstanding' of musical performances – the way that a direct on-the-spot evaluation is made of what is happening, what the significance of it is, and what response is required. It's a very complex social-aesthetic process that all enact in the time and space of the musical event. Appreciation is, that is, a necessarily aesthetic interpretation, but with the aesthetics/ethics ellision that this whole project illustrates – leading to the key question, *What is good musicking?* We will return to this at the end of this book.

27. SMART Music's 'Improvisational Attitude'

As SMART Music matured between 2005–7 it became clear that an overall attitude had emerged as a guiding force – one that matched (and perhaps was at the root of) the aspects we've discussed in the previous few sections. This was an *improvisational attitude*; a way of working and thinking that is confident enough to 'go with the flow', to trust that people and music will lead.[15]

This attitude (which to an extent is also SMART's as an organisation) contrasts with many other environments where people with mental health problems go to seek help. An organisational response to mental distress is often to attempt to find solutions through regimes of control and authority, which include specific protocols or interventions that are directed by doctors or therapists. In contrast, a core precept deriving from the Nordoff Robbins tradition of music therapy (and developed within the Community Music Therapy movement) has always been what we've come to call an *improvisational attitude.* This originates in the practice of musical improvisation proper, pointing back to how Paul Nordoff approached difficult situations with clients musically through his skill as an improviser – listening first as a musician, responding musically and creatively (within musical parameters) to anything that he could that characterised and called to the person he was trying to

[15] A range of interdisciplinary theory is now looking at the processes and virtues of an improvisatory attitude. See Richard Sennett's (2004) book, *The Craftsman*, and its section on 'craftsman improvisation' (p. 235ff).

reach.[16] He was essentially starting from the premise that he couldn't 'see through' [*im-provisare*] to the end of the human situation or the musical utterance, and just had to follow his instincts and musical sensitivity to guide him. This strategy proved vital in the sense of establishing and developing contact with the disturbed and hard-to-reach children who were idiosyncratic and unpredictable in their responses. Nordoff would musically follow them, then allow the music/client to lead, then follow again, establishing a responsive communicational milieu that often swiftly led to musical rapport and encounter. Importantly, this approach gave him the flexibility to make music '*from*' people, not impose music on top of them (as had been the case before in using music within special education previously). This basic improvisational situation in music also became a model or exemplar for a wider attitude towards working musically with people and situations – a stance that was prepared and comfortable to follow freely where people and situations lead. It stands for a confidence and competence to search and find within this flow of musical, personal and communal experience nascent possibilities for contact, relationship and collective action.

But of course an inevitable consequence of such an attitude (in music, in life) is that it's *messy!* Not knowing where you're going exactly means that direction, intensity, timing and spacing must be constantly *negotiated* and *re*-negotiated. It will work sometimes, but not always – and will require the messy ongoing process of correction (self- and relational), negotiation, tinkering and repair. It will require an overall ethos and aesthetic of non-perfection: the confidence and tolerance that things will usually work out well and good through the very process of keeping doing something with awareness, sensitivity, responsiveness and a tolerance of not knowing exactly where you're heading.[17]

This 'improvisational attitude' comes strongly through the data in how the micro and meso aspects of the on-going musical work emerge. And *emerge* is perhaps the key word. Musical things – songs, improvisations and later broader events such as gigs, parties etc. – start somewhere but don't always go entirely to plan (if indeed there is a plan!). This is because of how people want things to go sometimes quite differently (style, speed, key, inflection), or simply because they 'go wrong' (people forget the next line, the tune, or don't manage to 'bring it off' in the way intended). Within an improvisational attitude held as the frame for the whole enterprise the ongoing musical-personal-social work is all seen as

---

16 See Ansdell (2014), Chapter 6 for more on this.

17 It's of course possible to unnecessarily reify this distinction between 'improvisation' and planned action – whilst in reality there's a natural continuity between them (see Benson 2003). But such 'improvisational attitudes' do stand out in contrast to approaches and treatments in healthcare and education where methods, techniques, formula, procedures, protocols etc. are ways of determining or controlling set responses to certain problems and troubles.

contingent, and subject to being repaired, renegotiated in the ongoing creative flow of the larger picture – which is that we're all cobbling it together, trying to make it work.

In any given musical situation (dyadic or communal) this entails participants roughly knowing where they're going, but importantly, *not knowing* exactly how they're going to get there. This tolerating 'not knowing' gives space and time for the contingent, necessarily emergent needs and possibilities of these people, here now, in this place – emerging on the second-by-second crest of the present musical moment happening. Neither problems nor solutions can be entirely pre-planned (though strategy and forethought and preparation helps in a way). Rather any outcome needs the courage from all to follow the trajectory of current possibility, to tap into what could and might happen just now; to midwife the creative present moment into being. This is something shared by everyone, and something that everyone has the responsibility for (response-ability) – given the right conditions, attitudes etc. In this way there's also an 'attitudinal improvisation' going on too. In the process of improvising the musical moment and the musical future we are also crafting *how* we should think about the given moment – by allowing it to happen, valuing it, assessing where it could/should go, and being prepared to collectively support and contribute to this. This is serious creative *play* – playing in and *with* the present moment – the thing that music does best.

This interfaces with the aesth/ethics theme in the sense that all the above needs a parallel 'attitude of judgement': that *perfection is not required!* Only by acknowledging and being able to tolerate the necessary 'mess' of the on-going emergent assembly of the socio-musical reality is an improvisational stance possible. To put it the other way: the desire/need for on-going perfection, order, predictability and control will kill creative, improvisational play.

Part of our on-going research interest is how the music project has been able – for members, staff, visitors and others – to model an alternative aesthetic/ethic of life and health, an 'improvisational attitude' fostered by this musical culture. Think again of the fashion metaphor that we discussed in Section 12 above. There is, or there should be in aesthetic/ethical life no 'one size fits all', no 'model' way of doing/being to which everyone feels they 'ought' to conform. Instead, the improvisatory aesthetic and the widened musical community that this aesthetic fosters in turn allows for an expanded awareness of how it is possible to approach 'trouble' through not necessarily 'fixing' once and for all, but rather through tolerating the disjunctions, and the uncertain messiness of following and discerning sometimes emergent (and inhering) for-the-time-being solutions that are locally and situationally defined, managed: tinkerings, adjustings of things and attitudes etc. – as musically modelled in this case. Troubles/problems x, y, z are not necessarily fixed or resolved directly, but rather transfigured (if only for a time) through the fluidity of musical situations and 'musical solutions'. And this transfiguration is one that spills out from SMART Music's aesthetic practice and judgement in ways that are socially activist. Making things 'fluid' means making things malleable in other words.

28. Musical Flow

When Gary first talks about bringing more music to SMART in 2005 Dave the manager then imagines it helping with the problem of the static nature of the cafe for much of the week. SMART at that time had two basic constituencies: people well and willing enough to do the active projects they organise (catering, computer, floristry), and then a group of people with more long-term mental health problems who sit around the cafe most of the week – often in the same chair, the same configurations, talking and complaining about the same things. Energy and mobility was low said Dave, and somehow because the cafe was central to SMART this infected the mood of the whole. Perhaps said Dave, music could both stir up the energy, and break up the immobile and static patterns of the cafe. In the next five years it seems to do just that – certainly on the music days, but arguably amongst both members and staff in the place as a whole. One of music's chief social processes is to add flow and energy, to mix up what's become fixed and static; to move people – on, in and around, through …

Music as a 'fluid object'

An ecological perspective suggests thinking of music as a 'fluid object', and musicking as a 'fluid process'. This helps to get beyond the traditional closed boxing-up of music, people, situations, and rather notices how there's a flow and a constant metamorphosis and interpenetration laterally *across and between* these seemingly different things. The 'musicking' concept partly mobilises this deconstruction, but it needs to go another stage beyond the formulation that music = process. The concept of a musical ecology takes this further, theorising and demonstrating how musical action distributes and metamorphoses between and across musical people, musical things, and musical situations. We see in the data just such a fluid metamorphosis at the levels of people, music, ensembles and combinations, occasions, spaces, transformations ... Indeed the *point* and the positive outcomes for SMART people and the place in general comes by virtue of such musical fluidity and metamorphosis. Within the overall concept of 'music and change' and the musical basis of wellbeing we're looking at how musical transformation leads, accompanies and evidences personal and social change. Musicking allows such fluidity, a safe level of indeterminacy, shape-shifting, becoming else and other.

The significance of thinking about music in this way for the SMART environment is that music helps afford such transformation in a setting (and with people struggling with what they and/or others perceive as pathologies) where the opposite is often the norm: stuckness, impediments (other people, tasks, lack of resources and skill, impossible expectations, frightening situations, long-term forms of dependency), rigidity, lack of flow, over-investment in unchanging identity, perseveration and stasis. In contrast, musical fluidity and its ever-potential metamorphosis affords an 'ontological openness'. People say that one of the key things about mental health problems is that they often isolate you within your own problems, pain, distorted perceptions and judgements etc. In periods of illness people move away from the kind of fluid openness that allows 'things' to change us (to ameliorate a mental or physical state, the quality of a situation etc.). Eloise said that mental illness leads to people 'curling up like hedgehogs'.

What musick(ing) seems to help with is a compensatory openness to flow and fluidity; 'going with the flow'; allowing things to become other than they are … as the musick(ing) does just that within and around you. Improvisations are amenable to high degrees of mutability – they welcome it, in response to an immediate action. A tap on a woodblock leads to changes of texture, volume, instrumentation. One person can influence the course or interpretation of a musical event through the rapid incorporation of a gesture or idea, be it creative or subversive. A song starts this way, but then veers towards something different, metamorphoses in a way that incorporates something or someone else; changes pace to pick someone up or to latch onto their current action or pace. Individuals flow into each other as they musick together – taking a part within the texture as it too changes shape and assembly. Groups regroup and realign, situations mutate quickly or slowly. Nothing stays the same – nobody steps twice into the same musical river. If you feel stuck, or isolated this can be an advantage. Can you let yourself become part of this musical flow – even if just for seconds at a time? This 'ontological openness' works in the opposite direction to most pathology and its impact. But it coaxes rather than forces; its perhaps a safe and gentle form of return to the inevitable and necessary balance in physical and mental life between form and transformation; between identity and relationship; between security and creative insecurity; between being and becoming …

So 'openness' can be enormously helpful as a resource for pathway building and free improvisations, in as much as they may take the form of non-songs (seemingly 'new' and 'can go anywhere' structures), can offer participants openings, less rigid and less demanding formats than can more familiar 'songs' with all their cultural heritage, familiarity, stylistic implications, and, often, baggage. 'Songs' come with a host of contextualisation cues where free improvisations say, 'make of me what you will' and in real time. They say, you can participate peripherally because here there is no fixed melody, no required homophony but rather – we're channelling Adorno here – simultaneous multiplicity. They say 'we' can make this go where we like, where our sounds take us: there are no prefabricated 'right' ways of musicking. In addition, and because of this open-endedness, improvisations and their fluidity, open up space, make it less purposeful, less resolute, even for those who don't contribute directly to that flow.

For example, Tia remembers one of her earliest visits to SMART Music in 2006, watching a restless woman in the middle of the room who repeatedly left the room, perhaps five times in five or six minutes (to smoke, go to the toilet, go out to the corridor). It was as if, during the performance of solo songs, that she simply could not settle. Then, when a song finished Gary began to improvise something slow, quiet, open-textured at the piano and people offered muted, tentative musical contributions. The woman visibly relaxed and while she did not take part in the improvised music, she remained in her seat, quiet, less agitated, still. Tia's reading of this situation (and one that she also experienced) was that within these musical conditions there were no implied stylistic or rhythmic responses, no sense of having to become 'like' the music but rather a desultory or ambling form in which it was 'ok' not to be active, in which even 'non-participation' (just sitting back and listening, or dreaming) was a form of participation. If anything, the music became less like 'music as we know it' and more like an ambient condition – a 'gentle zephyr' for example. It was possible, in other words, for this non-participating member to 'fit in' with this music since its shape was undefined, rather as one might close one's eyes and turn one's face to the sun and simply bask in music.

So something between being and becoming, the attitudes of which become established in most sessions of SMART Music by around the end of the project's second year. Here, for example, is a complete session from that time which, we think, works like a snapshot of both the group and the individual members well on the way together in the collective musical journey of this project. It also has present many of the 'cast' of the on-going story we've been telling so far. You will notice music, people and echoes of situations we've described in the previous pages within this average session on an average Thursday afternoon …

29. SMART Music – Session 66, Thursday 1 November 2006

Present: Bobby, Daniel, Ella, Eloise, Jane, Brian, Giles, Barbara, Kathleen, Tony (for first time), Moussai, Simon, Mary, Vivienne, Selima, Roger + two music therapy visitors (Mercedes & Juao).

As Gary and Sarah are setting up Viv comes up to them and says in a very heartfelt way (with tears in her eyes) 'I just want to say thank you to both of you for what you do with the music here ... It really helps us'. She touches her heart as she says this. Gary replies 'well, thank you – you know we enjoy it too ... ', And she says, 'yes, I know that ... that's what really helps'. Viv has been coming to the Wednesday SMART Singers group recently and clearly values the combination of the Wednesday and Thursday groups.

At the start of the session there's lots of background noise and chat; people greeting each other ...

'We had a party yesterday' Jeremy tells me, ' ... it was very good ... did you hear about it? No pianist though!' he says and laughs ...

Introductory Improvisation

Gary starts improvising on the piano, a gentle jazzy lilt, and instantly a drum joins in, picks up and emphasises the rhythm. This is Brian, a new drummer in a red shirt, who's been working with Sarah doing music therapy in the day hospital.

He's making his first appearance at SMART today – a pathway for him. He's participating in the first minutes of the event. Bobby, a regular drummer is also here, and Gary looks round to see how Bobby reacts ... but it's immediately clear that he accepts Brian as another drummer, not a rival.

The improvisation gathers music and people together without the need for verbal instructions. People take places at the tables, select instruments, and in a few minutes you can hear drum, cymbal (Eloise), tambourine (Barbara), clacking sticks finding a place within the texture. Whisps of a harmonica (Roger) tentatively creep in, getting more confident, receding ... Gary sings as well, the music inflects into a Blues (clear in its structure and musical expectation for these opening minutes of the group) and the harmonica finds his voice, waa-waaing in the rhythmic gaps ...

Suddenly there's a moment of crisis ... *'Leave me alone!'* shouts Tony, a blind man who has come to the group for the first time, and has been frightened by someone well-meaningly pushing an instrument into his hands (he can't see them coming and gets scared). Gary says a few words of reassurance to Tony at the same time as carrying on the Blues piano. All is ok, Tony calms down quickly, and the music carries on ...

The improvisation broadens as people find confidence to elaborate their parts (Brian starts playing more complex drum rhythms around the basic beat). Gary cues in various people for solos, calling their names out – 'Roger ... .', who goes up to the microphone and takes a solo on harmonica. Gary then cues in Tony who plays a melodica in close musical dialogue with Roger for a few minutes ... so that now individual people, duets, are being balanced out within the overall communal music. The improvisation moves towards a climax, followed by whooping and clapping, and thanking of the key solo players. This opening number has instantly both reflected and created the social-musical shape of this group of people this afternoon – with freedom, opportunity and a subtle balance between the whole and its parts.

Eloise Suggests Autumn Leaves

Gary says that we're working from the yellow songbook today, and would someone like to suggest a song to start with. *Autumn Leaves*, says Eloise. People look for page 30, and Gary says 'nice and gentle this one', thinking of encouraging a contrasting mood to the improvisation. As he plays the introduction someone lightly whistles along (Mary?), and the drummer provides a light rhythmic tap ... Gary cues the first lines of the song – people gradually enter, as do the various instruments (harmonica, shaker, cymbal, melodica ...). 'OK, Tony solo on melodica ... ' and Tony gradually finds the right key (with a few quickly self-corrected notes ...). People listen carefully to the musicality of this new member, this solo giving him a platform to show himself off as a musical person. The solo ends and Gary cues the group back into the chorus ... then changes the rhythmic character a bit, adding a more South American rhythm, leaving gaps for instruments to have a short 'say' ...

Jeremy Sings a Tribute …

'Time for a solo I think', says Gary, 'Jeremy?'. And indeed Jeremy has something prepared, words written out in a spiral notebook. 'I have a little tribute' says Jeremy and looks towards Dave the manager who rolls his eyes and says 'I'll stand at the back … '. Jeremy does a little speech about the history of the song and singer, Bob Hope, with rhetorical questions for the audience, which he then answers himself, accompanied by good-natured heckling from the audience. 'This is called *Thanks for the Memory* … Do you know it? Do you?'. Jeremy tells Gary that he's not got the music so will do it unaccompanied. He launches straight into the song, and Eloise provides a little tinkling cymbal in support. Jeremy slightly gabbles through it, seemingly trying to get to the end … Chuckles come up (Peggy?), but people listen carefully. Jeremy gets nearly to the end, but cuts the last two notes/words and goes back into speech, asking Dave whether he liked it. We later find out that this is a premature tribute in that Jeremy, but not most of the rest of us, knows that Dave is leaving SMART soon.

Continuing the Mood, Brian Sings Blue Moon

'Let's stay with that era' says Gary, and everyone looks in the songbooks for something that will follow on. There's discussion, suggestion of *Blue Moon* and various people trying out the tune. 'Number 15, in the Red Book', and Sarah comes to the piano, as Brian has previously done this song with her in the hospital setting. At first he can't find the pitch, and Sarah's subtle attempts to orientate him with both her voice and piano accompaniment don't work at first. 'Instrumental!' calls Sarah, to give Brian a break and time to tune-in to the key … and when he returns to singing he's bang in tune.

'Something which we could all try together … ?'

Viv suggests 'number 8 in the Yellow Book – *Night and Day*', saying it'd be a nice one to sing together. A few people try out the rhythmic riffs, Gary says 'we'll need percussion for this one' and gets drums and tambourine playing as he starts the piano introduction. But people don't know the verse to this, so it ends up with Gary singing solo, with whisps of harmonica and then a flute coming into the texture, as Selima suddenly appears, playing her flute as she walks into the room. The texture is messy, clarifying slightly when the chorus comes and a few more people start singing. But as the song goes on its clear this is better as an instrumental number, so Gary encourages Selima to take a flute solo – which she does, gradually finding the right tessitura to play the melody. The other instruments blend around her sensitively … 'Well done Selima!' people call out afterwards. People's individual musical contributions solve group problems!

A Few More Solos – Mary and Ella …

Two people who we've seen tread musical pathways in this project ask to sing solos. First Mary, who sings one of her 'signature' songs, *I don't know how to love him.* This naturally makes a nice calm contrast to previous numbers, and Gary instructs people to let Mary sing the verses solo, but to join in together on the chorus. Mary stands up before the mic with dignity, taking deep breaths to calm herself. When she sings her inimitable voice fills the room – its unique mix (as Rob has commented on before) of strength and vulnerability, fullness of sound that feels it could just crack any minute. This voice, and Mary as performing person, commands people's attention and collective support throughout the song. It's one of the SMART performances that feels like a gift to everyone, though it's not entirely clear what exactly is given …

Mary tends to sing 'her' songs in much the same way each time. In contrast, Ella is clearly experimenting with her performance of *Summertime* – bringing it into a slow and sultry rendition, which takes a few bars to find its groove, but then stabilises nicely. Gradually other instruments around join in – drums, flute, harmonica – adding to the sense that this performance is unique to these people and this situation – it's never been heard *this way* before! Ella's voice opens up, she makes slight improvisations on the melodic line, and at the end of the verse she says 'instrumental'. The players oblige and there's a creative weaving together of flute, melodica, harmonica, piano, drums – kept together by the clearly known shape of the song's harmonic structure … Then Ella breaks this by coming in for the final verse … ending confidently with a half-spoken '*Don't* cry … !'.

A Musical Tea-Break

Unusually Gary accidentally leaves the tape on over the tea-break, and it catches something particular that's begun to be a feature of recent months of this group: how the tea-break allows a kind of 'fringe event' to happen within the main structure of the afternoon. We hear this:

> People are chatting, laughing, joking … cups clatter, chairs and tables scrape, a short buzz of feedback comes from an amplifier as an electric guitar tunes up to notes from a piano …
>
> A guitar fiddles around with fragments of riffs and scales, bending notes Blues-style, then a gentle harmonica emerges from the blend, leading to a few minutes of loose dialogue between harmonica and guitar …
>
> Across these sounds, a sharp voice chimes: '*Did you know it was Sally's birthday yesterday!? Did you? Did you?*' It pierces the atmosphere, then disperses rapidly …
>
> Attention returns to the music as the piano produces a sequence of jazz chords – bits of this and that, tryings-out, soundings … and the guitar recognises

> the chords and joins in … as does the harmonica, but in the wrong key. *'E flat? No? B flat … got you!'*
>
> Then unexpectedly there's a lull in conversation and people are listening, and the players orientate to their newly focused audience, swiftly choosing a song. The piano offers an introduction and the singer leads with authority …
>
> *'I Left My Heart … In San Fran … cis-co … '*, his voice stylishly curling over the room, commanding attention. There's a slight discrepancy between singer and pianist over the tempo, but soon all the players fall in with the singer, weaving their own melody lines and rhythmic elaborations into the mix. Within a few phrases, the chatting crowd turns into a listening audience – there's a gathering of attention and focus, someone quietly whistles, a few people sing snatches of the melody they know … [18]

Here is musicking amongst this group of people of a more spontaneous and messy kind. It's the kind that happens when the main show is 'off-stage' … But it's equally important in showing what's really happening here …

This music ends up with Daniel singing and Simon accompanying him on piano, the music ending by segueing back into the second half of the session – the liminal character of the interval having had its own musical/social character.

The Band Guys Do An Improvised Blues …

The main personnel of the interval music are guys who've previously played in bands, and who are part of the emerging SMART Band. Often these musicians turn up at the Thursday event towards the interval time, and do one or two numbers, shifting the soundworld to wired guitars and blues/rock 'n roll. Today Daniel picks up a guitar, people shout 'rock 'n roll!' but Dan says he can't remember any songs, so Gary says 'let's just do a Blues'. Daniel on guitar/vocals, Brian and Bobby (drums), Gary (piano) set off, and others join them in this improvised musical collaboration (otherwise known as a *jam*). *'Everyday … . everyday I have the Blues … '* sings Daniel, and it has real edge and groove – heads nod, Eloise in country headscarf and tweeds energetically beats the rhythm out on her small cymbal. This music is both stylised and authentic at the same time, and it collects together in such a powerful way all the disparate voices in this musical community. There's a solo break, with room in the music for antiphonal responses, and suddenly there's Tony the blind man on a melodica answering a riff from Daniel's electric guitar … and then the *waaa-waaaing* of Roger's harmonica … Driving towards a messy, collective finish. 'Some nice drumming there … tribal rhythmic stuff' Roger says to Brian, who says 'we've got some real *talent* here, I'm really glad I came … '.

---

18 This is an excerpt from Ansdell (2014), p. 24.

Tony Plays Pachelbel's Canon *on Melodica*

Gary announces 'and now for something completely different', and introduces Tony, saying that he's been working with Tony for years, and Tony is particularly good at playing tunes on the melodica. Gary suggests the Pachelbel to Tony as he knows they can carry this off together (even though they perhaps last did it 15 years ago).[19] Tony gradually elaborates his melody around the basic piano chords of the canon, with Gary playing a counter-melody. The room hushes to listen to this unusual solo. Gradually other musical voices steal into the background – whisps of harmonica and flute ... and all share a finely placed cadence. Tony gets a generous clap, and goes back pleased to his seat, now known by everyone for the musician he is.

Viv Manages a Song, With a Little Help ...

Viv has plucked up courage to sing after months of saying a polite thank you when her friends suggested she had a go. She picks *Life is a Cabaret* today, and appeals for everyone in the room to help her through it. Gary asks her who she wants as an accompanist – by this time in the afternoon there are no fewer than four pianists who could manage this ... She asks Gary, and throughout the song he works hard to point-up in his accompaniment the melody and the main structural aspects of the song, to keep her comfortably on the rails ... Everyone provides subtle support for her, morally and musically. It's a triumph for her.

Mersad is encouraged up from the back of the room to play ...

Lurking around the back of the cafe is a man who is on the periphery of this community, using SMART over the previous months to help his transition back to health. He took part in Sarah's performance group in the hospital, and a few times in the previous months has played in SMART Music. Several people notice him, and he's fairly easily encouraged up to play. He takes one of the electric guitars, Gary helps him to tune up, then he plays one of his own pieces in rock style ... People listen respectfully, add a bit of light percussion. He does a second number, this time singing too – a love song. 'Thank you!'. His ability and his recovery are witnessed by others here, some of whom have known him in a quite different state of mental health.

[19] Here's a musical pathway of a different sort – Gary worked as a music therapist with Tony many years previously and had recently helped find opportunities for Tony to play in a musical group again. SMART Music seemed ideal, and was hospitable to musicians coming from all kinds of places. This is Tony's first day at SMART Music – which he's settled down to well after the initial upset in the opening minutes. For more of Tony's story see Ansdell (2014), pp. 29–30 and 217.

Mercedes asks for New York, New York ... *which Daniel gives his own spin*

One of the visiting music therapists, Mercedes, asks for this song, and people suggest that Daniel sings it. 'It's a bit hackneyed, isn't it?' says Daniel, 'I'd rather do *What a Difference a Day Makes ...* ', but, given this was a request by a visitor Daniel generously concedes, to appreciative noises from others. But his compromise involves hamming it up to begin with, in a very good mock-Brooklyn accent! Daniel's musicianship takes over from the parody in a few lines, and we have a spirited performance ... including the usual intuitive negotiations needed for the various singers to collaborate in order to keep the song on the road given that Daniel is singing laid-back style, just behind the beat, and others are singing *on* the beat. Paradoxically, this actually keeps everyone on their toes in the musical moment ... Which is further needed when Daniel forgets the complex middle section of this song, covers magnificently and propels the song into its final climactic section ... The other singers join in more ... we're all there together. A big climax, shouting and whooping ... 'I *hate* that song!' says Daniel with a big grin.

This song functions well as a final number, so Gary brings the afternoon to a close. Most people help to clear up: Eloise collects together and counts the songbooks; others put back the instruments, turn round the piano, and restore the cafe to its usual configuration. The energy of conversation is quite different from a few hours ago. People look better, and say that they feel better.

After the members have gone Gary has a debrief with the two music therapists who've been participating. One of them is puzzled by how this event can be called 'music therapy' in the usual sense. Sarah and I say 'you should ask the members'. Mercedes comments how diffused the group is in contrast to the tight group of people music therapy sessions usually construct. Here in SMART Music there's a very different kind of focus and social formation – how it remains both a cafe but also a performance venue; transformed and remaining the same ...

30. Interlude

In 2007 the project took a great leap forward. The Nordoff Robbins charity sponsored Sarah to work one day at SMART to add to Gary's day. Initially she used this to co-run the Thursday afternoon SMART Music open group in the cafe, and then to come in on a further half-day on Wednesdays to help form two additional music projects at SMART. These projects increasingly feature in the narrative and were key to many of the developing musical pathways we describe.

SMART Singers grew out of a need expressed by some members for a semi-closed group that was more intimate than the Thursday afternoon group, but that also had more of a 'learning focus' than the Thursday afternoon's get-up-and-sing approach. Some members were both too scared to get up and sing on Thursdays, but also wanted to work on their voice, and on certain songs they wanted to sing. Sometimes they would also come to SMART Music, but SMART Singers gradually developed musical pathways of its own as a group. Sarah ran this group, which consisted of an average of six to eight participants, who met on Wednesday afternoons for a couple of hours, doing singing warm-ups, working on songs, with a tea-break and chat. The atmosphere is intimate and very mutually supportive, reflective and run by Sarah such that members themselves make all decisions, and discuss any ongoing difficulties.

SMART Band grew out of a similar desire of a group of musicians within the SMART community who initially came along to SMART Music Sessions on Thursdays. Many of these musicians had played in bands at a good standard before (sometimes decades before) but had typically not played for years as their mental health difficulties had interfered with their ability or confidence to play regularly. SMART Music gave them a way to start playing again, and to feel needed as musicians. But the group's very broad constituency and range of types of music requested and tolerated meant that this group of popular musicians wanted and needed more in the way of musical opportunity at SMART. Essentially they wanted to play as a band again, but needed both musical and personal support to keep doing so. When Sarah joined SMART she again followed this need, supporting the set-up of SMART Band. This met weekly after the Singers, and gradually developed its core membership, repertoire and activities. Its atmosphere was totally different from the Singers, however – these guys wanted simply to plug-in and play. Their progress in the subsequent years was turbulent and often difficult for all involved. They were reluctant to discuss process or problems, but also needed Sarah's on-going support to stay together and get past difficulties. Sarah used both her skills as a music therapist and mental health advocate to encourage the Band to take responsibility for their own development, and to deal with difficulties in a more productive way. The Band and its members have had a vibrant musical pathway over the years 2007 to the present.

A valuable part of this overall set-up was that it formalised to some extent the informal musical bridge-building that had gradually developed between 2005–7. Sarah still worked three days at the mental health hospital next door to SMART, and now with a music therapist role in both organisations she was able to work more actively and systematically in helping people bridge between care in the hospital setting and their transition to being members of SMART with all that this offered as a further transition to life back in the community. Sarah could help people forge musical pathways.

31. Ella's Musical Pathway

Ella talks of being surrounded by music and musicians as a child, as her mother ran a record shop. She felt at home in music, but her mother told her to stop singing at a crucial point. Ella lost her voice after this – sometimes literally, sometimes it felt to her that she'd lost her *musical voice.* Somehow this loss became implicated in her increasingly difficult attempt to maintain her mental health as an adult. Ella's tale is exemplary of what we've identified previously as the *music-health-illness narrative*: the close and paradoxical connection for some people between music and their best and worst experiences in life. Music is attached to their health *and* their illness in ways that cause distress, but also consistently show a healing path. This is the second strand of Ella's story – how music stands for (and indeed is) the source of what touches, elicits and helps flourish, the *wellness* in her – and through this supports what she currently sustains as recovery from her serious illness.

At a later stage of her life music leaves Ella, or she leaves music. She boxes up her records, she stops singing, her spirit leaves her and suicidal depression sets in for a prolonged period of her life. She ends up in hospital, and comes into contact with music therapy. When she's on the ward she doesn't remember that she has a short course of individual music therapy, but as she recovers she gravitates towards Sarah's small performance-focused group in the hospital, which works on songs and arranges small-scale musical events for patients to perform to other patients and staff. Ella's therapeutic work is consistently focused on her voice, and coming back into a creative and healthy relationship with the musical repertoire that's both central to her historical experience (presumably going right back to her childhood – jazz standards, 1960s–1980s pop), but also to something like her 'musical soul' and the social opportunities to share singing and musicking with others. In short, she finds music and her voice comes through again (for herself and others) – something she acknowledges as being due to the professional facilitation of Sarah and Gary. She says that she couldn't have done this herself, the force of the illness was too strong.

Ella's story mirrors the story of the musical pathway of the project itself during 2007 onwards. In parallel to being in Sarah's hospital-based rehearsal/performance group Ella starts participating in SMART Music on Thursday afternoons. When Sarah then starts working at SMART too – co-leading the Thursday group and doing SMART Singers and SMART Band on Wednesday afternoons from April 2007 – Ella increasingly becomes involved in all of these different musical formats.

In February 2008 Ella agrees to be interviewed by Gary in more depth about her 'musical pathway'. The following text is an edited version from that interview.

***

Gary: Some people here seem to be using music as a transition between illness and health ... ?

Ella: I'd phrase that as not so much a 'transition' but as the building-blocks of getting back into the community. They talk a lot about getting back into work, and getting back into the community ... because mental health issues are very isolating ... but actually singing ... and music ... seems to be another language altogether ...

G: I'm thinking this is really a way of you somehow performing your health and getting somewhere else in your life ...

E: … .which in a million years I'd never have thought was an avenue for me! But just *doing it* … just stepping out into the world through a musical avenue … where there are no … you don't have to explain yourself … you don't have to qualify … you just have to *be* yourself to the best of your ability. Nobody questions anything about you, or your background … it's … . I don't know what the words are … it doesn't fit into boxes … .everybody can relate to music – that's another way of saying it. You can just *relate*, and be out there … and when you finish you go back into your world … but when you come out you're in a *larger* world … and nobody's asking you any questions … nobody knows that you're on benefits … nobody knows that you have a mental health issue … you step into another *opportunity* … and you have a chance to reveal or explore another dimension of yourself …

***

E: … When we're in SMART Music, and I'm doing something … you'll *carry* me … so that if I miss a note … it's the *co*-working together … at least at this stage of my development. When I talk about SMART … I'm talking about the open-mic session [Thursday afternoons] … that has a different flavour … it's not a contained thing … it's a very *open* thing … and to get up and to walk to the microphone … and to put yourself on the spot … I don't know whether you remember … but when I first started coming to SMART I had a very quiet little voice … I sang in tune, but I didn't sing very well … and most of the time I *lost* my voice, because I was very nervous … . I don't think I've lost my voice in the last year … and it's got bigger and bigger … SMART has given me the platform for me to come out of myself … to emerge … that's the best way I can put it … and, um … . and this is actually hugely important to me … and it's not just through *music* … it's through personal confidence … being able to go up to a microphone and speak … to get myself back into mainstream life … and it's *all* helped … it's probably been the *single* most therapeutic catalyst … for my recovery … .that I can actually name … and I really *mean* that!

G: Can we just re-wind a bit? Because I'm interested in the actual narrative of the stages … I know this may not be very comfortable for you … and tell me what you don't want to talk about … but I'm interested in the story going from the very worst times for you when you were an inpatient in the hospital, and things were very bad for you … through to the move over here *[SMART]* and then doing the gig, and really connecting outside again … Do you mind doing this?

E: No, no … and it's interesting that you say this … because when you become ill … and I can't speak for everybody … but I can speak for my experience … you forget who you *are* … Because your immediate experience is so extreme … and so awful … that then this year of experience … where … it's a bit like a plant …

it's under the earth ... you've sown a seed in the ground ... and it's germinating ... but you have no idea what's going on there, because it's invisible. But once that shoot comes up through the earth, you can begin to see things visibly growing ... so if you take that year ... in the last year ... and you consider that I'm a little *shoot ... [both laugh]* ... and I've actually appeared ... *visibly* ... and I'm developing a bit here and there ... with a little bit of water and a little bit of sunshine ... you know ... .which is a way of saying ... with all the help and the love and care and energy holding you and Sarah provide ...

Well you're *very* different to Sarah ... you and Sarah are *quite* different ... Sarah can't do what *you* do ... and you don't do what *she* does! [laughs]

G: Well that makes a good partnership, doesn't it?

E: *Very* good! It's concomitant ... if that's the right word! It's the *and ... and ... and* ... every person in that ... .plays a part, so it becomes the holistic ... context ... or process ...

So as this little shoot is coming out ... what it means for me ... should I become *ill* again I now have something *completely* different ... in the dimension of myself ... that I know innately ... and that I have experience of. And it's in my *molecules* now ... .because it's coming out of me in my own expression ... that I have this voice inside of me ... or that I have this music inside of me. So should I become ill ... I can hold onto that ... in consciousness ... and *know* that this is a part of me that is *alive* and *well* ... no matter how ill I am.

G: That's beautiful ... I understand ... that's very clear. And that's the music, and the voice that you *can* hold onto ...

E: A while ago when we were talking over lunch we talked about how the universe *can't* be soundless! So if you would say that who I am ... molecularly ... represents the universe ... in that, every single molecule has a sound ...

G: So very practically ... .when you were last in the hospital ... was it about a year ago?

E: I was last in the hospital ... last year ... 2 February until the end of April.

G: Let's just take that bit first. What did you do during that time which was musically connected? I'm interested in what the role of the music was in each bit of your recovery ...

E: In that 3 months I was an in-patient ... and I did *nothing* musically ... there was no provision[20] ... it was ... I couldn't listen ... No, that's not true ... I had a small player and I played CDs ... and I had the radio on ... so there was something ... and at night ... when it was really awful ... I'd go to sleep with music on ...

G: Music you knew ... or just what was on the radio ...

E: Um ... both ...

G: Did you do any music therapy then ... with Sarah ... or ...

E: No ... I was too ill ... I've never done anything one-to-one with Sarah ... just the groups ...

G: So did you do a music therapy group ... ?

E: Not as far as I can remember ... but part of the illness is that I do blank out memories ... so I might say that I didn't go ... and I did, but I don't remember ... What happens after the hospital stay is that I came out and went home ... and was *very* ill at home ... with suicidal depression for about 4 months ... right from April to the end of August ... But I didn't stay at home all that time ... I was coming back to music ...

G: What was music at this point?

E: SMART [MUSIC] and Sarah's group up there *[hospital performance group]* ...

G: So you were a day patient ... or an outpatient going to the day hospital and ...

E: The day hospital to *me* was music ... was Sarah! And *is* my only connection to the hospital now ... but at the time I had to go to pottery as well ... I had a little programme ... But music ... it was the 12.30 on Wednesdays group ... I don't know what she calls it ... something like 'Willow Singers' or something ...

G: What do *you* think of it as?

E: *I* just think of it as Sarah ... Sarah's Singing ... that's what I also write into my diary ... I wouldn't go to the Monday group *[Sarah's hospital based open music therapy group – held in the day hospital, but attended by both inpatients and day/out-*

[20] This isn't factually true. Ella actually had individual music therapy sessions during her inpatient time (with a music therapy student on placement there). She also possibly attended Sarah's ward-based music therapy groups. But as Ella says in the interview, when very ill she is often unable to remember experiences.

patients] because that involves a lot of percussion ... and it's like ... too much ... but I'd go to the Thursday singing ... There's no holding her *[Sarah]* back ... she's like 'let's do a concert' ... and we did a concert ... and I remember being very ill the day I was supposed to turn up ... but I remember thinking *I have to turn up* ... because I'm scheduled to sing half of the songs. People were marvellous ... so supportive ... I know that I was in physically not in a good state ... the audience were mainly staff. Sarah organized a few of these events three months apart ... But even then ... the concert when I was ill ... I remember my experience as that the voice will *still* come through ... even if you see the illness as well ... you know that I'm not well ... but in the *midst* of that ... if you have the ears to hear it ... the voice will still come through ...

G: Do you think of the voice as the health ... bit of you ... when illness is surrounding you ... or even overwhelming you?

E: My answer to that is ... my voice comes from the *core* of my being ... and that can *never* be ill ...

G: I really believe that! You've named there my fundamental belief ... because I've seen people so ill ... whichever way, physically as well, but the core is never ill, is it? And that's where music comes from ...

So ... then ... SMART MUSIC was parallel to working in Sarah's group in the hospital setting? You'd also come to this too?

E: Yes, that's the open-mic session ... .and it's really interesting ... because the dynamics are really different ... when you come to that ...

G: Can you tell me how?

E: Yes ... some are to do with social dynamics ... like you don't want to be too pushy ... I'm very sensitive to everybody getting a chance ... to have their go. It's really important to hold back ... it would be really easy to impose myself ... I'm very enthusiastic and out of my own keenness I could override things ... or I could discourage people because they'd feel their voice wasn't very good ... all these personal dynamics ... I'm very sensitive to those ... and I know *you* are ... and I pick it up in the invisible conversation if you like ... I really appreciate that ... and I find that *caring for other people* in that room ... very much a part of what characterizes SMART MUSIC ... the love and care for one another. *You* inspire that, and you encourage that ... and it's encouraged between us as well ... so I think that's a very valuable dimension ...

G: Well ... we're not working towards anything, are we? That's a difference between that and Sarah's performance group ... .whereas the open-mic group is literally for anyone to come in and to feel OK there, and to feel OK there with their music ... so it's very different. but I can see why you'd want to ... you felt that the two groups were complementary ...

E: I didn't think about it … But the other thing about SMART MUSIC is that you've got a ready-made audience. The other thing about Sarah's groups is … they're not *always* heading towards a concert … but you're a very small group of people and it has a completely different feel to it … you learn songs there, so you've got a lot more individual time … so everyone gets a lot more singing time … .and you can explore things which you can't do in the group *[SMART]* … because you have to be sensitive to the whole all of the time … So it's quite different …

But in SMART you have an audience … and you know they're going to be *kind!* And the thing I always used to say about the open-mic session … .the thing I loved about it most … was that *anyone* could get up … and it *didn't* matter if you couldn't sing … or that you couldn't sing in tune … Everybody would support you anyway … and *that's* what gave me the courage to keep on stepping up … there was this compulsion to do this … but all these things stopping me … I didn't have to be good there … I could just get up and sing … and gradually that worked its way through. And now I'm quite fearless about getting up in front of a microphone … *anywhere* … so it's … um … .so *there* is evidence of a shift … through … um … a dissolving of fears … of the inhibitions I suppose … that accompany you when you … need the courage to get up and … . There are still people in your audience who have yet to come up the microphone …

G: … after two and a half years … and who may *never* … because their role is to be an audience … or there is a lady whose role is to play the tambourine … you know who I mean?

E: … I do … but there's another lady who has taken a step to join Sarah's *[SMART SINGERS*] group … who's been sitting there *[in SMART MUSIC] longing* to have what it takes … to have the courage to get up and sing something … because that's the longing of her heart … But it's evolving for her … and that's a real joy to see … And I know that I play a part for her … because she always looks to me for encouragement … so I have another part to play … *that's* what SMART MUSIC means to me …

G: I know that you do that kind of invisible communication that you were talking about earlier … I know that you're often helping *me* to help others … and I think lots of people do that. It's not that one person leads it … I don't think I *lead* it … I kind of allow it to happen … but it also happens between people, doesn't it? … it's almost a shared agreement that something is going to happen …

E: Perfect! That's it … And you're not leading it … but you *are* the focus of it …

G: … and it's my responsibility if it goes wrong!

E: It *can't* go wrong … it can just change in what's happening … it can't go wrong … you'd never let it …

G: But it would be my responsibility if there were something unsafe about it ...

E: Yes ... .but that's hardly likely ... and it's not happened yet ... and I'm very sensitive to safety, so I would have picked it up ...

G: So we got to the point when we were talking about you doing the two groups in parallel ... Sarah's Willow group, and coming here to SMART MUSIC ... and then we realised that it wasn't quite enough just to do the drop-in group because people said from that that they wanted to rehearse songs, and the band guys ... its wasn't enough not to be able to set up a proper band with them ... so we got the opportunity from Nordoff-Robbins to set up the Wednesday groups, which were designed as spin-off groups from Thursday ... to cater for people who have more specific musical needs ... and we're testing to see whether that works ... So could you take your involvement from that point ... when we set up, nearly a year ago, those other groups ...

E: Yes, that's been *hugely* developmental really ... because first of all what emerged was not just the Band ... but in my case I was asked whether I'd like to sit in their sessions and do some of the vocals for them ... or with them ... or whatever ... which I was very chuffed to be asked ... and I said Yes ... I don't know how good I am ... and I think that there's some way to go before something really coheres there properly ... but the longing is there ... everyone's very keen to do it ... and to meet the musical needs is a good way of putting that ... but I think there's some more to come from that ... .that's a growing situation I hope ...

But what has *really* meshed ... really well has been the *SMART SINGERS* group, which is a forum for people ... and nothing to do with the hospital ... for people to come and sing *properly* ... not just from the books *[meaning the repertoire books we've assembled for SMART MUSIC over the years ... also used by Sarah in the hospital]* ... but we're beginning to learn ... thanks to Sarah ... *how* to sing properly ... .she's beginning to introduce music theory ... .it's not exactly theory ... music *basics* ... to us ... scales and things ... and proper warm-ups. I think she understands that we take it *seriously* ... it's not just a recreation, it's for people who really want to sing. And this is a great entrée ... and she's marvellous ... she's so mild in her manner, and so inclusive ... And she's very proactive ... she'll suddenly out of nowhere say that we've got a possible gig there, and a possible venue there ... So there's something to *aspire to* ... it's not just to *work* towards ... but really you're aspiring to something greater than you can conceive of your own ability. To sing in the Atrium *[of Chelsea & Westminster Hospital next door, who have booked the group to sing in one of their lunchtime music sessions in June]* is to me ... *huge!* For *me* to go and sing *there,* in public ... it feels *huge*! *[D makes expansive gestures ...]*

G: It's like the size of the Atrium ... almost you expanding within that setting ... .

E: Yes, that's a good way to ... you're almost stepping into something larger that *you* have to fill. Somehow you sense that you know that you can ... but you're not there yet ... you're traveling along the path to that point. And you know everything will come into focus ... the pressure will come, because you only have so much time left to do it ... it'll all take its natural unfolding pathway ... but just holding that thought ... you ... I suddenly feel *larger* ... because it's being considered seriously ... Now another way of describing that is that the BBC people are coming tomorrow ... the *BBC!!* So suddenly you're in contact with something that you'd never have conceive of or have imagined ... that you'd be in touch with in a public way ...

***

G: Forgive me for saying this ... but people in this community who have recently seen you as a singer and musician have mostly seen you just as a patient before. This relates to one of the problems I see with medical settings is that you somehow you get *reduced* as a person ... to being the patient ...

E: ... and I think that probably the most significant thing that you could take from our conversation ... is the fact that in this forum ... whether it's with Sarah or with you ... there's no mention of mental ill-health ... there's no discussion of what's wrong with you ... *this* is something that's totally *transcendent* ... that's the word that I was looking for before ... transcendent ... we're on a transcendent plane with one another ... and that's what the music does for us ... it takes us to that level ...

I think that because you create a safe context and allow people to come into that place ... and do something ... which may be a bit clumsy ... initially ... but because the care and support is there ... it actually *causes* them to get better. That's the therapeutic part ... you are trip-wiring a mechanism that already is inherent in the person, to become well again ... through song or music ... .*[becomes emotional]* ... You're trip-wiring that innate mechanism that's already there ... [...] So if you create that context ... then it's possible for people to become weller ... .it's not when they get weller they do better ... it becomes *causative* ... it becomes a *facilitation* ... that's the word I'm looking for ... a facilitation towards wellness ...

G: And part of this is this going *outwards* ... because as you were describing earlier ... when you're very ill you're necessarily in survival mode, and thus confined to being very involved in yourself ... almost folded in ... then as you become weller ... that impulse to become weller ... *is* of going outwards again ... of connecting to people ... in relationship again ... but also being in community, in public spaces where you feel you can be yourself ...

E: *You re-connect to life* ... that's a bit of a dramatic statement ... but that's actually what happens ... instead of being in a downward spiral process ... you actually reverse that ... and you reconnect into the life-giving upward spiral ... .

G: OK, last bit ... or rather the last stage for you ... though I'm sure we've not got the full story yet! You managed to get back into singing again, and performing again ... via the gigs here ... and then you went and did you *own* one a few weeks ago ... not as part of any medical services ... or with anybody else facilitating it for you ... So ... *this* is Ella's musical pathway ... *so far ... !*

E: It's amazing to think about that ... I'm really glad that we're finding a language for it ... because I think that the way that we *language* these things is also a really healing influence ...

G: So can we pick it up again in another 6 months?

E: Oh, absolutely! Keep me away!

***

As this interview shows, Ella has a gift for being able to describe her experiences of music therapy. She mentions that the BBC are coming the day after the interview, and they do so for a special edition on music and health for Radio 3's *Music Matters* programme. They pick Ella to talk about her experiences of the project, and again she gives a moving and persuasive testimony:

> People think that mental health somehow affects your intelligence ... it doesn't! It may affect your ability to remember things, or to function ... but your innate intelligence never goes away ... and your innate music doesn't go either. So once it's been triggered ... it's a life-enhancing thing, overtaking the illness. It's the stronger force in me ... it's the wellness in me ... I think that ... not just music ... but what Gary & Sarah offered ... *that* triggered in me the wish to sing ... and that triggered in me a healing process from within *me*. So that, yes, it was being facilitated by them ... and *needed* to be facilitated by them for quite some time ... .before I could stand on my own ... .little vocal chords, if you like, ...and start singing for the joy of singing myself ... and carry my recovery beyond the state I was in before I fell ill nine years ago ... .to a level of wellbeing that I haven't had perhaps for thirty years ... .

The last phrase of this is picked up by Lord Howarth and put in a speech in the House of Lords on Arts and Health in 2008. Ella's story becomes something of a 'musical parable' that gives further shape to Ella's music-health-illness narrative, but also serves as a resource for others as a template for 'how music helps'. Gary checks in with Ella a year or so later, asking her whether I can put a quotation from her in my new book. She emails back, elaborating on the quotation:

> It is the 'wellspring of wellness' within me and consistently identifying with this that brought my recovery (with the aid and assistance of music and the catalyst of the expression of myself through singing that you provided – and which I still miss so much). I am now very well. I have been in remission for three and a half years and have a normal life. See how the seeds of your music therapy brought me back to life! You have touched a most genuinely sensitive spot in me, and if you can convey in your book what we so clearly KNOW in our deepest selves, and in our experience, that will go out like a carrier wave into the world I was taught a very long time ago never to underestimate the power of the Truth in expression. If there is anything I can do to be of further help to support/enhance your efforts to 'proclaim your message' and to awaken health professionals to the fact that the answer lies in drawing people into the experience of being 'truly whole', then please do not hesitate to ask.

Ella eventually became well enough to move on, literally moved out of the area, and was able to take her musical pathway further – joining classes at a local college in jazz singing and sight reading. She resumed her professional life, and is active in local community issues.

32. Musical Bridging

> *'Pathway people':* With each of these people their relationship with music is intense, necessary, often difficult in some way – in relation to their history and illness narrative and the present circumstances, and the immediate context of SMART as a community. This makes their stories fascinating but often problematic. For each musicking is simultaneously the bridge *and* the destination. [Gary's log, 7 May 2008].

A key component of the project has been the practical and conceptual theme of 'bridging'. We began this account with Bridget, who physically treads the path between the mental health unit and SMART. More symbolically she bridges between the medical model and more a social model of mental health understanding and intervention, and also between an identity as 'a patient with medical problem' or, alternatively, 'a musical person with problems in living' (more on this topic in Part III).

The practical origin of the project lies in the experience of the two music therapists feeling the need to form a 'musical bridge' between a music therapy service in a hospital setting and the wider community. SMART represented a 'half-way house' in this vision, where a variety of bridging could happen, depending on people's ambitions and capabilities: bridging-*between* (hospital and SMART), and bridging-*out* – from SMART towards mainstream cultural resources (people feeling confident to go to concerts and gigs, to join things such as Morley College's 'Can't Sing Choir'). This bridging project was considerably helped when Sarah joined fully in 2007, when she could herself act as a 'musical bridge' between the hospital where she worked three days a week, and SMART where she worked a day. People with severe mental health problems inevitably have a pathway that is partly determined by their illness, going back and forth between medical and non-medical settings and care (at different rates). It's of great importance that there's music at both ends of the bridge, and that they associate music with a particular person – usually a music therapist who is able to hold both an understanding of their 'musical self' and history, but also their illness and its challenges to their musical self.

The bridging operates at several levels simultaneously: between physical sites and buildings; between types and models of care; between practical forms of care such as music therapy professionally defined; between states and stages of illness across short, medium and long-term spans. Illness and recovery is a process involving many transitions, but often these involve problematic gaps that often remained unbridged, and are therefore risky for people, and for carers. Medical services traditionally stopped at the hospital gates (in asylum days there *was* no bridge!). The last 30 years of developments in psychiatric care have involved many practical and theoretical models to try to 'bridge the gaps' – with 'community care teams', day care centres and so on. Hospital settings are increasingly for acute treatment only. Our impression, however, is that whilst bridging is an ever-present rhetoric in mental health services, the continuing picture is of only bits of the bridge being available to people – it is often at best a bridge with gaps – and as such doesn't always afford safe passage in either continuing care or progressive recovery. Is this because there's uncertainty and confusion as to what stuff actually *builds* such bridges? Is it purely structural ('get the right services in place', 'the right care package', etc.) or is it an aspect that simply doesn't get much thought? The precise way, that is, that the bridging material relates to the personal, social and cultural material of our lives. The SMART Music Project was in its modest way an attempt to look more closely at the meso-level of constructing and maintaining bridge building.

The music project at SMART is based on the simple idea of 'musical bridges', in all the interlocking dimension described above. People often described their own lay music therapy practices as music 'holding their hand', providing continuity, or helping with safe passage on the risky transitions involved in recovery from a mental health episode. Music therapists often build on these benefits, adding a personal therapeutic relationship to the relationship with music itself that people have established. This combined relationship (to music/to a person associated with 'musical care') then affords the ideal bridging potential for people. It eases the passage between physical journeys and more subtle metaphorical passages of personal and social recovery. Bridging and pathways are of course interrelated:

the complex pathway work that Tia DeNora (2013a) describes in *Music Asylums* via projection and introjection socially construed is also a form of bridging. But although a bridge is part of a pathway, there's also specificity to a bridge and bridging. You need a bridge when the terrain below has a gap in the territory; when without the bridge the path is impossible.

There are problems of course. Daniel remarks that the bridge needs connecting at both ends! For him the bridge-out offered by the music project is partly a frustrating journey – it gets him so far, but there's no reliable connection to the 'other end' beyond SMART and into the kind of musicking he wants to do, relieved of his identity with mental health services. Effectively, he says, he has to come back each time, retrace his footsteps back into SMART. What kind of bridge is *that?*

For others (Henrietta, Ella, Simon, Carolyn) music and music therapy in this project achieves bridge building more satisfactorily for them, in ways that are scaled to the limitations of their illness. Music helps provide a bridge to both musical and paramusical outcomes: to other musical places and their social opportunities away from mental health settings; to learning opportunities that afford development of skills, confidence and new identities not reliant on a patient/illness identity; between physical sites of care and their confining identities and roles – where the passage is often fraught with anxiety about losing current security and support. Music seems to be able to offer something of a 'transitional space' and a 'transitional object' that can be held onto, and travelled with. Music therapists of a psychoanalytic bent are fond of quoting Winnicott's theory of transitional objects in relation to music, and there's some truth in this formulation. But it perhaps needs extending away from the primary care relationships and its therapeutic relationship equivalent, and also animating in line with a specific musical phenomenology. David Stewart (in Pavlicevic and Ansdell 2004) refers instead to '*transformational* objects', a more dynamic formulation. But we need to remember the full complexity of a musical ecology with its ever-active interpenetration of musical things, musical people and musical situations. This whole package is what does the bridging, which in the SMART situation comprises a trusted set of musical relationships within a particular space and opening-up of new pathways. For example, Sarah often physically accompanies a patient from the hospital the 10 metres to SMART, a journey that bridges the sometimes-huge symbolic distance between the two forms of care, and the two identities the person has within them. Sarah acts here as a *therapeutes,* in the original sense – a person who walks besides, accompanies, shares the transitions between critical states and stages of a person's existential voyage. It's just that without music the patient may not want to make the journey at all, or trust Sarah in a particular way, or have a glimmer of the view of 'the other side' of illness. This is where a 'musical bridge' is both specific, and particularly helpful.

33. Henrietta's 'Musical Hand'

Henrietta is the other person interviewed on the BBC Radio 3 programme about the SMART Project, and she's equally eloquent about the relationship between music, music therapy and her experiences of health and illness:

> **Henrietta:** I suffer with personality disorder ... so often interacting with people can be quite difficult ... my mood changes very rapidly ... so when I'm using music to help me it's a stabilising influence ... because it's something very constant and very stable ... that I can enjoy and build something around.
>
> **BBC interviewer:** So has it had an effect then ... in the rest of your life, in negotiating those relationships with people ... the experience of making music with other people, and what's happening at SMART today, has helped?
>
> **H:** Yes, definitely ... it really is ... this is *so* crucial. Without the music groups I probably wouldn't have got out yesterday *at all* ... had it not been for the music group. And likewise today ... I probably wouldn't have been able to get out of the house had I not had this group to actually *want* to come to, and enjoy, and meet people and talk to people, and have contact with the outside world ... which is *so* crucial in recovering and *maintaining* recovery. Mental health can be incredibly lonely ... it's an incredibly isolating condition in its broad spectrum ... so to have something that everybody can come together and have contact with a couple of people twice a week, once a week ... whatever it is ... is absolutely crucial to maintaining it ...

Henrietta then wrote the following in the SMART Newsletter that month:

> When I heard about Radio 3 coming to do a programme on music therapy in relation to health I was thrilled. I've always found music an integral part of me but never thought of it as therapy until I started the music group here at SMART. Meeting with people to work on something that we all share in common is an uplifting experience. Being able to tell part of my story, and how music therapy continues to support me, was important to help ensure it will be there for people who will benefit from it in the future.

Henrietta's is a particularly strong example of musical bridging and the importance of the *continuity* of support afforded both by her own relationship to music, and the more professionally-mediated relationship to music that music therapy could provide through the SMART project. In May 2008 she does a long interview with Gary about the specifics of her musical pathway, and after checking this and approving it for research use she returns it, asking for the following summary to be added:

> Music's been the constant companion ... But it's also something that has grown with me ... and I've grown through ... to get to where I am now ... And hopefully to get even further ... to the point where now I'm doing voluntary work at the hospital now ... admin ... working and helping out with the Open Day on Saturday ... I mean ... four years ago ... I couldn't string two sentences together, and I was catatonic because they had to put so many drugs in me. So music's been the constant support ... just in the background ... always there ... and having the specific support of music therapy ... and growing with ... and moving on with ... my pace at every single stage ... it has just been there ... and it's been something which has given me a crutch ... not in a bad way ... it's just always there ... It's bridged and supported every step to enable me to progress – in a way that no other therapy has managed in such an all-inclusive way. [Henrietta, June 2008]

This is interesting in framing this 'musical companionship' as stretching further back (and hopefully forward) than just music therapy or the SMART project. In her interview Henrietta tells a tale of a relationship with music that's always been both personal and broader than this. There's clearly an important familial level to this – she tells the story of the frequent family car journeys between London and Cornwall where there was an unbroken family performance of songs for six hours! Music is an important part of family mythology, as well as part of Henrietta's personal life course, leading her through school – where she was not chosen to sing solos – and to her early adult life where music continued to be both comfort and connector as she seemed to literally lose the sense of herself through her illness:

> **Henrietta:** Music's always been an integral part of my life. My whole family's very musical, I've been brought up with music and stuff. So it's a core thing that's been in me ... whatever state I've been in my head. So to be able to actually *access* it here in the hospital when I was first in, and use it in whatever way I did use it ... whether it was just sitting and listening in a group ... or physically participating using instruments or singing or what have you ... it's a constant ... throughout the whole thing for me, personally ... that I was able to go back to. It was like re-zeroing ... whatever else was going on the music was going back to something that *I* knew ... that I felt safe with ... that I understood ... and felt some sort of connection to be able to do *something* ... or even just *be there* ... and not totally inside my own head ... and going *aaaaaaaahhhhhhhhh!!* [makes comically pained face].

As we discussed above, Henrietta is one of those people for whom music is like Winnicott's 'transitional object', a source of comfort, but also an enabler – something you literally clutch onto – within difficult personal transitions. But having said that music literally holds her hand Henrietta corrects this and says that she needs a metaphor that's more *active,* as she's experienced music as something that inwardly and outwardly connects things together and provides forward momentum and hope.

In a very practical way music connected and bridged Henrietta's progression from being an in-patient and day-patient in the hospital to her transition to SMART, all of this within a fairly long-term and winding path to recovery for her. As she herself says, music and music therapy has ' … tracked all the way through my recovery … I've been through all the variations of the music here!'.

At first, in her stay on the hospital ward during the worst period of her illness, she was only really aware of music therapy as something peripheral, but despite this it was one of the few things that connected her to something she felt good about:

> So it's always been there … the music … and to have *that* in the ward … in such an *alien, terrifying* … environment … it had something … it was almost like a comfort blanket in a way … .you kind of know what it's like, you know it's smell, you know what it feels like, and it's *there.* And that was great … that was so good …

Henrietta remembers occasionally participating in a music therapy group on the ward that involved playing percussion instruments and some singing. But what really caught her was when she became a day patient and had access to a new group that Sarah had set up in the hospital for patients who wanted to work on songs for small performances within the hospital. In the autumn she worked towards singing a Christmas carol.

Gary and Tia remember attending this event – a very small-scale performance in front of about 15 people – other patients, a few staff and friends (Henrietta was unknown to Tia). She sang the less well-known setting of *In the Bleak Midwinter*, and her voice was small and intense, with a paradoxical quality of beauty, fragility and strength in her performance that was witnessed and understood by all. Henrietta cites this musical moment as the advent of her recovery. At this point she knew that she could find the will to get better:[21]

> **Henrietta:** I was terrified … absolutely terrified! Kind of the … guts to get up and do it … that confidence that had been given to me by doing the music therapy group. I'd performed in groups throughout my life at school … but to actually … I'd never actually managed to pass an audition to do a solo at school … I could never do it, because the nerves got me … I couldn't *do* it. So using the progression of getting better … and support with the music … kind of built a slightly different strength in me … found something that wasn't there before. A confidence that I lacked somewhere else in myself maybe … to actually stand up and sing before 50 or 60 people … and that was … I *did it!* And it's kind of *try and hold me back **now!*** [laughs]

---

[21] Henrietta sends Sarah a Christmas card that says 'Thank you for all your support and helping me back to music … '.

She says this to Gary in the interview that took place at the time she's into the next phase of recovery, having made transition from medical services to SMART. But this wasn't an easy one, and music was helpful again in the transition:

> **Henrietta:** I had occasionally come down here to SMART and realised that the music group was here too ... I think that at that point I was quite frightened of stepping away from the security of a secure unit ... the medical support unit there ... to being in a community project really. But again the music was the continuity to help make that transition ... [...] And so being able to go and make *another* step to a *different* place ... but with the continuity of the music ... um ... I think unknowingly has probably made it what it *is* ... the fact that it *is* a different location ... [...] so it's been little baby steps ... kind of coaxing out ... and having something with the music ... again it's that continuity and having something at the next stage up ... It was still the music, it was still Sarah ... I knew her and I knew some of the people in the SMART Singers' group, again in a slightly different setting. But it was still *safe* ... but unknowingly kind of moving on, and moving up and *away* ... from the Mental Health Unit ... so it's that next progression ... [...] because Sarah's seen where I've come from ... where I've got to ... and kind of knew where I was wanting to go *to* ... and that's always ... I think that was very key as well. I think that with any care and support it's the continuity ... it can *bridge* it ... can kind of link different parts of it ... You can go to one part of it ... and then the next one ... and link it through ... so that music is giving that continuity even if the medical services can't ...

From April 2007 Henrietta becomes a key member and stalwart supporter of *SMART Singers,* lending her organisational skills to organising the music and helping with other practical matters. For Henrietta this weekly semi-open group is exactly what she needs to support her recovery, and to help direct and structure her musical pathway (which is also increasingly her recovery pathway):

> **Henrietta:** Sarah said that you were thinking of developing a new group for people who'd gone from being in-patients ... then out-patients no longer day-patients ... so to speak ... and actually work on specific projects. Actually have a specific goal, as opposed to going to a group once a week ... which *is* a goal of course! But depending on what stage of recovery you are, the goals differ. So just turning up to a group once a week often is a big goal anyway ... heaven knows! [laughs]. So it was an opportunity to set a different goal for me ... a slightly *further* goal. So, OK, we're going to a group once a week ... but we're actually *working on things* ... regularly ... with a view to doing something *with it.* And again, it was actually feeding on that little bit of confidence that'd been given through singing in the hospital singing group ... those little performances in the hospital dining room, what have you ...
>
> So actually working together as a group ... to actually put things together ... to perform *specifically* ... to actually go out and do things ... .for example on the

> older person's ward ... and bits and pieces ... And it was that ... it's the different level of goals that feeds through from being on the in-patient side, then to the day-patient ... then to being an in-patient. And it seems to be set so perfectly that the goals are just that little bit further up so that they're attainable ... for *everybody* ... no matter what level of recovery ... Because if they are not able to *make* the performance, and do it in front of other people ... they've done all the work, and are working up *to it* ... and they *will* do it at some point down the line ... when they're ready and they can ... Which is great ... because nobody is excluded, and everyone has the chance to have that voice ... and find it in their own time. Which is crucial ... .because you can't just shove someone in and say 'OK, you're in this group, we're performing in 2 weeks time, we're going to sort it out'. It doesn't work like that! [laughs]. And that's the whole thing with therapy ... it's *working* on things, and finding out things about you, and what makes you tick in certain ways.

In the following years Henrietta takes part in, and supports, many of the *SMART Singers* events, and the other occasions in which Singers and Band perform in. She goes from strength to strength as a singer, announcing at the beginning of one group that she's found a singing teacher to work on technique. She then begins to forge a musical pathway for herself away from SMART, singing solo in a play at Kensington Palace, which three of the SMART Singers go to hear her perform. Ella, one of these, specifically cites this evening as proof to her of how music helps people's recovery:

> **Ella:** I just went to see Henrietta performing at Kensington Palace on Monday evening. I looked at that girl, she was absolutely magical! She sang a solo as the entire audience swept through the State Apartments, looking up the stairs ... . She sang there looking sublime in her evening gown ... and I said to myself 'nobody in a million years would know that girl has a mental health problem ... and I thought, isn't that just marvellous! I just don't have the words to capture the wholeness of really what that must mean for Henrietta ... but as an observer, and knowing her ... and we're friends ... just to know that she has that *dimension* in her life ... which probably ... . I'm guessing ... would not have come about but for the encouragement of Sarah ... . whether in SMART or upstairs *[in the hospital]*. It's been a catalyst for that ... she wouldn't have had the confidence otherwise ...

Henrietta comments about herself in this performance:

> **Henrietta:** I surprised myself ... yes! And it's still hard to get the connection with the fact that I actually *did it* ... but again it's something within the music, and within the context of having gone through the groups and stuff that kind of gets that bit more connection. And that sort of reinforcement from people that you know and that you've worked with ... and that's something to do with the group

and the people you've worked with *in* the group ... you ... they acknowledge the progress you've made by coming to see things like that. Or you go off and do something with them ... or you go and see a concert together that you'd never been able to go to ... because you'd never been able to be in a room ... but music has kind of linked it together ...

***

Two aspects seem key to what Henrietta finds helpful about music in terms of her recovery. Firstly, the learning-focus of *SMART Singers* – the working-on musical material within a supportive environment. Secondly, the challenging, but rewarding opportunity to perform music publically, and to have this performance witnessed by others. Both these factors somehow link her musical and personal aims. Henrietta is especially eloquent about this relationship between her experiences of illness, health, recovery and musical performance, and helps us understand the nuances that are often overlooked in the traditional line that performance is therapeutically unhelpful within music therapy.[22] Henrietta explains the logic to Gary in her interview:

Henrietta: I've had a great problem with actually having a connection with anything that's been happening ... So even this morning ... at the community meeting in the day hospital ... I know I *have* been there ... but it was sort of it's like watching it through a video-camera ... it's not actually *me* doing it ... So with the *SMART Singers* group and the way it works ... working with projects to attain goals other people have done with you ... and they can kind of corroborate in a way that you ... it's proof to yourself that you've done it ... even if you can't quite grasp the concept that you *did* sing at something ... there are other people that sang *with* you ... that say you *did!* So there's that kind of back-up ... that reinforces and starts to try ... you start teaching yourself to recognize that you *did* do something ... and it *was* you doing it ... And that's the thing that ... with these sort of goals of doing little performance projects ... it's a real way of ... sort of ... group photos show me that I actually *was* there! And that's something that I've only just started to realise! Um ... and start to work through ... at all ... or to realise that that's what's been going on ... and I'm *not* making it up ... I've not just fabricated it to fill in a space in my memory ... there are other people there with me, and apparently I enjoyed it!

So it's starting to get two points together and make them into a line ... because at moments it's just dots all over the place ... So it's like a join-the-dots puzzle ... of memories and events ... and actually knowing you're there and

[22] The Community Music Therapy movement has in the last 15 years given adequate counter-arguments and evidence to this belief, but it's still to some extent prevalent in therapeutic dogma.

trying to connect the two [points]. So I've got point A, and I've got point B ... and it's starting to get the lines from each end to try and meet in the middle. And for me ... working on those [singing] projects ... and going through from the beginning stage ... here ... with people ... you come every week ... and ... [hesitates] ... coming back to the word *continuity* ... it's bridging something ... um ... that for me my brain doesn't seem to have the capacity to *do*! But through the group, and through the singing, and through the music and stuff ... it's starting to build those bridges to try and connect the two ... If that made sense! [laughs].

G: It does ... but I suppose the obvious question is 'why *music?*'. I mean, would anything that happened every week do ... like a gardening project? Is it music because music for *you* is particularly important ... as you said at the beginning of this interview? And music has continuity through this music therapy project?

H: Because of this total disconnection ... usually the only things that I find given me *any* connection are pushing myself physically to the limit ... to get any connection. So whether it's self-harming ... or bulimia ... or what have you ... it's pushing my body to the absolute limit ... and only *then* do I have get a connection ... that I'm not a robot ... But with the music it's actually ... it *is* pushing myself to a limit ... but it's not that physical limit ... So there's some sort of connection ... Whether its performing and being scared *witless* ... but still doing [it] ... because it's pushing me to *a* limit there is some sort of connection ... you still feel that kind of adrenaline going in ... which you get self-harming ... or what have you. But it's in a productive, constructive ... non-*destructive* way ... It's a *healthy limit* ...

G: ... and it's a limit together with other people ...

H: Exactly! There *is* support ... you're not doing it totally on your own ... which is ... what most sort of manifestations of what I do ... they're very ... er ... isolated ... totally alone. It's a very singular thing ... So to be able to actually push yourself to ... that kind of gets that same physical connection ... but with a group of people ... it kind of starts to break it down a bit ... So again that kind of performing ... or trying new song and desperately trying to keep harmony ... .even *that* ... I'm thinking 'Oh my God have I hit a wrong note?' [laughs] ... it's that pushing a limit somewhere in you ... and ... [hesitates] ... it's quite hard to explain ...

So ... unwittingly ... challenges have been set for me ... and I'm not really knowing they've really been set. Like a new group that's slightly outside my comfort zone ... or a performance when I think 'Oo, I'm not sure I can do *that'* ... but then there's the support of Sarah ... and the group around you ... and the whole way it works ... and your realise that 'Aah ... *not so bad* ... maybe this is actually quite *good* ... ' and then you realise that you *can* do things ... and that sort of ... um ... aids the recovery ... Because I think 'well, if I can do that in *music*

> ... and sing in front of x people ... or sing in the group and do a new song ... well then maybe I can do that in my illness ... and actually attain levels in my illness ... and say, OK ... this is what I need to do to get better ... this is what I need to do to become more stable ... whatever level, whatever step it is ... If I can do it in *music* ... then ... for me ... maybe I can do it in that as well. So it's realising ... finding out ... that pushing yourself isn't so bad [laughs] ... and that it's *good* ... and that it's *productive* ...

****

As with many people, Henrietta's recovery path is not a linear one. In 2010 Gary comes across Henrietta standing at the outside door of the hospital. It's just after SMART Music, and Henrietta asks Gary how it went. She apologises for not being at SMART Singers for a few weeks, says she's 'had a bit of a blip' in the last few weeks. She knows when she's not coping, and has been admitted to the hospital to help her stabilise her mental state again. The good thing, Henrietta tells Gary, is that when she's back in the hospital again, music's there too, and so is Sarah, who she knows and trusts as the music therapist working in both sites. 'And I know that when I get out' she says, 'I can go back to *SMART Singers.* It's the continuity that matters … Music's still there, even when you have a blip, to hold your hand … '.

34. Event and Ritual Along the Pathway ...

Henrietta's story seems to revolve around a sequence of musical events. She talks about the more public musical experiences as being equally important to the more intimate aspects of music therapy (in the broadest sense) in her recovery. This balance between the more intimate and more public aspects of musicking seemed to characterise most of the 'pathway cases' we explored.

Musical situations or more specific events are a key aspect of what makes up a musical pathway. This could also be said not just for the evolving personal musical pathways of individuals, but also of the evolving music groups themselves. As *SMART Singers* and *SMART Band* matured from 2007 onwards, so their pathways led out and around from SMART, motivated by the needs and ambitions of their members, but often catalysed in their development by the power of a musical event. There's an increasing intermingling between individual musical pathways and the collective, collaborative pathways of the three music groups. The development of these pathways is chiefly motivated and mediated by a sequence of particular musical events.

What is a musical event?

> ... an event is thus *the effect that seems to exceed its causes* – and the *space* of an event is that which opens up by the gap that separates an effect from its causes. (p. 3, emphasis in original) [...] event is not something that occurs within the world, but is *a change of the very frame through which we perceive the world and engage in it.* (p. 10 emphasis in original)
>
> Slavoj Žižek (2014)

> The 'musical event' is ... an indicative scheme for how we might begin to situate music as it is mobilised in action, and as it is associated with social effects [...] The *musical event* consists of a specific act of engagement with music. (p. 9)
>
> Tia DeNora (2003)

Žižek's notion of an event, and the *space* of an event as being something where the effect somehow exceeds its causes links with the ongoing theme we've been developing of musicking being always to some extent *transformational*. There's a time-before, of expectation, risk, hope, possibility and belief ... leading to a live and present process that is mobilised within particular *musical* qualities of time, space, and action ... resulting in a time-after where there's a condition (personal and collective) that is somehow different from before. This of course sounds just like a ritual process, as many theorists (Turner 1982, Schechner 2002, Small 1998, Dissanayake 2000, Ruud 2010 Aigen 2005) have described in relation to musical-social and music-therapeutic processes.

Such ritual process of a music performance event often functions, as Žižek suggests, to *change the frame* of our perceptions – of people, of an environment. In the SMART project we see members involved in the events transform into performing musicians, as able and capable, and so on. They also begin see themselves in this way through the mirror of an event, and are able to begin countering the stigmatised identity many have.

Music has a particular ability to create an event; to support an event; and to transform time, place and people through an event. DeNora's (2003) empirical schema for studying musical events provides a useful framework for ensuring that we don't just focus on 'before' and 'after' only, but attend clearly to the 'time between and within' of an event's happening, where its transformations show up as visible and audible.

Eventfulness is central to the SMART Music project – both to the regular 'mundane' event of the regular weekly SMART Music sessions, or the *SMART Singers* and *SMART Band* rehearsals, as well as the 'special' occasional events both inside and outside of SMART.

The regular 'uneventful events' of the groups and rehearsals are both similar and dissimilar to regular music therapy conventions, being supportive and constant over time for attendees, but also to varying degrees performative and based around an 'enhanced' sense of action, collaboration and 'result'. These non-conventional features are further emphasised in the 'special events' – where something 'out of the ordinary' is planned and happens through performance. But these events, like more conventional therapy, often have strong paramusical outcomes related to members' health-related challenges and aspirations. For example, Henrietta says the following at a public workshop that *SMART Singers* put on for members of the local mental health community:

> **Henrietta:** We are *SMART Singers*, a group of people who are brought together by our love and enjoyment of music. The group has come together to sing and to bring music to others. *SMART Singers* is also equally about contact, continuity, and community; a place that is safe and friendly. To be able to do something we all relate to on our own levels, and on levels of aspiration ... whether it's just to get out of our homes once a week, or whether it's to enable us to succeed beyond our expectations. The confidence and sense of self-worth that it gives is often plain to see ...

This description again characterises conventional therapy aspects (continuity, dependability, support), but also more social dimensions – 'to bring music to others' – and acknowledges a place for clients' musical aspirations, and acknowledgement of the personal fruits of succeeding beyond expectations through performance.

***

Add music, performance, food and drink to a gathering of people and it becomes more than a gathering – it becomes an occasion, an event. Not something abstract and general, but local and timely – at this time every week (between 2–4 on Thursdays for SMART Music, for example), with roughly these people (who become 'regulars'), in this place, doing these kinds of (usual or unusual) things, with these supporting things (instruments and paraphernalia). There are rituals of preparation and greeting, rough times of engagement and conviviality, rituals of parting and dis-assembling – all of this peppered by an accumulation of customs, habits, norms and prohibitions etc. SMART Music always feels an event – even when at its most 'ordinary'. There were plenty of times when it felt extraordinary, but all its occasions shared something that is both grounded in the everyday, but also lifts itself (and the people involved at any level) somehow out of this everyday. This seeming paradox is at the heart of how music helps people, personally and socially, within this community.

In terms of the other music groups at SMART (*SMART Singers/SMART Band*) there's perhaps more of a 'mundane/special' quality to them, as they more closely resemble rehearsal events than the Thursday group. But in terms of people's every week social experience the Singers and Band *are* indeed special occasions too.

When people feel bad these groups may be their only social event of the week, they get people out of the house, meeting other people, doing something and feeling good for a change. The 'special ritual' of these groups maintains people's wellbeing (as they continually tell us).

Perhaps this blurred boundary between mundane/special within the SMART musical community is key to its process and success. This between category of the 'mundane special' ensures easy access to the special for SMART musicians (in contrast to their real or perceived exclusion from many of the more culturally enhanced opportunities that preserve a clearer boundary into the 'very special' – e.g. the Royal Opera, Westminster Abbey, an O2 rock concert – all of which make 'problems with the threshold' (physical, symbolic, cultural) for people with mental health problems. In contrast, musical events associated with SMART gently elide the mundane and the special within an occasion, therefore making the threshold more porous, habitable and hospitable.

We mentioned earlier (Section 13) parallels between musical/music therapy events and phenomena described by ritual theory. We often saw in all categories of musical event at SMART key elements of transformative ritual – often no less than a transformation of consciousness and action for people, with musical ritual acting as an 'emotion transformer' (Stige 2010) as well as some of the more communal outcomes of ritual events such as feeling an enhanced sense of belonging or identity. This returns us to Christopher Small's basic description of the function of musicking as a ritual that enacts and symbolises the overarching pattern of ideal relationships that we want and need in our personal and social lives:

> Such ideas held in common about how people ought to relate to one another of course define a community, so rituals are used both as an act of affirmation of community ('This is who we are'), as an act of exploration (to try on identities to see who we think we are) and as an act of celebration (to rejoice in the knowledge of an identity not only possessed but also shared with others). (Small 1998, p. 95)

What we so clearly see in the musical events at SMART are the overlapping affordances of affirming, exploring and celebrating within the community – both within the diurnal pattern of each subsequent year, but also in the often unexpected but necessary fissions in the social fabric (good or bad) that create an event that often needs music's help; that becomes a *musical event.*

Researching musical events 2007–11

We identified 47 musical events during the main research period. An analysis of these suggested seven basic categories, where events afford a variety of functions for people and places:

A: Celebrations of public secular and religious (mostly Christian) festivals that naturally and historically involve music in our culture (singing Christmas carols, 'end-of-term' events at Easter and summer), but also public anniversaries that may only be significant for a sub-set of SMART members (e.g. VE day)

B: Marking and celebrating people's key personal events: birthdays, anniversaries, presentations, high-points – where a momentary or longer event is collectively musicalised and ritualised for the sake of that person, affirming their value and place in the SMART community. Along with these personal events, there are also the more public side of anniversaries: helping-with, oiling the wheels of public and formal events that are to do with marking, profiling/promoting or celebrating the public life of SMART (organisational anniversaries, presentations etc.). Music helps these events along – involving and 'displaying' people/groups, preventing attendees getting stiff and starchy, projecting an (aural) image of the best of the place etc.

C: A 'usual day' becomes eventful by a visit from a 'special' individual or group (e.g. the exchange between two similar music/mental health groups – *Musical Minds from East London* and *SMART Music),* or an organisation (BBC). Alternatively a social outing by a specific or ad-hoc group of SMART Music members to someone else's event, or to witness something (Henrietta singing in *Dido*), or to a film or concert, or to buy music.

D: Marking, coping-with, 'processing', getting-through the sweet, bitter, or bitter-sweet (or sometimes plain difficult) person-based, or more general transitions in the life of a small organisation such as SMART: when, for example, a staff member arrives or leaves, when there's a difficult situation to navigate publically (a resignation, redundancy); when there's a death and the need for a memorial/celebration of a life, or simply when there's a 'difficult day' (or week/month!).

E: More formal memorials and tributes for SMART members (especially those closely associated with the Music Project) who have died. The need both to help everyone get through an upsetting time, but also to musically create something that is 'fitting' to that person and their place in SMART/ SMART Music project.

F: Events within SMART – music for the community *by* the community, mostly involving the Singers and Band – that are planned, rehearsed for and tied to a particular circumstance – which might be exclusively for the group (a one-off gig), or be tied-in with an already-happening event (such as a regular summer party, Caribbean evening, club night etc.). These provide a motivational focus for preparation, and then a public platform for performance, appreciation, contribution etc.

G: Similar events *outside* SMART ('away gigs'), where there's the added bonus of the Singers/Band being booked to do a gig (could be literally a regular performance, or joining-in with/creating an event in another health or social setting). With these events there's greater potential reward, but also greater pressure and greater potential for 'trouble' (musical and otherwise). Such away-gigs advocate for SMART's profile as an organisation, and for the Music Project. They also often involve additional interesting issues of identity, stigma, and social negotiation for members and staff.

35. Music for the Community by the Community

One of the cultural changes at SMART during the years of the music project which is in step with policy directions in UK mental health philosophy is a necessary move from a friendly but slightly care-providing attitude towards members to instead a philosophy in step with the recovery model – an assumption, that is, of mutual help and development between service-users and professionals; an expectation (with appropriate support) that members participate in as many aspects of SMART's communal life as possible, providing for each other, using their own resources and talents. A concrete example of this shift is that when Gary started the music project in 2005 and suggested that members participate in the Christmas party entertainment this was seen as unusual, since it was always the staff who had always entertained the members at such events.

By the second year of the music project, and with the new management of SMART very much championing a recovery-model approach, things were really changing. Indeed Amelia the new Chief Executive was clear that the music project had been a guiding light for what she wanted to see happen at SMART overall.

A series of musical events recorded in the data increasingly depict a picture of music being provided for the community *by* the community, mostly involving the Singers and Band – who from the second half of 2007 are up-and-going and ready for opportunities to show what they can do. Some of these were when the Band or Band/Singers provided party entertainment for seasonal events or already-existing SMART traditions (the SMART Summer Evening Party, and Summer BBQ in 2007, the Caribbean Night in 2008). These events functioned on many levels: partly a straightforward opportunity for the musicians to give something of their talent and energy to their own community, and to enjoy being appreciated. They were a motivational focus for planning and rehearsing, and then a public platform for performance, appreciation and contribution. On another level these events provided a safe 'testing ground' for performance and repertoire in the early days of the Band and Singers – when things were sometimes rocky especially when a performance event added extra pressure and exposed fault lines. The musicians really wanted to perform again (having mostly not done this for many years), but also often had problems with this (both individually and within the groups). In-house events were a good way of test-running whether more ambitious projects could be planned outside of SMART, and were a safe way of finding out what happens if things go wrong, what needs to be worked on further, negotiated further, understood more by Sarah and the staff:

Friday 27 July, 2007 – SMART Summer Evening Music

SMART cafe is set out beautifully, with dimmed fairy lights, candles, tables and chairs moved back for dancing – a special atmosphere has being created.
But before the gig the Band are wound-up and in various states, the musicians are snapping at each other, there's conflict about the running order that we'd set, someone flounces out, then returns a bit later to take part after all. But all's well that ends well! – there's dancing, a good crowd of members coming from many different directions and networks : 'we've never had a Friday night like it' says one person. So a triumph, but how difficult it is to ensure that everyone is included, and we do what we plan to do! [Sarah's log, 27 July, 2007]

The opening set is by the Band, it's been prepared and rehearsed. Seems to go well at first with some rock numbers, appreciated by the crowd. But I have the feeling that some musicians have high performance anxiety, and there's a moment where it all goes a bit pear-shaped when the Band seem to just go with the flow despite the running order. A musician literally goes up to another and pokes him, saying 'this is my one'. There's an altercation, but looking around the room I'm not sure most people know what's going on. It's all quickly back on track, another musician grabs the bass and there's an increasingly nice atmosphere.

As the evening gets less planned, suddenly there's a 'Band B', comprising Simon on piano, Andrew (dressed up in smart suit) on drums. In contrast to 'Band A' they're are a bit lighter, jazzier. They do *Twist and Shout* and everyone gets up dancing, with Barbara prominent in this.

By default it all works – everyone is accommodated. Tony gets up to do a solo spot melodica, with me on piano, Simon on violin, Robert on harmonica. We do lovely expansive version of *Amazing Grace*, which nicely shifts the mood of the room for a while.

Serendipity, and an improvisational attitude has saved and made the day. There's perhaps a natural process of rupture and repair in this kind of musicking event. The evening certainly hovered on a knife-edge at times, but as such is a proper musical community in action. [Gary's log, 27 July 2007].

***

There's somewhat of a repeat of this pattern at the next event, SMART's *End of Summer BBQ* in September, when another one of the Band threatens to pull out at the last minute. This time it's about money – he wants paying as he thinks the Band are working as 'proper musicians' now. The other members persuade him to stay and play, reminding him that there is after all free food!

Looking at the list of people and music for this event it's clear that it functions somewhat as an enhanced version of the normal Thursday afternoon SMART Music Session. There's a broad, eclectic range of performances, a convivial feel and a freedom for members to simply make the music they want to make, and to be appreciated for this by others …

> **28 September 2007 – SMART End of Summer BBQ**
>
> The usual pre-party panic, as it's raining and the barbecue is wet. One musician had an issue about paying the 'proper musicians'. Another Band member persuaded him to stay.
>
> When it gets going there's a nice adult, intimate atmosphere. The event is important symbolically – for SMART staff to show that SMART can still put on a quality service for members after recent management upheavals. Some guests from the mental health services from the hospital who come to this event witness their former (and some current) patients in a different environment, being different – and these people also want to be witnessed being well.
>
> First set by SMART Singers (Ella, Michael, Mary, Jeremy), then some rehearsed items by Band members. Ella is carefully dressed up, does *Those were the days*, and *My baby just cares for me.* Mary is surprisingly focused and in voice with *Moon River*. Moussai is bizarrely but carefully dressed up in kilt and a pile of hats on his head! His song is accompanied by Sarah, Daniel and Robert. Simon plays interval music requests on piano. He's appreciated for the quality of his jazz playing.
>
> Anthony, finely dressed in suit and tie, comes up to sing *Berkeley Square*. He sings it better than I've ever heard him do before, with sensitivity and inflection. Someone later says about this 'perhaps it's because he really did feel it was like a proper nightclub at that point'. He's also going on about how he sung at the Dorchester Hotel – it was like he was there. 'It just makes me cry, listening to him', says another member.
>
> Evening ends joyous and freestyle – the music follows the flow: blues, rock 'n' roll, with dancing from Peggy, Anita, and Dave behind the bar. This really could be anywhere where people enjoy food, music, and dancing – it's so normal and so enjoyable! [Gary's project log – 28 September 2007]

36. Musicianhood, Ambivalence, and the Trials of Performance

More challenging aspects of the music project began to surface as the two newer groups (*Singers* and *Band*) started to mature, and as musical events started to develop within SMART. In short, trouble started to brew – alongside acknowledged triumphs of the project.

As music therapists working within a Community Music Therapy approach Gary and Sarah take the view that conflict and 'trouble' is not something either to be avoided or to be concentrated on in work of this type. Rather, they try to use their therapeutic perspective and experience to help 'work through' difficulties, balancing the needs of individuals against the needs of the community as a whole. Their overall attitude is that the powers of music, health, illness and everyday personality issues are all likely to come into play in a sometimes volatile way in a context such as SMART. When the stakes become higher – in performance situations, for example – specific problems are likely to surface. When they do, Gary and Sarah's aim is not to act as therapists for individuals, but to help manage the overall situation such that the best possible outcome can be reached for everyone: that everyone can be heard and respected and can contribute to a resolution of problems, and that where possible, everyone can feel understood even if they are personally unhappy with the solution.[23]

From many discussions at the time, and from an analysis of the data, it's clear that one of the particular difficulties that occurred both for individuals and for the SMART community and music project more generally revolves around the issue of being and developing as a musician. This issue is focused by the ambivalences of performance.

Daniel's story is a good example of the trials of what we will call 'musicanhood':

Musicianhood

For some people, music is life defining; it is their primary attachment and way of making meaning of things, and of finding their place in, and their way around the social world. *Being a musician* is then a role that is performed and elaborated across all aspects of the self – with both positive and negative aspects. It concerns both how 'musicians' experience themselves, and how they experience others' perceptions of their talent and accomplishments, and their social role. Stan Godlovitch (1998) suggests the term *musicianhood* to characterise this type of all-encompassing musical identity. Like personhood, musicianhood is partly a status *attributed* to someone by others. But it isn't merely the social category 'professional musician', nor is it just about talent or the quality of performance. Musicianhood, rather, registers when there is a particular match between how a person experiences themself in relationship to music, and how this comes to be recognised and acknowledged by others. As such, musicianhood is typically long lasting, but it can also be a transitory yet key happening in a person's experience (it does not need, that is, to be a prolonged state to be significant – as many examples from music therapy could attest). But the value of this state of musicianhood accounts for both its ecstasies and its occasional

[23] For more on this theme see Section 44, *The Therapy of Non-Therapy.*

agonies. There are, that is, times when this particular identity is a burden for people, or it invokes conflicts within the psychological or social ecology of lives (when, for example, illness or disability interferes with the natural functioning of musicianhood). Musicianhood is a strong and mostly helpful identity, but – like any strong identity – also a potentially vulnerable one. [adapted from Ansdell 2014: 133]

In most communities of people we could think of a continuum stretching between those people who are 'music lovers' and those who are 'music needers'. Daniel is someone strongly on the latter end:

> Daniel asks Simon to come up and play piano for him. He sings *What a Difference a Day Makes,* perhaps for the hundredth time at SMART Music. He sings it (they perform it) with style and elegance, as good a jazz rendition as you'd probably find in London that month. It's Dinah Washington in stylistic delivery, but it's also 'Daniel's song' as a jazz singer, and it's also Daniel, here and now, feeling good, or not good, in a mental health community setting, concretely or symbolically travelling from here to there, wherever that might be. [Gary's log, 15 January 2008]

***

Daniel describes music as providing the best and worst in his life. Daniel craves and needs music; he has a passion for it; he's attracted to all variations of it; he cultivates every single practice around and about it. In an interview in 2008 Gary asks Daniel to complete the sentence 'Without music … ', and Daniel answers 'be dead!'. He goes on: 'Music's a kind of sixth sense in me … without music I'd lose one of my senses'. To others around him Daniel often looks transported and 'sent' by it. But the 'comedown' from this high often brings trouble for Daniel, and then just as he's feeling so good he also often feels the worst about himself and his life situation in relation to his illness. This means that overall Daniel remains somewhat ambivalent about music, and the music project at SMART. His story is a good example of how an attachment to music and 'being a musician' is necessarily constructed, maintained and negotiated in concrete social and cultural contexts, and interwoven with personal factors such as illness. It involves Daniel's long-term musical life course – his cultivation of his talent, skill, preferences and then the sites and opportunities in which he can perform both his music and his musicianhood (the early gigs on the London jazz scene).

Then there's the confrontation of this aspect of personality and professional identity – as a musician – with the realities of an emergent chronic illness diagnosed as paranoid schizophrenia. As with many of the people in this community, the worst phases of the illness takes them away from music, or the music is somehow invaded by the illness. Daniel tells Gary how, at the point when the music project began, he'd not played guitar for four years (though he had listened to music). At SMART he talked about music to those people he'd known for years, and had sometimes previously played music with. The music project activates Daniel's active passion for music; and he becomes in many ways the figurehead for the project and the SMART musical community. When Sarah helps set up *SMART Band* this is just what Daniel has been dreaming about for years, and he's the dominant musical personality in the set-up of this group. But over the years Daniel goes in and out of the Band, and there's continued trouble both for him, Sarah and other members in relation to his ambivalences about playing in this group, or in SMART overall. Of course this is partly typical of what bands do – dis-band! But in this particular small context the disappointment and hurt feelings of real or threatened disbanding seem worse than most. Many crises are weathered over the years with different groupings of the Band, and an experiment with more than one band. Overall Daniel is an honest and generous man as a musician, trying to reconcile the conflicting aspects of his relationship to music, and to being a musician in the SMART community. But it often seems that he's left the most hurt as a result of what happens.

Daniel is admired as probably the best musician in objective terms – it's clear that without his problems he would have no problems making his living from music in the wider world. But illness and other factors get in the way. It seems he can't motivate himself, or keep himself in music making for enough time to make a go of it. And here comes the main dilemma both for Daniel and the music project at SMART. It gives Daniel a way of 'being a musician' again; it gives him a platform for his musicality and musicianship to bloom again; to be admired for his talent. At times Daniel is exceptionally generous, musically; inspiring; his performances are raw and moving to people. Just like the most authentic Blues man, he sings out the excruciating truth of how beauty, truth and suffering puzzlingly blend; how transcendence is always a phrase away; how hope can always be found even as you face the wall. Many in the 'audience' know this reality only too well. Daniel's song articulates it for them eloquently and directly.

While the music lasts it's transcendence for Daniel too. When it stops it can flip to hell. He looks around and realises where he is. It's not the 101 Jazz Club in central London, it's SMART, a day centre for people with mental health problems. His admirers are not jazz aficionados, but fellow sufferers. It can be a big come down, and Daniel retreats often to beat himself up about this gap between fantasy and reality. He appreciates what the project is doing, and in moments appreciates what it's done for him too. He wants and likes his music inspiring and helping others; he wants to help others to make music too … But … here's where the shadow falls; frustration and disappointment get the better of him. This is not right or fair that he should be making music here, with us.

But Daniel's story is also a very important corrective within this project to the increasingly common rhetoric in popular culture during the last ten years that music is an unproblematic panacea for people in health and social settings. Rather Daniel's story clearly shows that any talk of 'how music helps' must be nuanced and bound to the real situations and dilemmas of individual people and communities. Likewise his story cautions any too pat conclusions of our own on the 'musical pathways' and bridge-building theme. 'The thing is', Daniel says to Gary one day, 'but it's *not* a pathway for me, because I get half-way over the bridge there's no connection with the other side!'. He's right in a sense, we're operating on different levels of what pathways/bridges mean or entail for people. For some project participants it's a modest journey, from the hospital to the music groups, then to an external resources such as Morley College's *Can't Sing Choir.* SMART likewise does support Daniel over the years to do various musical bridge building, on the back of his newfound confidence from playing again in the project. He goes to a music technology training but it's too basic. Other stuff is out of the borough and they can't find funding.

But however unfortunate these episodes of 'musical trouble' seem, Daniel always returns in some way to the project, and to the music. We say simply 'He just can't keep away'. A true music-lover and music-needer, the passion to keep playing and singing is always more than anything else. If music's there, Daniel needs to be there too.

***

In different ways related to personality, ambitions and limitations, something of this pattern is present for other participants in the music project also – this struggle between musicianhood, illness and circumstance. Placing all of one's identity eggs in this one, musicianhood, basket is risky as the stakes are raised, emotionally, socially and professionally. We saw earlier how emotionally risky Simon found being a musician again within the music project, and how he had to carefully 'titrate' his participation. In a different way, musicianhood was crucial for Ella because of her core identification with music as something precious, and her need for her musicianship to be recognised and appreciated by others.

Musicianhood therefore becomes a key dimension of the music-health-illness narratives of these people, and of some others within the project. The dilemma is that musicianhood is necessarily a fragile identity, and one that can be easily interrupted or spoilt through personal or social circumstances. There's a paradoxical connection between how music is attached to their health *and* their illness in ways that cause distress, but also consistently shows and builds a healing path. Music is the source of what touches, elicits and helps flourish, the *wellness* in these people. Perhaps what the project, and its gently therapeutic perspective has been able to provide for these people is a safer framework and a longer dependable time-frame for the paradoxes of musicianhood, illness and health to be grappled with, and hopefully for some sort of balance to be reached in relation to the continuing ambivalence surrounding music's help.

***

Types of sometimes challenging behaviour during the music groups – especially SMART Band – arguably have their origin in these 'problems with musicianhood'. As an identity that verges for some people as a condition of personhood, musicianhood is vulnerable to the affects of chronic illness, and distorted by an 'illness ecology', with knock-on effects on how musicians feel about themselves (and even potentially losing a feeling of themselves). It's a vulnerable status of personhood that risks becoming a ‘spoiled identity’ through the impact of the illness in terms of how musicianhood is something on-going that needs to be cultivated, sustained and continually proved. This in turn requires a suitable place, people and occasion – in order that the social recognition and attribution of musicianhood can happen.

For those SMART members who have cultivated musicianship through training, and long-term serious engagement with music there's an ongoing ambivalence and frustration about the gap between their musical status and their musical situation – and how other members of the group, or particular heightened circumstances such as public performances become a target for this frustration.

***

The positive side of these dilemmas of musicianhood is that exploring them has reinforced the importance of the ‘music-centred’ philosophy of the music project at SMART. This puts music’s capacity to help at the forefront of therapeutic action, and it puts the musicians in the SMART community in a position where they can be musicians again, using their talent and skill to help themselves and others – despite occasional or ongoing problems, despite ambivalences. As Daniel says:

> ... you know, there are three or four really, really decent musicians here. They are mentally ill ... but at the same time they are musicians first and formost, and you will judge them by how they play music. And no other factor! If you’re gonna talk about bridge-building, in some ways I am a complete member of society, I have a full life in many ways. But in other ways, I need help. I do need help, to bridge that gap. And this will be an ideal way, a halfway house ... [Daniel, interview with Gary, October 2008]

There's also the opposite end of the spectrum found within the project, where this sense of musicianhood as being a socially bestowed and appreciated aspect of personhood is also seen in the project in people who are not trained musicians with a long-standing identity. Something important can happen also for people who 'become musicians' unexpectedly through cultivating and then being witnessed in their musical performances – and for whom this is a particularly positive experience of a shift in identity.

Tim, for example, successfully plays his part on the metalophone in a Christmas concert and says afterwards: ‘I've always been told I'm an idiot – but after yesterday I think I'm a musician!’. This man has suffered decades of being confined to a negative and stigmatising identity within old-style psychiatric treatment, and moves in one experience to a benign identity that perhaps stands for everything he longs for as a status of personhood: recognition for doing something well and beautiful, with others, towards something that was a success.

Other of our pathway cases have come to think of themselves as musicians in various ways that are less common in our culture today, where there's such a sharp divide between people who are seen as musicians/not musicians. People in the SMART project discovered instead that they were certainly musical *participators*, making their musical contribution in a way that was original, recognised and appreciated by others. Rather than musicianhood exactly, this is a kind of more modest change of cultural status and identity in relation to music: people 'finding' themselves *musical*, and this being a state and status that is pleasurable and often helpful to re-establishing and maintaining their wellbeing, and to being more comfortably in community with others.

The unusual thing about the music project in SMART is that it managed to cultivate two communities at the same time: (i) a *musical community* which is democratic, based on 'core musicality', in which anyone can participate on equal terms, but at the same time (ii) a *musician's community* – where skilled players are given space within SMART Music for recognition of their musicianship, style and success of performance, and the mutual offering of musical help. It's a challenge to maintain both types at the same time, and the project has not always succeeded. But sometimes it has.

37. 'It's Music That Will Get Us Through ... '

More collective troubles and challenges inevitably hit the SMART community at various times during the decade of witnessing this project. There were several deaths of well-loved people in the musical community, but also rocky periods for the organisation for one reason or another, and simply those bitter-sweet transitional events that a stable community can find challenging, such as when well-loved and trusted doctors or other staff retire or move on. Sometimes people with mental health problems can find these occasions difficult given their own 'problems in living' have often been crystallised by difficult events and transitions in the first place. SMART understands this, and does its best to help people cope. But it's also true that SMART members, and the community as a whole has an unusually good understanding of, and sensitivity towards, 'difficulty'. They tend not to pretend that everything is ok when it's not, and can offer valuable mutual care to each other through challenging times.

It becomes widely acknowledged that music helps with many of these moments and times, and that one of the key benefits of the music project was that it had given members confidence again to use music to help with troubled times.

***

Sometimes it's just a difficult day (or week, or very occasionally month) at SMART:

Session 89, July 5, 2007

Ongoing uncertainties about the future of SMART as an organisation are hovering in the air. There's an atmosphere of uncertainty and tension, although I'm not sure whether the members yet know exactly what is happening. The stance that Sarah and I take is simply that it's our job to keep the music going whatever – this is what music therapy does anyhow, for people: brings music to help in various states of difficulty and crisis. Community Music Therapy is just an extension of this, in how it broadens music's help to a place or community in crisis. Music is important in a crisis – personal or institutional, because it doesn't just build community, it helps sustain community when times get rough.

In this way, this afternoon's music group seems most helpful for the staff today – Dave the manager was teary at the beginning, but soon cheered up and joined in the singing. Other staff now often sit for a while with a cup of tea in the music groups, listening to the Band and commenting on how they are improving. The crisis that SMART is in encourages public recognition of the music and the music project. It takes a crisis sometimes to see things clearly! [Gary's project log – 4 July 2007]

***

This organisational crisis resolves, but involves a challenging transition of staff and culture. Music comes to help in a more focused way when two staff who have resigned ask to have their leaving party within the Thursday SMART Music Session. There are mixed emotions and loyalties, as some members are very attached to these staff, so the event is potentially a challenging one. Sarah is asked whether the music groups could help, and she carefully plans and thinks through – with her therapist hat on – just what would be the best way to manage this – musically, practically and emotionally – so that the best outcome is likely, and the worst prepared for and hopefully avoided.

***

SMART Music Session 103, November 29, 2007: Staff Leaving party.

This afternoon is precarious in 'political' and emotional terms, with both leavers saying that they were dreading it. It really needed music! 40 to 50 people crowd into the cafe space, and about 40 stay the whole two hours. Sarah had planned the event carefully, preparing a structure such that the very personal contributions of members could be contained/balanced within the general musical/social flow of the afternoon (as a way of managing the emotional aspect – preventing anything from getting 'too much' for anyone). The structure was: a warm-up period to gather people; leading to a 'special items' period with prepared songs & speeches. Ella had prepared in SMART Singers some well-known songs with personalised words for the occasion – *You will Survive*, and *Leaving on a Jet plane*, supported by the Band members. Then there was a tea break, and then the usual SMART Music stuff – with the aim of normalising the event for people again. It worked perfectly! – I congratulated Sarah for this architecture, and how it helped to modulate the emotions of this event in a helpful and appropriate way. Everyone had a tricky job, but the music served it perfectly, as music *can* do, and is perhaps *designed* to do.

There were moving moments of people expressing their sadness, but also humour and passion in many ways, so it all seemed manageable. Very much a *ritual occasion*, with all the features of this, and showing how music can carry and help such rituals.

Also a wonderful showcase of what we've been doing this year: showing the sub-communities of musicians at SMART, and how they can feed back into large events like this, and feel good about it ... [Gary's log]

****

Several other events shared both similarities and differences to this especially tricky occasion. The data has a series of less dramatic but equally bittersweet events that involved the transitions of people out of the overall community (defined as the larger hospital site, and as the people whom SMART members were involved with, or had been involved with in the past). Music again shows itself in action, smoothing the path, focusing the celebration, and usually getting the pitch just right ...

As with the leaving party for the SMART staff written about above, over the years there are several other tailored events for retirements, with individually crafted material by SMART musicians. Each time this is for people who are liked and respected within the mental health community. Sometimes it's of course difficult to pitch such events right – staff will have had their ups and downs with individual patients/SMART members, and there's always some kind of hierarchy lurking in these services. But again this is where music helps, oiling the social wheels of the occasion and creating musical *communitas* to level everyone for just a few moments inside music.

***

Dr B's Leaving Party – Thursday 15 May 2008

Once we heard Dr B was leaving a music event seemed like a good idea. He's always been a supporter of music therapy, loves music, and we all knew that he would find the goodbye difficult, so to have something organised would work better ... [Sarah's log, May 2008]

As with some of the earlier Christmas events, Sarah co-ordinated the musicians' group on the hospital site (*Sounds of Willow)* along with the now strengthening *SMART Singers,* and set up a lunchtime concert in the Day Hospital. Most of the musicians were keen to work on this project, some having known Dr B over a period of more than 30 years, going back to the days of the older psychiatric hospital in the area. Interestingly, one singer did still have some unresolved issues with Dr B as his psychiatrist, and after talking the dilemma through with Sarah decided to act as the group's 'roadie', helping set-up equipment rather than singing.

The event took place in the Day Hospital dining room and was attended by Dr B and his wife, outpatients, inpatients, daypatients, staff, and doctors. It was quite crowded in the room 15 minutes before the concert. The musical programme included:

New York, New York – sung by all
Ol' Man River – Tim
When I'm 64 – Jim
Divine Mercy – Jim [original composition]
These Foolish Things – Jeremy
Wonderful World – Ella
Steal Away – SMART Singers
Shalom, Shalom – SMART Singers
Dancing Queen – All
All You Need is Love – All

This programme shows up the musical network operating at that time: the connections between the different geographical sites, and the close relationship between events, SMART Music Sessions, and the musicians' personal musical pathways, repertoires and preferences (people give their music as a gift for this event, and to Dr B that day).

At the beginning of the event word-sheets of *New York* are given out to all, with the wording slightly altered to 'Start spreadin' the news … *He's leaving today!'*. Then a group of musicians who Dr B had been professionally involved with for many years sang an individual solo, each presenting something of their personal relationship to him through their musical performance. Ella had substantially re-written *Wonderful World* in a witty way for the occasion:

Don't know much about stethoscopes
Had enough of those long white coats
Talking groups may have their place
But neuroscience won't win the race

Cos I do know one and one is two
And it's music that will get us through
What a wonderful world this can be …

We end by singing *All you Need is Love* together, a maxim proved by the feeling in the room. But overall the concert has managed to avoid excessive sentiment, balancing heartfelt feeling with humour and quiet, reflective songs. Dr B and his wife look very moved by this musical offering, and overall it's a great success. Sarah comments in her log written soon after:

> This was a tricky event to co-ordinate, and I think the first where I've been so aware of the audience's emotions and possible reactions. It felt like I needed

> simultaneously to manage how it was for Dr B, for all the 'ex-pats' coming to say farewell, sad staff and long-term colleagues – incorporate possibly rambly speeches as well as my musical performers, play the piano and compère ... a tough gig! A perfect example, however, of how music can facilitate an occasion, can enable people to express difficult emotions or previously unsaid sentiments within a safe, structured, expressive and interactive shared event. [Sarah's log, May 2008].

This event, and Sarah's account here, gives a good picture of the type of therapeutic thinking and working that the music therapist adds to the event, which complements the contributions all others make. And it also shows up – as Ella's perfect phrase expresses – 'it's music that will get us through ... '.

38. Performing the Soul of SMART

Music of course 'gets us through' in a variety of individual and communal and ways during the course of the phases of the members' and the organisation's life that we tracked over the years. These events also demonstrated something important about the relationships between the 'personal pathways' of the people involved in the SMART project and the broader developmental pathway of the organisation and social context. Both dimensions are interdependent, as people and the place shift and develop. Strengths and vulnerabilities are demonstrated; networks (hidden and apparent) are lit up by patterns of collaboration, invention and possibility during events. The culture of SMART undergoes an important change during the period 2005–7 in its style and philosophy, adopting a 'recovery approach' linked with current thinking about mental health support. This chimes in well with the developing music project, which in many ways exemplifies this attitude and ambition in a very concrete and practical way (we will talk more about this in Part IV). In short, the emphasis is less on containing and managing people and their illness, more on providing opportunities, resources and support for members to demonstrate and perform their wellbeing and recovery at different paces (and to help build their pathways towards and around this). This thinking and practice becomes increasingly visible (and obviously suitable) through public events that 'show-up' this inter-relationship between the development of individuals and of the organisation as a whole.

***

SMART's survival in the last five years has been precarious, but survive it has. In June 2011 it celebrates its 25th anniversary with a formal occasion, one that showcases where SMART currently is, and appeals for help to pursue further developments. Music, as ever, is a key part of the event, but it's also a showcase for what the music project has managed in the five years in alignment with SMART's philosophy:

> It's an event for supporters/fundraisers this afternoon, with SMART members providing hospitality in different ways (this inevitably caused some disputes in the planning, but everything was resolved for most people, and today everyone looks happy with their roles). Sarah was asked to provide entertainment from the music project. It turned out to be a significant event, both in terms of members' experience (combined Band /Singers), and public perception of the integral nature of the music project within SMART, and how this incarnates its mission and ethos. The place is poshed-up, everyone in formal dress-up mode.
>
> A new publicity film is premiered, portraying SMART's mission and achievements through moving personal testimonies of members telling stories about their mental health and how SMART helps, and then through the various projects, including music. There's beautifully shot and edited shots of Sarah working musically with both Band and Singers. There's a lovely sense of her really *working* with them; a learning focus there, and humour, and the musicalising of people moving/talking/smiling, within and alongside music – *being in music*. Humour, soul, musical life, commitment, participation, performance – all of this conveyed in images, with the separate soundtrack of the finished song they were doing. This beautifully conveyed the multi-levelled and fluid activity (musical/personal/social) that's this project. Michael talks about the influence of music at SMART on his life and mental health. People are very moved by this film.
>
> The Singers and Band provide party music, a half-hour set with varying combinations and some lovely new material as well as regular stuff from Gary M, Jeremy, Roger, Henrietta and Michael.
>
> In small speeches at the end of the set Henrietta thanks Sarah and me for making music available to them. Roger grabs the mic and says 'I just want to say music therapy works. You've seen and heard the evidence'. People laugh, but they also firmly get the message. Dr B, founding director of SMART, fan and supporter of music therapy (and also long time psychiatrist for Roger) smiles and says to me 'this is Roger's campaign against evidence-based medicine'.
>
> The evening is a triumph, with the music firmly in the centre of SMART, its mission and soul, and an indicator of its success and benefit. The music was one of the most moving sequences the film, and the party without the music would have been stiff and starchy. Somehow the music *performed* the soul of SMART, with some of its 'pathway people' (Roger, Henrietta, Michael, Gary M) being witnessed by their medical consultants in the room (who were very moved). This was a performance of health and well-being – for these people, but also collectively for all of us I felt – a reserve of hope and inspiration for us all. [Gary's log, 30 June 2011]

Just as with the celebration of individual anniversaries, so with this collective celebration there's a focus on appreciation, recognition and a certain kind of proof of something through its being displayed and performed in front of eyes and ears, not just talked about as theory or policy. A threshold is crossed – for individuals, for the community – each time an event like this takes place …

39. Christmas 2007 and the 'Ripple Effect'

Another direction of travel was happening by the end of 2007 and accelerating during 2007–11. This was partly by design, and partly due to keeping to our core philosophy of following where people and music led. And, as we've seen already, with music the direction is often *outwards* ...

The 'ripple effect'

' ... music naturally *radiates,* like dropping a pebble in a pond, and seeing the waves of energy spread out in concentric circles' (Pavlicevic & Ansdell 2004: 16). This ecological metaphor of the ripple effect has become something of a core image for the Community Music Therapy movement (Pavlicevic & Ansdell 2004; Stige et al. 2010; Stige & Aaro 2012; Ansdell & Stige 2015; Wood 2016). In conveys the sense of how the very physical attraction and energy of music permeates spaces and boundaries and then often attracts people's attention, gathers and connects people together. The physical and socio-cultural aspects of the ripple effect therefore merge into each other. In terms of Community Music Therapy, the metaphor has been used to promote the idea that music therapy can appropriately work 'outwards' towards community, as well as bringing community inwards for people who may be isolated; it can take people towards community, and create community within a building or site. This encourages us not only to think of individuals of groups developing 'within' themselves, but also how people and places develop between, amongst and beyond themselves. Community Music Therapy projects often generate networks and catalyse ecological processes, where the ripples from a single event ('pebble') reverberate across a whole environment, causing changes for individuals, groups and physical spaces at the same time. The aim of Community Music Therapy therefore matches the basic eco-phenomenology of music: it's about mobilising and supporting purposeful movements, directions, transitions and pathways ...

The beginning of being able to see the ripple effect at work in the SMART Music project is well illustrated by what happened around the Christmas period in 2007. By this point the three music groups were beginning to work in themselves, and several in-house events during the autumn of 2007 had shown how the musicians could also work interdependently. Sarah was also working fluently between the hospital and SMART, and we were seeing a satisfying musical-social flow between the two sites. Quite naturally the music groups and their musicians were starting to ripple out between and amongst the various venues.

Christmas is often an ambivalent time in such communities. For some people it is a seriously challenging time to their mental health, but at the same time it's not an option for an organisation like SMART to do nothing (although there are also religious and multi-cultural sensitivities to attend to). On the positive side from the music project's angle, catering for the musical needs of the Christmas season was a way to focus the individual and group resources, to highlight collaborations, and simply help people to have fun, and cope with the more difficult aspects of this holiday period.

***

SMART Singers and *SMART Band* are keen to use Christmas as a focus for working towards performances. This follows on from the first successful 'outside gig' for the combined forces of Band/Singers earlier in the summer when they are invited to provide music for the elderly persons' ward Summer Party. This is successful for all, showing what's possible from 'in-house entertainment' (the ward manager says 'we normally pay £100 for outside bands, but you lot are better than any of them!'). On the strength of this the SMART musicians are invited back to this ward for the Christmas party, and want now to build on their first ‹outside› performance event. The only slight problem is that the Band is too loud for the older people›s party (indoors this time!). Sarah negotiates and a compromise is found: for the ward party *SMART Singers* will combine with Sarah's hospital-based singing group *Sounds of Willow,* and SMART Band will be the main musical focus for SMART's own Christmas party. Then through the link of one of the Singers the group is invited to provide Christmas entertainment for the outpatient mental health service's party at another venue, located five minutes along the road. Finally, a small group do informal carol singing around the wards of the psychiatric hospital:

(i) 19 December (mid-day): SMART Singers & Willow Singers at elderly persons' ward Christmas party.

A group of SMART musicians gather late morning: members of *SMART Singers* (Ella, Henrietta, Michael), *Sounds of Willow* (Brian – with djembe, Csezlaw, Paul the nurse, two ambulance crew with good gospel voices, Sarah, Gary, two junior doctors. Instantly there's disaster – the patient's Christmas lunch will arrive 1.5 hours late! There's staff stress, patient disorientation ... so the performers quickly re-plan and get on singing to cover the gap. They're admirably calm and professional, making last-minute decisions on the running-order. Members of the ward staff say they recognise some of the singers, it's nice to have people they know do the music – an event for this community by the community. It's also nice to see all the varied people in the group – the combination of staff and patients:

> Fantastic to have such massed choirs! A real joy to see a large group of people who share commonalities – from SMART, elderly persons' ward, hospital, Gary, myself ... but with vastly different experiences and reasons – coming together to make music and share that with others. I admit I was a little surprised by the enthusiasm from staff, their willingness to commit and participate – in an NHS climate now of stress and pressure

> on time and paperwork. Perhaps that's why musical opportunities were a temptation, staff got something out of it themselves, and were with their clients directly, rather than abstractly through forms and policies! [Sarah's log, 12 Dec 2007]

Photos of this event show the performers have carefully dressed up for the occasion, with sprigs of tinsel round their necks and heads adding festive effect.

The music starts off with a performance of *Mary's Boy Child,* sung by Jim in a strongly-inflected Polish accent, but with energy and warmth. He's accompanied on an equally energetic djembe drum by another patient, and the chorus come in vigorously on *Hark now, hear the angels sing* ... Immediately the musicking is inclusive and encouraging. As the song goes on there's a tendency for the soloist to get faster and more excited, to which the drummer responds by elaborating the 'fills' of the song with increasingly florid rhythmic patterns. Sarah hears this, and pulls back the song to safer territory through her piano accompaniment. It ends well, the room and its various busy and still people pulled towards the music. The programme is a mix of prepared solo and group items from the Singers (*When A Child is Born, O Holy Night, We Three Kings)* and favourites for all – *Jingle Bells, Rudolph, White Christmas, Rockin' Around the Christmas Tree ...).* There's a lovely introspective contrast to the mood when Henrietta and Ella sing a unique unaccompanied version of *In the Bleak Mid-winter.* They've rehearsed this for weeks, and unusual it certainly is: the two singers found that they knew different versions of this carol (the usual and the Harold Darke), and that if you put the two melodies together they (sort of) fit! So that's what we get today, a trick perhaps only noticed by the cognoscenti! But it creates a beautiful point of stillness.

Throughout the event there's increasing conviviality, and a visibly changing relationship between people through the combined effect of music, food and a bit of dancing.

As the performance goes on there's also an increasing fluidity of personnel, with informal staff and patient interactions happening at all levels, afforded through singing together: staff sharing song sheets with residents; an old lady conducting *Silent Night* with a spoon; an OT doing a verse on her own; a few of the doctors getting mixed up with it too. There's central and peripheral participation – or rather the whole range of possible participation types. The outcome is a sense of mutual respect, and mutual benefit – the musicians seem to grow six inches taller over the course of the hour. Henrietta comments that her voice gradually frees and gets louder as she sings with the others and finds herself absorbed by the energy of the music and other people.

The musicians are competent, professional and they cope so well with the unforeseen, and seem comfortable improvising, and adapting to the circumstances. Henrietta says 'we know these situations when people can be difficult ... it's different from getting in musicians who don't know this kind of setting, and these people ... '. The SMART musicians rise to the situation – and this is in marked and sometimes amazing contrast to the current difficulties some of the individual people are currently struggling with. Staff witness them here not just as 'people with problems'. but rather as the musicians of the community, achieving something for the benefit of others. From this comes value, respect, recognition of skill, dignity.

(ii) 19 December SMART Christmas Party (evening)
This was never going to be an easy one! Only a month before there had been a difficult transition as some staff, unhappy with the new culture, have resigned and left. The mood has been difficult since, and everyone was left a little anxious about the 'traditional Christmas party' and how it'd come off this year. In previous years it was the staff entertaining the members at this event, but this year there is to be a shift, with members more involved in entertaining other members – a shift signalled by the planned contribution of the newly-formed *SMART Band*. The event proved somewhat of a mixed experience, with Sarah's log recording a combination of musical triumph and trouble! In contrast to the meticulous preparation and rehearsal by the Singers for the afternoon's event, the Band have been reluctant to plan or commit – when they play they just want to play! Sarah has helped them to prepare a draft running order, but when it comes to the evening there's the tendency to just go with the musical flow. All well and good at one level – the proven virtues of an 'improvisational attitude' are part of the philosophy after all – but there are problems with collaborative, more public events. The first set by the Band is good in getting the energy for the party going ... but then the relentlessness of the amplified sound is too much for some members. Sarah engineers a break, and negotiates with everyone a second performance set, but this time with only acoustic instruments. This works better for this occasion – both in terms of volume, and breadth of cultural reference. Jeremy does a solo, Leslie arrives in suit and tie to do one of his typical guest performances – he does two Christmas songs with panache and style – and the whole room refocuses to listen to him.

By the end of the evening all is well, a good time has been had, dancing has taken over, and the Band have relented on their initial refusal to play 'naff Christmas songs'. There's relief from the SMART staff that conviviality has replaced awkwardness, everyone has felt included, and celebration has taken over, despite any other feelings.

(iii) SMART /Willow Singers – carol singing at Chelsea Chambers

The next day sees the third Christmas music event, when the mental health community outreach team ask whether 'Sarah's music people' could do some carol singing for their members' party. It's useful that we can almost do a re-run of the event in the elderly persons' ward the day before. The musicians set off mid-afternoon in a caravan of people and instruments (loaded in a supermarket trolley), travel five minutes up the road and set up shop in Chelsea Chambers around the Christmas tree. A photo shows that quite a few members seemed to have themed their clothes in Christmas red and green! The group provides about an hour of music as people arrive and settle at the party. The event works well in the space there: people gradually gather around the musicians, listen and join in. There's a nice intimate acoustic and social feel, with an increasing informal exchange between musicians and party-goers, who interact by joining in the singing, applauding, making a request, chatting, eating and drinking. The quieter songs like *Silent Night* are especially effective here. An unexpected moment happens when after listening carefully to the music one of the members of the audience asks to say a prayer, and improvises a prayerful thanks for the staff who support him, for his friends and family, and for peace in the world. It's a moving benediction to this event. Again, it's obvious that this is not entertainment *for*, but 'between' ... Partygoers and musicians know each other because they come from the same mental health community. But all the same their roles within this event are subtly different. The musicians feel good and proud about their performance and social-musical function here: and there are generous comments about the musicians' professionalism, focus, attitude; their musicianhood is acknowledged and witnessed by fellow patients, but also by staff who'd previously often seen them only as patients. Here again is music *by* the community *for* the community – recycling resources, developing capabilities. The musician's sense of achievement is added to by getting their fee of £10 each that Sarah has negotiated. But they›ve not done it for the money, but rather for what this represents in terms of acknowledgement and appreciation of what they can and want to do.

(iv) Christmas Eve – Carol singing around the hospital wards

Only a few of the musicians are still around by Christmas Eve, but those that are say they'd like to do some low-key carol singing on the hospital wards. Henrietta, Carolyn, Gary, Sarah and Paul meet and wander around for an hour, armed with guitar, a few instruments and carol sheets. Most people on the wards know either Sarah or Gary from music therapy ward groups – so it's different from just a load of strangers turning up to do this. People request carols – we're surprised when one lady asked for the plainsong *O Come Emmanuel* (but this

> is Chelsea after all!). Lastly we go down to the elderly persons' ward when there's rather more of a captive audience. The music is really appreciated there, and the good feelings are reciprocal – the musicians also feel good to be appreciated. It's a nice coda to the year's work: mutual benefit, recycling of resources, moments of achievement, joy and hope within this circumstantial community ...

40. Performing as Advocating

The outwards trajectory of the SMART musicians' work continues during the following years. Each time Sarah lets the members decide what they want to do, why and how. As we've said previously, it seems natural for musicians at any level to want first to work on learning and mastering musical material, and then sharing it through performance with others. As SMART *Singers* and *Band* developed over the years they also cultivated and experimented with ways of taking their music out towards others – either independently or through joint-events. Partly the motivation was simply to have a stage to perform on, to demonstrate the fruits of rehearsal, and to feel good about being seen as musicians. But there was also often another agenda as well, one that resonated with the situation of these people: to advocate for SMART as an organisation, but also for an understanding of mental health recovery, the idea of mental *health* within illness. This could come from getting people in the wider community to witness their musical competence and talent, and quite simply from getting the chance to do something positive for other people (rather than always be 'the helped'). The various 'away-gigs' proved to be crucial in the development of individuals, groups, and also the philosophy of the project overall. Not that they were always easy, or straightforward.

***

These 'away gigs' originated in a booking just for one of the musical groups, or else by their taking part in an event with others – both in medical/mental health settings and regular cultural venues. These events held the potential for good experiences for the musicians, but they also inevitably involved greater pressure, and possible 'trouble' (musical and otherwise). They sometimes catalysed dilemmas and conflict around identity, stigma, and social negotiation for members and staff. This proved important and interesting in terms of our attempts to explore all angles of what 'musical pathways' could be within a mental health context, and how we could best navigate challenging aspects for people and places.

The year 2008 saw two key first time performance experiences for Band and Singers away from SMART: the Band at a Mental Health Users' Conference in a church in Notting Hill; and the Singers' first lunchtime concert as part of the concert series in the atrium of the adjacent large general hospital.

SMART Band at the Mental Health Users' Conference – 22 April 2008
First away-gig for the band, at a church in Notting Hill. Pickup of equipment fine, setup okay, short warm-up.

We're introduced as the SMART Band. Daniel takes the role of compère, skilfully and confidently. Instant hit with the audience, who joined in, clapped, sang and applauded vigorously, and wouldn't let us stop. Music was the most coherent, warm, intuitive and interactive I've ever experienced playing with them – certainly the best performance ever given. Stuck to the schedule, no problems.

After performance went for a cuppa tea, everyone very pleased with themselves, glowing and feeling good, especially the audience reaction. This music was the only user-led part of the whole day – ironically, the rest of the conference was presented by professionals to passive service users! Our guys were also rightly pleased that they›d done something as users, and been paid for this.

Sting in the tail of the day: the guys swan off to the pub, leave a few to pack up – then it seems the bass guitar is stolen (it wasn't – somebody else from the SMART staff took it home in a car but forgot to tell me!). This is the strain with this work for me – managing what other people can't seem to do, needing to take responsibility for almost everything! [Sarah's log, 22 April 2008].

I get there lunchtime, and it seems a dreary event so far, all talk, with mental health professionals quite patriarchal towards the users. The SMART Band guys all dressed up – Bobby in spivvy costume and trilby hat. They look ready for it, and have really collaborated in preparing, collecting instruments and setting up, etc. – level of professional responsibility.

Audience of about 60, service users mainly, but some managers of local centres and services, plus supporters from SMART, and Dr B has come specially. The band look professional on stage, as soon as they start there's a great leap in energy in the room, clearly welcome contrast from the mornings talking, and seeing service users confident and in charge.

Aint no Sunshine to begin; Daniel sings, laid-back and confident. Then Ella belts out *Leaving on a Jet Plane*, with style and panache. Bobby moderates his drumming – good collaborative musicking happening within the group, not just Sarah directing. Mussei does reggae number, *Wisdom of the Temple*. He produces his costume just before going on – spectacular multicoloured jester's hat that has us all smiling. Robert does a Blues solo on harmonica, then there's *Roll over Beethoven* sung by Daniel, with a big jam from everyone to finish.

Great appreciation from audience, and after the gig the band really generous to each other – lots of mutual appreciation and congratulations. Although seemingly stolen bass is okay in the end, it

> highlights some of the problems the band still has, and the strain of these events for Sarah. [Gary's log, 22 April 2008].

These log excerpts both make it clear what the benefits and the challenges of 'away gigs' are. The event is empowering to the musicians, and the process of working on the programme and performing within a context where their standard of performance counts and is acknowledged serves to raise their game as a band. The public nature of it, albeit still in a mental health context here, also serves to enact certain messages about stigma, capability, talent and the ability of users to provide things for each other (something that stands in contrast to the overall culture of the day in general, which retains a real us/them feel between professionals and users). It's music that breaks down the barriers, roles, stigma and prejudices. SMART Band experience themselves as *musicians* first and foremost – and are appreciated and perceived as this in return by fellow users and mental health professionals.

***

These issues of identity and stigma are also strongly shown up by the other first outside gig by the *Singers*. The concert series in the atrium of the nearby general hospital is a long-running event at 1pm on Wednesday lunchtimes. Through an informal contact with the arts co-ordinator who manages the concert series Sarah gets an invitation for SMART Singers. They prepare and rehearse with great seriousness and application for this important gig for several months before, and it gives an important focus and impetus for both rehearsing and for getting their standard up to a suitable level. It really matters to the group that they come over at their very best. Related to this attitude, an interesting dilemma arises amongst the Singers when they are asked to confirm the publicity material for the concert. The performers at this lunchtime concert series are a very mixed bunch usually – students from the nearby Royal College of Music, professional and semi-professional soloists and small ensembles ranging over classical, folk, jazz and world styles. The conversation amongst the Singers – which gets heated at times – is how to describe themselves: as just 'SMART Singers', or as 'SMART Singers from the mental health charity SMART'. Some members want their performance also to be an exercise in anti-stigmatising, an advocacy for the capability of people with mental health problems to perform in regular cultural venues. Others – who are in the process of recovery and nervous in case their mental health status prejudice future employment – are less sure they want the label 'mental health' stated in relation to the performance. In the end suitable reassurances are given to the musicians that individual names will not be used, and the billing in the Spring/Summer Hospital Arts leaflet is as follows:

SMART SINGERS – The singers from St Mary Abbot Rehabilitation and Training community mental health project meet weekly to explore singing together; learning new songs, enjoying singing old favourites, writing their own songs and performing at local events.

***

SMART Singers lunchtime gig in the hospital Atrium – 19 June 2008

It's been a big build-up to this one – the first 'non mental health' performance in SMART Singers' history! They've worked progressively and steadily to build up both repertoire, and the performance standard ready for this concert. Members have themselves selected solo and group items. It's probably the first group of its kind that this hospital concert series has seen – amateurs who are also facing another challenge in their lives.

Gather at 11.30am in Willow for warm-up. All of us smartly dressed in black-and-white dress code, with polished shoes ... fantastic! Last-minute tensions and flaps over music folders, where to stand etc., but this is usual to any choir. Take ourselves and equipment over to hospital, set up the performance space under the escalators – a challenging very public space with a bad acoustic, but loads of people naturally passing by. Audience gather – hospital patients, visitors and staff, Willow and SMART staff, users and friends (Tia also there). A man on the bed arrives from a ward with his wife. Then we're off:

Anything Goes – lively group number with semi-improvised humming to begin with – so we can warm voices up, test the acoustic and deal with performance nerves. Works fine, but projection is difficult without amps and the background noise, but we manage. We realise that we need to get closer together as the sound basically goes straight up the building! At the piano I find it quite hard to hear the singing and the audience were hearing more piano than singing! So we rapidly adjust to this environment with a bit of quick cueing ...

Dona Nobis Pacem – this quiet, unaccompanied two-part round is difficult in this environment, but also makes people listen differently. I look over and see the old man in the bed mouthing the words – 'give us peace' – his wife holding his hand. An impossibly moving moment!

In *Steal away* and *Rhythm of life* everyone in the group has a bit of a solo role.

Streets of London – Roger does this solo, with harmonica break, which wafts around the lofty architecture and attracts more people down and round the performance area.

Michael sings one of his own songs, accompanying himself on the guitar. A fragile feel to his performance, but interestingly this is where wider participation seems to start. He encourages audience to do an offbeat

> clap, Ella picks this up and amplifies it, and a few other people pick it up too (especially a man with a little daughter who's had a medical procedure that morning). Michael gets big applause, something's happening now ...
>
> There was an important sense today of 'we're doing this for ourselves, in fact we've already done it because we've prepared for the occasion' followed by 'this is for everyone else, we've made an effort for our audience'. How extraordinary when I'm so aware of the medical system in mental health where everyone is viewed individually – how they function, behave, etc. In contrast, there's a special phenomenon when I try to encourage people towards each other, so as not to be functioning just individually. This creates not just cohesion, communication and community, but also individual self-development, and autonomous decisions and actions too ...
>
> It's a triumph – everyone's happy and proud – because of bringing it off, but also for me because of the quality of the music-making ... [Sarah's log, 19 June, 2008]

***

> The programme is eclectic and varied – style, performers, degrees of seriousness, and cultural reference. Despite all of the challenges of the situation, somehow it really works with this audience, this place and time – they both listen and join in. I can see and feel a *gathering process* happen – people stop and stay for a while, come out of doors (and presumably listen upstairs from balconies). There's an audience of about 50 people eventually (I learn later from the arts coordinator that this is more than usual). She also says that the style of participation in our concert is different from usual when they have students from a music college, or semi-professionals. Partly the greater participation comes from the more informal and spirited performance style; partly I think it's a response to the fragility and 'incompleteness' of the performance, and this gives permission for other people to step in, help out perhaps? [Gary's log, 19 June, 2008]

***

Tia has described the same event in detail from another angle in Book One of this triptych, *Music Asylums* (DeNora 2013a, Chapter 7). She remembers the moment, over lunch, after the main concert, when the Singers were discussing their amusement that an audience member had mistaken them for a choir of hospital staff. The irony was rich and it was productive: mistaken identity proved that the Singers could 'pass' (and under conditions that might vex the nerves of any group of singers). That 'passing' was itself an object lesson. It told the Singers (and the rest of us) that wellness, the mien of confidence, skill and – especially in this performance situation – adroitness in reaching out to, and connecting with, an audience was in their gift, their gift to give. Tia has written about how this moment was both catalytic for the Singers' identity and self-perception (individual/collective). It also provides an incident that can be used to think about the question of what 'good music' might mean, where and for whom. At the time of its making, this was the best music there was because the situation it created (the 'fragility and incompleteness' that Gary describes above, which created an open-ended, participatory aesthetic) collected disparate bystanders; it created the possibility for something made together as opposed to something simply witnessed. The event involved some high stakes moments – skilfully scaffolded through by careful preparation. It was, arguably, a milestone, a way of marking off part of the journey and thus the path of this group and its members.

***

Directly following the concert comes another more spontaneous triumph for these musicians. Part of the agreement Sarah had made with the hospital arts co-ordinator is that after the public concert the Singers would go up to a few of the wards and repeat some of the song for patients who couldn't get down to the concert. So the Singers, and SMART 'friends' such as Gary and Tia trail up a few floors and begin on one of the long-stay medical wards:

> The Singers repeat bits from the concert, some unaccompanied, some with digital piano. This kind of work can be embarrassing as I know from experience – you go into a ward wondering whether you're wanted. But interestingly the Singers are more used to being in a patient role themselves, and at being in hospitals – so they approach the patients in bed in a natural, kind way, without embarrassment. I realise that *they* are the experts here!
>
> *First ward* – two very sick ladies respond well to us. In another bay we sing a single song to young man. At the third bay we sing a spiritual at the request of one of the men, after which one says 'the end of that sounds like *Swing Low Sweet Chariot*, and so we burst spontaneously into this – it's like SMART Music on Thursday transplanted to this ward. The other men start singing with us, and Tia says that she has tears in her eyes by the time we finished.
>
> It's somewhat of a revelation to me how professionally and humanely SMART Singers are able to function in this environment – their human touch, but also the kind of musical spontaneity and responsiveness that Sarah and I have cultivated professionally, but they seem to have naturally in a way.
>
> Overall the fascination of this event is how successfully the Singers were able to elicit communication and response from others – both in the concert and on the ward singing. They have a particular expertise – not necessarily conventional musical polish, but a spirit that draws others' response. Perhaps it's their very fragility and vulnerability themselves that creates this response

from others? But this is at the heart of a very human form and valuable form of musical communication. [Gary's log, 19 June, 2008]

***

Fast-forward five years … to **10 June 2013.** SMART Singers are back at this hospital for another lunchtime concert. In the intervening years they've done two recitals most years – just before Christmas, and in the early summer. Some of the Singers have remained stalwarts throughout this time, and have considerably increased their confidence to perform, in some cases their tolerance of a broader repertoire, and an increased ability to collaborate with the other singers in rehearsals and performances. They've also simply enjoyed both the process and the occasional successful products of their work. Others singers have come and gone according to the pace of their recovery, or how they've been associated with SMART. But like many other choirs and musical ensembles, something of the core style and spirit of *SMART Singers* is constant throughout the years and pervades their performances, even as the membership and repertoire shifts. Some of this continuity is of course due to the skill and ethos that Sarah brings to the group. It's another example of how continuity of provision in this area of helping people with mental health problems is crucial. There's also the ambassadorial function: SMART Singers have a local following, people who regularly come to the hospital concerts know them, and like them. They advocate superbly for the crucial notion of *wellness within illness:*

Before going to see the lunchtime concert in the hospital this Monday in June 2013 I've been ploughing through the 1500 pages of data about the SMART Music project – so both the project and the people are very much in mind! Although I'm not longer directly involved the project I have rich memories of people and events like the one I'm about to see. Preparing for the gig today has evidently been slightly fraught as due to various unexpected events it's already been cancelled once, but fortuitously it's also caught the best of the current grouping of SMART Singers – Sylvie, Claire, Liliana, Jeremy, Mario. They really go for it today! The continuity of both this lunchtime event, and the style of performance strikes me, coming in as I do very occasionally now. There are lots of old friends and supporters there in the 'audience' – Paul and Jo from Willow, Phil the psychologist, and Janet, Dr M's secretary.

The Singers really bring the concert off – both musically, and in the unique way that these people can do for a health venue in particular – they've got spirit and heart, and it communicates and draws others in.

There's also new repertoire, including a Coldplay song, *Viva La Vida,* and *We are the Champions* at the end. Sylvie later links these choices to the fight all of the Singers are having at the moment with the new government benefit changes, and their struggle to manage. The songs they sang, Sylvie says, are all about power and strength. And in itself it's a performance of empowerment and strength in adversity (as it also is for many of the people in this hospital – patients, relatives and staff alike).

As I'm sitting there in the audience I suddenly get the feeling that 'all the world' is somehow flowing by during this performance. There's a surreal moment in the middle of *Fields of Gold*, happening along the three sides of the hospital corridors which enclose the performance area, when I suddenly see simultaneously:

- A toddler in mum's arms clapping perfectly in time to the music, with other people noting this and smiling.
- An old lady in a wheelchair swaying her hand to the music, caught by the melody, transported ...
- A woman on a bed, wheeled by, with a newborn baby in her arms, an anxious husband in tow. She looks over towards the singers and smiles.

Each mini-scenario is captured and connected somehow by the music, and the energy and goodwill of this performance – all of us drawn together within this remarkable scene.

Mario's sister watches her brother singing with such pride. It's one of the few things he can do equally with others, she says after. Later, the new Polish lady, Liliana, in the Singers (a lawyer, amateur pianist) tells me of her chance finding of the group – through meeting another member. She said how she'd fallen into a severe depression a year ago, and that it's been the music that has lifted it, and taken her back into life again. And then through this experience she's dared to get back to playing the piano again, she's now playing in a trio with other Polish people. Depression, she said led her back to music. This, she said, was what she thought her depression was about ultimately – to show her that music needed to be in her life again, or else she'd become ill.

I see Sarah's amazing talent and technique anew today, in both the macro and micro aspects of facilitating this group, this music, and this situation. From, for example, coping with Jeremy's idiosyncratic timing to also mobilising these people in the music within this special occasion, with everything else going on in its gloriously messy but harmonious way.

I'm very moved by my return to this project today – seeing and feeling how the heart of the project beats in events such as this. The event is important in itself, for us here and now. But it's also part of something much larger and very fruitful that's happened over six years in this location, with this musical mental health community. It's exemplary of what can happen ... [Gary's log, 10 June 2013]

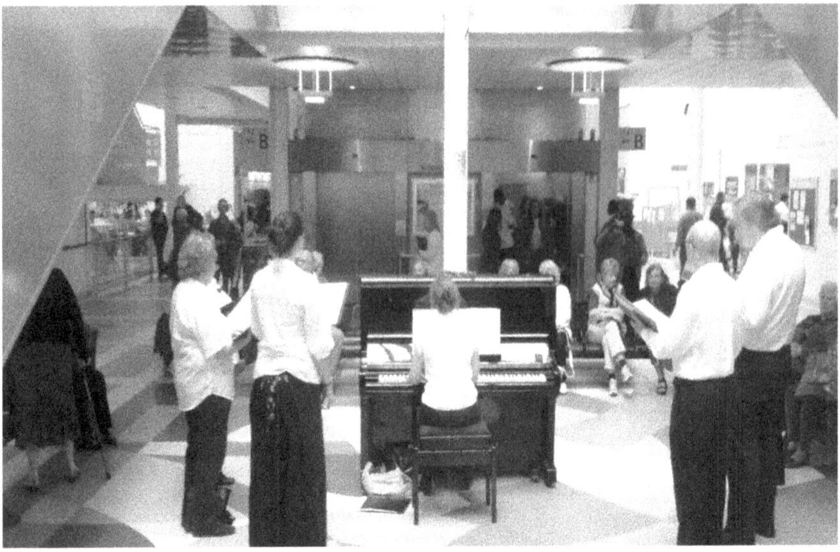

Figure 9 SMART Singers performing in the general hospital atrium

41. Interlude

The last four sections will step back from the action a little, and take a slightly more synoptic view of the music project. To an extent this has been a pioneering project, and we were honoured to receive the 2008 Royal Society for Public Health Arts & Health Award in recognition of this. Both SMART and the music project continue to thrive to this day (we will include a 'catch-up to date' section by Sarah Wilson at the end of this book). In addition to the valuable week-by-week practical outcomes of the project there have also been the substantial fruit of our growing understanding of how, where, and when music can help people in this situation. We've tried to listen to what the project and its participants have been able to tell us.

In our attempts to understand we've been continually careful to balance our own perceptions and understandings as practitioners and researchers alongside those of the project members, and to look for ways in which they can also 'step back' and make sense of the dense pattern that the project has woven over the years.

42. Exemplary of What Can Happen

Many of the musical events described in the last section showed up or exemplified aspects of the project at several levels – which is just what we'd expect and hope for from an ecological perspective. A musical pebble dropped into the pond – whether this is an individual gesture, or a collective accomplishment – often amplifies across several levels of the ecology. We find in this way that some of the key musical events:

- Exemplified SMART's overall values and virtues: of community and conviviality; creativity and collaboration; support and tolerance; spirit and fun; creativity and musicianship; respect, appreciation, passion, enthusiasm …
- Exemplified a staging-post in the developmental story of SMART Music and its three core activities (SMART Music, Singers, Band) in terms of how each group both performs its integration, identity and functioning, but then also demonstrates their fluid *interaction* for creative purposes – to support a song, to allow a members' song to be realised, to pave the next step of a musical pathway, or perhaps simply to create better music for that situation, there and then.
- Exemplified the musical-social aesthetic that the musicians, the audience and the situation co-creates: a musical party that is totally fun, and totally serious at the same time; that portrays the musical pathway building of individuals, and of groups …

As we've described previously, SMART underwent a significant change in culture a year or so after the music project started. A new Chief Executive, Amelia, describes to Gary in her interview for the research project how after a few weeks of witnessing the various groups of the music project she realised how they enacted exactly the kind of philosophy and value system she was looking for. It was there already – musically – and this could stand as an exemplary model for how she wanted the place to shape up overall:

> **Amelia:** I got into the job, and there was a lot of good stuff here … but it felt really institutionalised. Um, it felt like people were just sitting around not doing much. I was desperately looking for something that I could grab onto and build, and that's, when I first heard the first music session, that's when it hit me. That was the energy I wanted throughout the organisation … […] It was brilliant, it was an expression of cultures, and ideas and unity. It just felt fantastic, and that was the atmosphere I wanted, it felt liberating. And it didn't feel that the walls were confining, this space wasn't confined anymore, it wasn't institutionalising people. […] By grabbing onto the music and saying look this is what this can be, this is what we can do, it was much easier for me to make the changes. It was easier for me to understand people, and understand members, and kind of hook into that. […] When I saw the music it was, well actually, that's already doing it. That's doing the job. That's the draw, that's what makes people want to come here, and that's what stops it being an institution. And, yeah the rules are now really flexible. It feels like people can move in and out of SMART at their own pace, do what they want to do, drop in and out, but take something

> precious away with them and use that. And that musical pathway, like you say, we do get people in next door from the mental health unit. And I think maybe before they were coming here, but not as many as should have been. And then they were getting stuck here. And I think the music's kind of opened the gates on either side. [...] [So] bear in mind that my philosophy about this place has grown *from* the music, so I have taken my leave from you guys. [Amelia, interview with Gary, October 2008]

We think it's worth commenting here that just as SMART Music members themselves turned to music as an exemplar of how to be well, so too Amelia turned to SMART Music as an exemplar of what SMART – the wider organisation – could do well ('By grabbing onto the music and saying look this is what this can be.'). So the music project seems to exemplify: (i) an attitude about people in relation to their illness *and* their current/potential health; (ii) a practical way of working with and on this principle; (iii) outcomes that align with the principle. It does this, we suggest, through:

1. A clear 'therapeutic principle' – which is based on the Nordoff Robbins /Community Music Therapy belief that everyone has a dimension of themself that is still healthy (within seemingly quite severe illness or incapacity). This shows itself through a core musicality (a psychobiological capacity) that can be called-out and cultivated as a creative capability through musicianship (a socio-cultural facility), and further elicited in situations through active *musicking*. The 'therapeutic principle' is not one of treatment, but of 'guided accompaniment' (different with different people, problems and settings, but always based on 'being musicians together' and adding therapeutic judgement, intervention and reflexive thinking when/as required by the needs of clients/situations).

2. A genuine activity, which aligns well with SMART's core founding model of recovery through purposeful activity. This serves as a platform for working on inclusion, bridging and development – of people ideally flowing *through* SMART rather than sticking there, through being helped to access forms of social and cultural support and benefit in the wider community. Importantly, what happens in the three music groups is not artificial 'recovery activities' but things that members *want* to do, but which also involve the key factors of recovery: (re)making relationships and networks, (re)finding skills, capabilities and opportunities, performing and finding fresh confidence and hope.

3. Creating realistic and real outcomes – which are as varied in scale as not sitting in the same place all week in the cafe, doing something different through music, doing something different with other people, finding a sense of achievement and identity, making a bridge to a choir outside SMART, or having the courage to perform again in a jazz club.

As SMART becomes more like Amelia envisions it, and more in step with up-to-date thinking in mental health, the music project continues to be treated as exemplary. Amelia and her staff are up front about scheduling visitors and potential donors on a Thursday afternoon when SMART Music is in full flow. She wants them to witness the 'buzz' of this: the energy, involvement, commitment, self-advocacy and relative independence that this event mostly portrays and conveys to others. She treats it, that is, as exemplary practice.

Such practice aligns well with the increasing popularity of the development of the 'recovery model' in UK mental health policy and practice over the years of the music project. But although the fit is indeed good, there's another dimension that the music project exemplifies which challenges the reovery model in its more ideological articulations, especially as the practical consequences of this policy begin to show across the site we are researching. Within mental health services hospital settings are now almost exclusively for acute admissions, where high-pressure outcome-based work is done on symptoms to stabilise people to get *out* of hospital as quickly as possible. 'Recovery' work then becomes a way of keeping people out of medical settings and services, something that is good in itself but has consequences for a whole constituency of people who have been struggling with mental health problems over decades of their lives. There seems to be, that is, a 'missing middle' in the pattern of care for people who have a chronic illness, and who do not recover quickly and simply re-assimilate into society, but need an on-going supportive community within on-going mental health services. For these people such services are a benign and necessary form of asylum, maintaining their health and hope. The dilemma is how to keep within on-going services a way of still finding wellness *within* illness. This is 'health maintenance work', and we would suggest that the SMART Music project is a good exemplar of this: providing services whilst empowering users, helping keep people well, encouraging and supporting them to do the things that maintain and enhance their wellbeing. What we might call 'creative asylum' acknowledges the need for a place and activity that is both safe *and* challenging; that accepts the reality of chronic illness, whilst also paving pathways outwards and between (at whatever scale and scope individual people can manage). Such a service needs to be accessible and constant as a long-term, secure provision.

We feel that the music project exemplifies something of such a 'missing middle' model of services for people with enduring mental health problems in how:

- it doesn't over-pathologise people, but at the same time acknowledges their illness, and their struggle with recovery/wellness.
- works long term where necessary with people's long-term passion for / relationship with music (as one of the key motivations and resources that carries on keeping people well(er).
- helps assemble the practical and people resources for on-going and developing musicking.
- allows for long-term constancy in personal and therapeutic relationships and formats, and creating space for movement and development

- helps people *keep hold of music* even when they temporarily change venue or health status (going back into hospital, coming back to SMART etc.).
- helps forge and maintain recovery pathways which are real but also scaled and realistic.

We will explore this issue of the relationship between the project and mental health thinking and policy in more depth in Part III.

43. What is Good Musicking?

> When we get excited about something in music that we love, we are excited about what it affords, what it stands for, what it lets us be. Music is always even at its most apparently neutral, social performance and ethically charged. […] Goodness in music is goodness from music … ' [DeNora 2013a: 131]

> It's not just the noise and energy – it's also a sense of the kind of anarchic cornucopia of music – of all types, all standards, all going into some crazy music mix, which in this place is entirely natural (though anywhere else it would be odd in the extreme). I suppose I'm back to the aesthetics/ethics theme again – the 'good musicking' that happens overall, and seemingly incorporates and cancels out rather extreme contrasts, opposites etc. [Gary's log, Nov 5 2009].

What has the project shown us about music, and the vexed but key twin questions *What is good music? Good musicking?* And why do these questions matter in this particular context? Several aspects come under this general umbrella of the relationship between ethics and aesthetics (or *'aesth/ethics'* – though this is easier to write than to say!):

1. **What's good in music? Who says?** Two questions that are constantly considered, puzzled over, and negotiated within the musical activities of the project over the 10 years.
2. **What are the musical-social goods and values that flow from musicking?** such as appreciation, recognition, respect, support, belonging, generosity, conviviality, celebration, etc.
3. **How can musicking help with 'ethical life'?** the role that musicking plays in everyday social exchange, negotiation, conflict resolution and creative change in people and communities.

How do these three areas of question play out within the particular needs, challenges and potential exemplary conduct of the people at SMART, and for the community of SMART as a whole? Is music any different from any other ethical good?

***

> The music afternoon at *SMART* cafe is hosting a visit from a music group in the East End of London called Musical Minds. For the first half of the afternoon, each group has performed a set, with the other group as the audience. After the tea break, we revisit some songs from the first half of the afternoon, with both groups singing together this time. We then ask if anyone has special requests.
>
> Hester asks to sing a favourite jazz standard, *If You Asked Me I Could Write A Book*, and as the song is being announced, Luke pops up, enthusiastically says, 'I love this song', and is up at the front asking whether he can sing it with Hester. She seems fine with this, but because they are dramatically different heights there's some fuss for a few minutes arranging the height of the microphone they need to share!
>
> So there's some pre-negotiation and accommodation before starting the song, and then increasingly more negotiation is necessary as the song goes on. It's clear that, although they both know the song well, there's a basic difference in how they usually sing it. Luke has a 'laidback' delivery – strongly behind the beat – whilst Hester 'swings' it yet is basically *with* the beat. The first verse is somewhat awkward for both, as they realise what's happening, but they find it hard to change their style and preference and accommodate to the other to produce a single performance. Luke looks at Hester with puzzled sideways glances, drops out periodically for a phrase, then joins her again, catching up by pinpointing a particular phrase that they can more easily 'get together'.
>
> Gary is accompanying this on the piano as a kind of 'musical host', attempting to arbitrate the increasingly obvious performance-style differences between the two singers. In order to help this situation, he changes his accompaniment to a 'rhythmicised' delivery for verse two – which is a conscious move to subvert both of their habitual renderings of the song and get them to listen a bit more to each other (via listening to 'what's new' in the piano). To an extent this works, as both singers jointly converge on a third way of singing the song, which then allows others in the audience to more comfortably join in. Hester and Luke end the song together, shake hands, and smile towards the audience.

As the therapists, Sarah and Gary take overall responsibility for the afternoon going well, whilst not wanting to control it. Luke is also a member of the hosting group, but at the moment before the song starts Hester also becomes a host of sorts too. She's at the microphone first when Luke asks to duet, and she politely invites him to join her – though, of course, it would be socially difficult for her to say 'no' in these circumstances. During the song itself, there's a complex musical-social process of mutual attention, accommodation and response within the ongoing navigation and negotiation of the performance. None of us wants a 'breakdown' with its embarrassment for either host or guest, so we all try to keep the show on the road despite the emerging difficulties. Hester and Luke are helped in this on-the-spot musical repair work by the non-conscious, 'natural' process of 'collaborative musicking' that adjusts the intersubjective musical timing and spacing between them such that they (just) keep together. But there's also the more conscious musical strategy Gary employs to help this negotiation, using his music therapist's toolkit for keeping people within music.

This scenario highlights the ambiguities and complexities of musical hospitality – how something personal or social is usually at stake within musicking, and how this automatically brings ethics and etiquette into play too. Occasions of musical hospitality such as performing with others often involve tricky 'moral moments' when there's a tension between inviting others into a shared space, being open to what they have to give, and not losing your own needs, wishes or integrity. This vignette can stand for hundreds of similar moments where aesthetics and ethics jostle each other, but also often serve as a natural everyday template to reflect on the broader SMART ethos and principles of hospitality, respect, acceptance, negotiation and compromise.

Aesth/ethics

A postmodern view of ethics suggests that without firm, traditional religious or imposed political foundations, we need to improvise them ourselves, through dialogue and dispute about our values, and in response to those ever-fluid situations where we are challenged personally and communally to an ethical demand that we must approve of, and act towards. The paradigmatic ethical situation today is perhaps when we face someone directly, and face up to their claim on us, and our response-ability to them – framed by the questions: 'What is good, here and now, with this person? What then should I do?'. Cobussen and Nielsen (2012) talk of 'doing justice' to a person, a work of art, a situation – or the multiple relationships between these three. How do we 'do justice' in and through musical work?

Increasingly music has been used to provide a reflective template for ethical thinking (Cobussen and Nielsen 2013; DeNora 2013a; Sennett 2004; Becker 2000). For example, the jazz musician and philosopher Garry Hagberg writes that 'jazz underscores this fact of ethical life – the flux of our moral interactions with self and others' (2011, p. 282). The face-to-face spontaneous interactions of jazz players are backed up by a 'musical etiquette' that has evolved to guide successful playing together. This informal 'code' consists of an attention to the relational and social quality of the immediate and local situation:

'What, jazz improvisation asks, is happening in *this* moment, with *these* people, in *this* setting, under *these* conditions? Given that *this* musical gesture has been made in *this* circumstance, what is *possible* now? Jazz improvisation indeed shows within its practice how much attention we should give to the complexities of real moral questions, real moral moments, people, settings conditions, and circumstances.' (Hagberg 2011, p. 282)

Hagberg suggests that musical groups inevitably evoke 'moral moments' as players strive to:

- listen, attend, notice and acknowledge others and their gestures – both musical and paramusical;
- utter and answer (with responsiveness and responsibility) in order to help and support others, and to keep the performance going;
- demonstrate respect for another's difference and autonomy;
- attempt to understand others' immediate action: where they are 'coming from', are 'going to' (even when this conflicts with their own trajectory);
- remain authentic in gesture and response;
- attempt to balance self against others so that mutual respect is demonstrated in the balance and flow of the ensemble;
- tolerate and work with tension, conflict of direction, immediate confusion, and to trust in the emergence of mutual flow ...

Together, this is a tall moral order for any player. But this list of musicking virtues also underwrites the social values and principles of most participatory musics – and it contrasts sharply with those 'presentational' styles that are mostly concerned with delivering a perfect product. This brings us to the interesting territory of how ethics and aesthetics relate within musicking. A participatory perspective is by nature more interested in 'good musicking' than in 'good music'. That is to say, the goodness of a musical event is defined in terms of the quality of the relational experiences of participants and the overall social enhancement achieved. But is it too simple to separate out 'good musicking' from 'good music'?

A further step in this direction of musical ethics is the question of what musical conduct might afford the practice of moral conduct itself (not just the fact that to an extent it mirrors it). Is it possible that musicking actively encourages certain ethical attitudes and practices?

The sociologist and jazz pianist Howard Becker suggests that etiquette is 'particularly important when people think that everyone involved in some situation *ought* to be equal but really isn't' (2000, p. 176). Richard Sennett, another sociologist and amateur musician, makes this issue the central concern of his book *Respect* (2004), which tackles the huge dilemma of how to reconcile inequality and respect. In our age of centrally organised welfare and treatment, people often feel disrespected. The way that they get the help they need becomes part of their problem. The etymology of 'respect' tells us that it's to do with being *seen* in the right way.[1] But we might also think of the crucial aspect of how someone feels they are being heard or, more accurately, *listened to*. Certainly someone can diminish you by looking away, but the way you are attentively listened to is surely central to feeling really respected.

The 'problem' of inequality is structured into most of our relationships, both personal and professional. But in therapy or teaching such 'structural' asymmetries can be compensated by mutuality in face-to-face interactions. Sennett's point is that you cannot respect a person by just intending to do so; it's something that needs to happen in practice: 'Respect is an expressive performance ... in social life as in art, mutuality requires expressive work. It must be enacted, performed' (2004 pp. 207/59). Here Sennett draws on his experience as a performing musician, playing cello over the years in many chamber music groups. He asks us to imagine the problems the

---

1 From *respicere* (Latin) – 'to look back at', 'to regard'.

players have preparing Brahms' Clarinet Quintet for performance. The piece involves the rapid sharing of musical material between players, which means that the players must solve the problem of balancing the parts and co-ordinating the flux of musical gestures that weave in and out of the musical texture. How is this all worked out, 'made good'? 'They do so', suggests Sennett, 'by inventing rituals for performing together' (2004, p. 213). These musical rituals start in rehearsal when each player gives attention to both the notes and the gestures conveyed by the others' eyes and bodies in order to assemble their musical togetherness and shared understanding of the piece. These rituals are then carried over into the more charged space and time of the performance itself, where their respectful practice helps to ensure a 'good performance' for all.

This model of musical collaboration in action encourages us to think about the broader problem of helping whilst respecting, and how this might mutually be accomplished by *both* helper and helped if thought about differently than usual. Musicking is collaborative respect in action. The specifically musical phenomenology of respect involves the careful 're-*hearing*' of a person – in their wholeness and potential – and then the acting alongside them. It involves attending to all dimensions of a person, not just to first or surface impressions. This can allow a particular kind of freedom, for both helper and helped.

Adapted from Ansdell (2014a), pp. 11–14; 302; Ansdell (2014b)

A wide variety of 'good and valuable things' flow from the musicking in SMART: basic personal/social goods such as contact, communication, relationship and community – all of which we might group together under Simon Procter's (2011, 2013) term 'musical capital'. This necessary resource accrues particularly through musical *work* within SMART Music, Singers and Band. But, put the other way round, (and from a music-centred position) these 'social goods' come not because people *pursue* them – for example, coming to SMART to 'make a relationship' through music – but rather because they *ensue* because of the immediate demands of musicking with others. People are motivated to come and make music, and then the demands of good musicking involve modes of awareness, contact and negotiating relationship (entrainment, shared direction) and togetherness (synchrony). The musicking is in this way an *indirect means* to personal and social goods, one that for the people in SMART does not smack of the latest mental health treatment theory that promotes 'communicative behaviours' or 'bonding and bridging outcomes'. The purpose is simply to *make good music,* for oneself and others.

A 'secondary' menu of 'good things' then flows from the getting into musical communication and community: the social virtues of appreciation, recognition, respect, trust, support, belonging, generosity, conviviality, celebration, etc. None of these are exclusively musical, but as paramusical features of musical occasions they are potential entailments of *good musicking*. They are also directly related to basic human psycho-social needs, to the pleasures of living, but also often to some of the 'problems of living' experienced by people with mental health difficulties.

In this way the relationship between the music project and the wider ethical agenda of a mental health community such as SMART becomes clear. Amelia talks in detail in her interview about the connections between illness and behaviour, and how this relates to the everyday management of SMART as a functioning community. The organisation has a strict ethical code: you are responsible for your actions even when you're ill; and if you can't control behaviour that is unhelpful to others' mental health you must get medical help for your symptoms until you can. On the positive side, such an explicit code of ethical conduct is modeled and encouraged: people are at SMART to be good to each other. What helps this is in turn helpful to everyone's wellbeing. One of the reasons that Amelia clearly sees the music project as exemplary is in relation to this implicit and indirect modelling of being good to each other – music and musicking seems to help this quite naturally, and to communicate shared 'values' in an implicit way.

So 'good musicking' and 'being good' interact and often merge. But of course not in always unproblematic ways – there are conflicts about both 'good music' and 'trying to be good in/through music'. Musicking in SMART frames and re-frames ethical responsibility (responsiveness as a capacity and an action) in sometimes particularly useful ways – especially when the additional framing is a reflexive therapeutic one that is actively considering the reciprocal aspects of health/illness, history and context on the situation of the moment. What we might call 'ethical trouble' comes up in the music groups as it will in any interpersonal or social situation when there are 'demands for responsibility' (in a micro-moment of musicking, or within or a larger issue). Sarah, Gary or other SMART staff attempt to help the musicians work through these ethical moments – as far as possible in relation to the musicking itself. That is, they are treated as paramusical rather than 'behavioural'.

***

Bobby complains that 'it's just noise' in the Thursday afternoon session. He especially doesn't like Eloise 'banging away on the cymbal' when he's trying to do some more subtle drumming on the djembe. The irony here is that Bobby's own drumming is the source of aesthetic trouble within the early days of the Band – where his heavy and enthusiastic style overwhelms others' more subtle playing and annoys the others. So we see here how the statement 'That's not music!' is importantly not just to do with taste preferences (styles, idioms, repertoire) but also with *ways of playing* that are directly or indirectly related to modes of awareness, sensitivity, flexibility etc. (which may or may not in turn be related to illness states and/or substance misuse etc.). Then there's Daniel's 'that's not *good* music' issue, mostly with the Band, but relating to the whole of the musical situation at SMART. His high musical standards for himself also affect others. His frustrations with the Band are at least partly to do with Daniel's expressed opinion that if they're not able to make 'good music' then there's no point playing. Whereas for most of the other musicians the simple pleasure of playing together at whatever standard they can muster is the chief aim. A paradox here is that it's exactly the 'high standard' of Daniel's musicianship and performances that are inspiring and important to people in the SMART community. In the first round of interviews canvassing people's opinions about the music at SMART Daniel is probably the most cited as someone who is admired and who gives pleasure to others through his music. His 'good musicking' clearly does good many times over the years. But his often inflexible notion of musical standards is sometimes problematic in this context – for himself and others.

So we're back to the territory of 'good' in a fuzzy variety of ways: as (i) a value judgement of what's preferred/tolerated/appreciated, but (ii) in relation to modes of conduct that are related to the judgement of (i); leading to (iii) outcomes that are somehow a composite of aesth/ethics aspects.

In SMART we've seen many times a moral theme of people simply wanting to become better people. There's often a moral-existential force in their struggle with themselves, others and the world. Music can, and often does, help with this struggle. Making music is often a help in making something good, something better – for the sake of 'it' (music), but also simultaneously within ourselves, between ourselves and others, *for* ourselves and others. Roger's story is a good example of this:

Transcription of Roger's talk – Workshop at Mental Health Users' Meeting – May 2010

Roger: I want to talk about a few things ... starting off with early musical experience ... this is a little bit of my life! Paul Robeson, Billy Cotton, Frankie Lane ... and then in my teens, Elvis Presley, Jerry Lee Lewis, Chuck Berry ... in fact most rock 'n roll! School experience ... well, it was a very prescriptive regime – I was chucked out of the school choir because I tried to sing like Paul Robeson! I didn't want to sound like a girl you see! Music lessons were dictatorial and very old-fashioned ... there was no attempt to tutor or coach us in any way – music was treated as a bolt-on to the rest of the curriculum. The only music we were allowed to play was recorders – we sounded *dreadful!*

While I was staying at St Bernards Hospital – the mental hospital – in about 1970, one of the inmates gave me a harmonica. To my surprise I started to bash out a tune on it! I then spent the next 25 years searching through my record collection trying to find music I could play along with ... Scarcely ever during this time did I get the chance to actually jam with other people ... .

What does music therapy mean for me? I believe it's a way of discovering ... or rather re-discovering the innate properties and qualities of sound ... and therefore music. Also, the art of learning to contribute actively, and/or passively, to the making of music with others, and *for* others. As far as I'm concerned music therapy works!

How has being part of *SMART Singers* helped me? It has played a major part in my development as a human being ... I have noticed that I am now less self-seeking, and more able to listen and take a back-seat. As a result my playing and singing has improved ... .and I'm now a more confident person.

Thank you ... *SMART Singers, SMART Music,* Nordoff Robbins, and all the people that have played music with me!

This is Roger's testimony about his experience of the music project at SMART, given to other mental health service users as part of a workshop SMART Singers did at an event. Roger gives the basics of his musical pathway here, centring around his life-long love and need of music, but only lately flowering in a context where he and his musicking were truly accepted, and where he could learn to play and sing with others. In his interview for the research project Roger goes through similar territory, but expands usefully on a few of these dimensions:

Roger: Basically on paper, and in the world of socio-economic status, I hadn't arrived, I was going nowhere. And I think the music here at SMART, and then subsequently me playing in pubs and doing stuff, and putting on several parties at my place, and realising that yes I could do something. Realising on occasion that I could, dare I say, do it very well.

You're within the setting and I realised when I'm playing that sort of music ... and there's lots of people who can't stand some music but can stand others, but there is quite a lot of overlapping going on ... it reminds me of the Monty Python *Now for Something Completely Different.*

And it's so important to do something alongside what you're doing, so when you go back to say, as it were, your first love, you've been informed differently. And when I get on with the stuff in life that I'm doing normally, I'm probably doing it with more energy, not just grasping ... I'm doing it within a capacity in myself which wasn't, which is possibly better. Or can I say *definitively* better, can I be that brash?

... it took me ages to sing at SMART. I think I said to you 'I think I might want to sing sometime'. And it was *Knocking on Heaven's Door* by Bob Dylan ...

Gary: So you sang for a while on Thursday afternoons ... then Sarah set up the Wednesday groups. So tell me about what happened then?

R: There was the Band on Wednesday. Well there was a personality mismatch there, which I won't enlarge upon. And I withdrew, 'cos I thought this is doing more harm than good, and at the time I did have the outlet of the open-mic, I'd actually run a night at my local pub for some time, which became arduous, because people would turn up and its time to go home, and I'm loading the car up and unloading it. And I felt like a bit of a workhorse in the end. Because I was trying to not be upfront, I was trying to facilitate. And yes it worked very well sometimes, and appallingly the others. Because there's no recipe for deciding how things are going to go.

G: So then after the Band?

R: I'd already been aware that there's a singing group too at SMART, and then I thought, well I got used to coming along on a Wednesday, so I thought I'd come along earlier and I thought well give it a go. Because I was aware sometimes in

> like *You'll Never Walk Alone* … that final high note whatever it is, I don't think it's the highest note that I can do, it's just there was a dead spot and I'd go 'eeeurgh', you know, and I thought 'you gotta work on this' you know. This is acutely embarrassing.
>
> **G:** And that's quite a different group isn't it, from the others. So instead of just singing, you work on things, you work for specific gigs and little performances. Why is that particular group good for you?
>
> **R:** Well, it's good for me because we did get gigs, and to satisfy my sometimes rather energetic ego, I do like, as I call it, showing off in public, and I could give evidence … well probably as a kid I wasn't heard enough, so for me being an eight-year-old kid that no one listened to. But to actually do something quite well and having people, shall we say a number of people, listening, and apparently enjoying all this, is a very powerful connection, very powerful, and it's … it gives me a boost. I like standing up. Once again I have to, but I'm in danger of getting somewhat over-elated by that. And in danger of not entirely listening and hearing what other people are doing. And then, sometimes I go back too far in, and someone will say 'come on'. So I've gotta get that right. Because in playing with a group, this is where I'm sure even the most ordinary youth club/rock band goes on the road, they learn a lot about themselves, they learn a lot about give and take, and the overall flow, which is not always easy to get. Whether it's an orchestra or a group, sometimes it's not quite right. It sounds off, you know? [Interview with Gary, October 2008]

When Roger checked the transcript of the interview he asked that the following was added:

> I would like to firmly state that the process of music therapy at SMART – both Thursday afternoons and *SMART Singers* on Wednesday afternoons – have been immensely helpful and empowering to my personal development. My musical skills have improved – and with this my confidence and – dare I say it – my stage presence! There has also been a marked improvement in the way I 'perform' in a group setting – in the social sense! [2009]

***

A particular incident helps Roger compare his experiences in the SMART Music project with a similar yet different scenario:

> Roger tells us after the session today how he went to a community jazz venue last night for the first time with his harmonica. An established Blues band were playing in an informal setting. They eventually asked Roger if he wanted to join them for a number, but when he played it was rather more difficult than he had

> expected and hoped – he couldn't hear himself, and the band simply played their own routine above and around him. Roger says 'there was no musical generosity there, like there is here in SMART Music'. It seems that nobody in this established band was explicitly giving him a 'playing space', working with *his playing,* so he didn't get a good experience of doing it. Roger was rather conscious of being out of his depth with these musicians, and was embarrassed. The great thing was how he framed this to us – with a positive spin: 'It was good for me to have that experience' says Roger – 'I can be a bit full of myself sometimes, so it's good to be taken down a peg or two ... '. Rather than putting him off, he's realistic, realising that these people are playing a league above him, he resolves to go back and listen next time, see what he can learn. He makes musical friends with them anyway, chatting with them about music and gigs after the playing.
>
> This incident highlights some of our key developing themes – the *musical generosity/hospitality* of SMART Music – and the explicit provision/enactment of musical generosity towards people, and amongst people. This means giving musicians a musical/personal space for performance. Generosity and hospitality is a *specific* thing in music – not just an overall invitation to play (which is what this Blues band offered him). Roger's music pathway is not exclusively following his participation in the SMART Music project (he was doing some of this already). But somehow it's changed some of his attitudes towards himself and music. [Gary's log, 25 Sept 2008]

***

Roger's pathway story mirrors many of the others in its interweaving of several dimensions of the 'good musicking' theme: (i) his desire to *make good music* in relation to his taste preferences, but also the quality of his performance for its own sake; (ii) his desire to make *make good* musicking with others, in the sense of improving or repairing the quality of the enterprise when necessary; and finally (iii) to use music as a way of helping him *be good* as a person in the moral sense.

We believe that this theme of 'good musicking' is somehow central to the value of the music project. As Tia has written elsewhere in relation to thinking about this project and theme:

> From this perspective, goodness emerges as a way of life, linked to collective action and collaboratively, institutionally produced. […]
>
> Loving and caring about music is simultaneously loving and caring about each other, musically mediated: we hold each other dear in and through the ways that we hold our music dear. We love music because we love what it does, what it is about, what it takes and what it means (to us, for us, for its makers, for humanity). When we draw music into our environments, it is because we want to become what music can make us. Music is in this sense, actualising, transformative. (DeNora 2013, 132)

The SMART Music Project has shown us how we need a far wider and more flexible sense of what 'musical goodness' is, where and when it appears, and how it can be cultivated and helped to flourish. Being good, doing good and making good – musically conceived – needs, as Tia has written, 'multiple and local understandings of goodness' (2013: 124), and a notion of such goodness as being a 'locally situated, grounded, property that is performed and emerges relationally in the same ways as does health/illness'. So an answer to the ecologically-oriented questions: *Where and when is music good?* is simply that it's good when it turns out good! But of course *that* is relative to the immediate situation and the people involved in it. And it's a situation in action, in time and place, and where occasional 'trouble' may well also be part of the aesth/ethics story and its musical resolution.

44. The 'Therapy of Non-Therapy'

Is this project music therapy? Are Gary and Sarah working as music therapists? Some traditional music therapists would tend to say 'no' to both these questions based on the evidence we've given in this book. This is because music therapy in many professional contexts has in the last 30 years been based on an individualistic and psychotherapeutic model, in which the word 'therapy' means very specific things, and has very specific working principles, practices and constraints. To a large extent, however, the SMART Music project has been working within an alternative understanding of music therapy characterised by the international Community Music Therapy movement. This has been substantially developing since 2000, and is proving to be increasingly in step both with the needs of clients and the contexts of treatment and care they find themselves in. It also aligns well with a changing philosophical perspective about illness, health, recovery and the relationship between these and music, musical performance, social and cultural inclusion and quite simply the way that music is seen to work and help people (more about this in Part III).

The logs for this project are peppered with comments and reflections on the theme of whether and how this project can sit under the umbrella of 'music therapy', as Sarah and Gary wrestle with the questions and everyday dilemmas that arise from the project in relation to their role, responsibility, past experience and 'theories' of music therapy, and their developing understanding of what the project and its members are teaching them.For insights into this theme Gary and Sarah have necessarily relied on the mirror of other commentators to give reflections on how they came across, what they did, etc., (as they were by definition 'insiders' to their own practice). The 'outsiders' were SMART members, Amelia, and Tia – who characterises something important about the whole of the project in writing about a 'non-therapeutic therapy', or 'the therapy of non-therapy' (DeNora 2013, pp. 91–2).

***

When in 2005 Gary approaches SMART with the offer of establishing some active music they say yes please, but not music *therapy*, because 'we don't do therapy here'. This was perhaps a cultural and territorial thing at the time – 'therapy' being *over there* in the hospital, and associated with drug therapy and the psychiatric model. SMART was a haven from 'all of that', offering a social and occupational solution for members' mental health difficulties. Gary's solution was to say 'let's not call it therapy, let's just say it's SMART Music'. He was clear, however, that he would still be known as 'Gary the music therapist', partly because having worked in the hospital setting for the past six years, many members in SMART already knew him in this role. He also kept the role for professional reasons. Sarah and Gary were clear (both from professional instinct, and in relation to evolving thinking in the Community Music Therapy movement) that whilst the shape that 'music therapy' took was a variable feast according to need and situation it was important that they maintained their identity, role and professional identity as *music therapists.* This sustained a professional responsibility to help guide and facilitate the project in collaboration with members, but also to keep trying to understand what happened to it as a whole, and to individual people on their musical pathways – in order ensure optimal outcomes.

More specifically the role of music therapist carries responsibility for 'safety' as a first priority. Sarah and Gary are trained to facilitate the best and minimise the worst in relation to situations where music can both be helpful, but can also catalyse challenging responses. They don't always get it right of course, but they have enough training and experience to anticipate difficulties, deal with them as best as they can, and to hopefully make people feel some security based on their professional identity. This is confirmed by SMART staff who've said that they certainly want music therapists doing this work with their members (and specifically Nordoff Robbins as a credible organisation involved at first). Amelia has been clear that the professional aspect is key for her.

At the same time both Sarah and Gary have been very conscious of not hiding behind their role, especially in the way that had become almost the norm for some music therapists working within a music psychotherapy model. This tended to emphasise the role as a *therapist* first and foremost, and as an expert in treatment using music, based on a medical model. This typically involved drawing clear boundaries between music in everyday life and music therapy, and between therapists and clients (Darnley-Smith 2013). Gary and Sarah had felt that this was a professional cul-de-sac for some time, and in contrast, as the alternative conception of Community Music Therapy began maturing they had been travelling in the opposite direction – to make these professional boundaries and certainties less watertight – though still preserving the aspects that kept the work safe (for clients and therapists) and as effective as possible, using craft, skill and experience (Ansdell 2014c; Stige and Aarø 2012). The SMART project has been a continual testing, proving, experimenting with these distinctions, and with the idea of the 'therapy of non-therapy' – both within the immediate field of the work, but also in relation to ongoing disciplinary and professional shifts in music therapy and mental healthcare overall (Bunt and Stige 2014). Aspects of this theme concern how SMART members and professionals experience themselves, how they see the work and the professional role/identity in relation to the project as a whole, in that particular place.

***

Is it Therapy?

> **Amelia:** We've got this funny thing with members and non-members now, and it's good that the music caters for both. And looking to extend that as well to the cafe. But also, well what else? I mean I think that music does speak to everybody else, everybody. But could we do that with exercise? Could we open a gym in the space over there that's not being used? Could we do something with visual art? You know, more pathways ...
>
> **Gary:** Absolutely. Interesting that all of these things are, they're not *treatments* are they? I mean in the sense that, one, you probably know all my stuff about, you know, the problem with arts therapies. Many of my colleagues have these very psychological models, trying to make it a 'real' therapy – and then you turn the art into a therapy. Whereas, for me, the art is the art. You know, art is art, music's music, dance is dance. And then what a therapist does and what our specialist training does is to give ways to help give people access to it, and then help actually regulate it so that it doesn't go horribly wrong. But you know, it's the fact that things are allowed to be themselves here is good. You know, you're not turning them into something else all the time.
>
> **A:** I think that that's really interesting, I kind of knew you thought that, and that was your approach but I hadn't really realised it. I come from a self-help background, so it's, you may do something because its there and it feels therapeutic but it's not therapy in itself. Or no, sorry that's wrong. It is therapy, but it doesn't have to be delivered as a treatment, if you know what I mean. Yeah. I mean when I started doing it, all those years ago, I kind of used to look at research and interventions and be very scientific about it all, and then realised that actually, you can't be at times. Sometimes things just work, sometimes you have to feel your way. It's really intuitive. And music allows that. It's not like medicine, it doesn't target a certain point in the brain or a certain enzyme, it's broader than that.

As the definition of 'music therapy' has recently broadened and loosened it's increasingly made sense to others that not everything that is done by a music therapist needs to be *called* 'music therapy' (Stige & Aarø, 2012). To an extent this hands the baton to the service users, who can describe what it is to or for them and exactly *how* it's helpful to them. Many participants of the SMART Music project will say that the Thursday group, the Singers and the Band is 'therapeutic' for them in the common sense meaning, and is helpful in their coping with life alongside their illness. But as Gary and the psychiatrist John Meehan found out in a piece of earlier research in the hospital site (Ansdell and Meehan 2010) this does not necessarily mean that it has a direct effect on their symptoms or illness experience, though it may have an important benefit in simply going on living-with the illness. Given that 'therapy' is often experienced and understood by people with mental health problems as a verbal/conceptual practice, they often have problems seeing music therapy as 'proper therapy' in the first place. For some clients this is an advantage – giving them access to alternative forms of therapeutic help. The downside of this ambiguity of whether music therapy is 'proper therapy' or not is the loss of professional prestige to projects and therapists, with possibly an impact on how a project is seen or potentially funded.

An interesting and possibly important aspect of this theme of how the work is perceived is that there seems to be a greater congruence between client and therapist experiences and formulations (which is often *not* the case for other forms of music therapy, where the client thinks they're there to do music, and the therapist thinks that they're doing 'Therapy', and is disappointed when the client doesn't realise this). This finding matches recent similar studies in Community Music Therapy and mental health (Procter 2013; Solli et al. 2013, 2014; Solli 2015; Hense 2015).

Are They Clients?

What role and identity do people find themselves in when they participate in the music project? You will have noticed a subtly fuzzy description of people throughout this book: as 'members', 'clients', and mostly, as 'musicians'. This has been intentional – questioning as we go along what role the music project affords people (members and staff included).

At best what the various situations of the project seem to offer are opportunities to side step some of their usual roles as people with mental health problems. As Tia writes, observing people perform in the SMART Music session:

> The solo slot in BRIGHT's [SMART's] structure can thus be understood as a non-therapeutic therapy, the creation of asylum through musical furnishing/re-furnishing. The requirement for action that song performance poses is also a request for the performer to put him or herself in a situation where they must pull themselves together musically – they must perform and for real – in the shared, public, albeit safe, space of others. It is also an opportunity to stand outside the trappings of the therapeutic encounter, the sick role and the client-therapist relationship. The key issue here is that these community music therapy practices and the client-therapist roles they configure (deconstructing those roles in fact), highlight what all of us in the setting, irrespective of medical history,

> have in common: 'We are all making music here today and will do next week', for example. (DeNora 2013a: 91)

Are They Therapists?

How did SMART members and staff see Sarah and Gary? Mostly as music therapists in professional role and identity. This was partly based on the specific situation (that Gary had worked in the hospital, that Sarah had roles over both sites). This did not mean, however, that they understood Gary and Sarah providing 'therapy' in ways that they understand by comparison with other treatment they are receiving, or have received. An earlier example from Gary's practice with a patient called Clarissa illustrates this:

> [Clarissa] tells me that she'd like piano lessons from me. I explain that I'm a music therapist and don't do piano lessons as such. Clarissa is unimpressed. 'But I don't think of it as *therapy*, Gary,' she says. 'I just think of it as enjoying myself … I've forgotten all my piano … if someone asked me to play a perfect trill, I'd be quite hopeless … .' (Ansdell 2014a, p. 126)

At the same time there was nearly always an acknowledgement of Sarah and Gary as trained specialists – particularly as musicians. At times this perception of the role was used to shift back responsibility from the collective to the professional, as aspects of the projects became 'passed back' to Sarah and Gary to deal with when things got too hot to handle for other members. But in this way the music therapists' role identities provided a sense of safety and security to individuals, and to events and performances where a combined sense of authority, experience and reliability was invested in the professional role. This aspect was especially important in relation to the unique 'bridging' aspect of the music therapy role between the hospital and SMART sites. Gary (historically) and Sarah (from 2007) was known in both sites – in the hospital site in a much 'tighter' professional role (as defined by the medical structures), but as also being able to 'safeguard' people across the gap between provisions. People felt safe to make certain transitions because they were accompanied (both physically and symbolically – because of how Sarah knew/understood them and their illness in relation to music) between the sites. This was firmly part of the professional role and activity of 'music therapist' in this project.

Professional boundaries are certainly there – and have been tested over many incidents of the project, requiring careful action, reflection and consultation with others. Overall we could characterise the difference in our conception of these basic professional boundaries (especially the 'boundary of person') as 'ethical' rather than 'heoretical'. That is, how Sarah and Gary are as music therapists in a particular context is not prescribed by a particular theory of therapy (e.g. 'you need clear personal boundaries in order for the transference to take place' within a music psychotherapy model), but rather by the immediate ethical demands of a particular situation. So 'how a music therapist is', or is perceived within this project is grounded by a situation-specific judgement of 'what helps' musically, inter-personally, and socially – including what a therapeutic relationship is, and how it is helpful here and now.

Why is a Music Therapist Needed?

The descriptor 'non-therapeutic therapy' characterises perhaps how it's a light touch and effacing approach, attempting to intervene as gently as possible, and to allow members to generate their own musical and social resources in order to mobilise 'good musicking'. But as the data has continually shown, this is not to suggest that a music therapist is never required to help ensure that this is indeed what happens. 'Maintenance' work, and occasional skilled and clear intervention is also a characteristic of what the therapists do – in the groups, and within events and specific moments of musicking. This is where their craft, knowledge and experience come into play. It's where they exercise their professional responsibility and judgement.

When Sarah and Gary have done presentations on the project to music therapists they've often included a list entitled *Why does SMART Music need a music therapist?* (since this is a question traditional music therapists often ask – as sometimes do community musicians). It includes the following functions for the music therapist:

- listening
- 'hosting'
- compèring
- organising and re-organising
- accompanying (both musical and personal)
- collaborating
- 'orchestrating' (musically and paramusically)
- setting atmosphere
- noticing
- monitoring
- regulating
- planning
- holding history
- intervening

These various music therapy professional skills and foci have all been described within previous sections above. They describe how a music-centred music therapist informed by the tradition of Community Music Therapy will variously:

1. Help with the immediate needs/opportunities/demands of the current musical-personal-social situation (through trained listening, listening-in-

playing, intervening etc. – working from the specific affordances of the music and musical situation).

2. Help with the social-therapeutic needs of the immediate situation – compèring, hosting, organising aspects of the musicking etc.

3. Use his/her awareness, experience and understanding of how people are in music in relation to their problems/illness. This might either be in relation to someone they don't know, or alternatively, how they carry or hold such knowledge or history in relation to someone they have known and worked with long term (perhaps helping pave their musical pathway between sites, or episodes of illness/health). To put this another way, the therapist works in relation to a sensitivity to people's music-health-illness narratives. This allows the therapeutic functions of accompanying, noticing and when necessary helping regulate the *whole person* within a situation.

4. Accompany people – in the combined and often simultaneous musical/personal/social sense – through and across time, occasion and place.

5. Intervene when necessary – to midwife the best, or to prevent the development of the worst in any given musical-personal-social situation.

As an 'outsider' Tia has also been interested in the question of Community Music Therapy 'craft' (a topic which was considered in great detail by Simon Procter (2013) in his thesis). Tia's initial thoughts on this topic, via her conversations with Gary, were presented in Section 25 above. She has also discussed this topic in earlier writing (DeNora 2013a) where she gives a useful 'outsider perspective' on the therapist role and action within SMART Music in relation to a less secure performance by a member:

> Here is where we see the therapy of non-therapy. On these occasions, the concept of musical accompaniment is brought to the fore and it is possible to see Gary's considerable craft – both as a musician and music therapist – which enables him to move adroitly from musical foreground to background, to lend musical and social support when it is called for and to conceal the techniques which provide, as it were, a sheltered musical interaction. The appearance is, for all practical purposes, that nothing is happening except that people are making music and having fun. This juggling act is complex, virtuosic and self-effacing – as, to a much lesser extent, is our own as participant members of the audience, clapping, commenting, cheering, encouraging, with the promise of musical support (the chorus) always on tap. It is important to remember that the sheltering work performed by Gary is not a feature only of the community music therapy session: on the contrary, it is part of the everyday work of caring and is in no way linked to the specialism of mental health. As Goffman noted, this all part of how demeanour is ceremonially constructed and conserved. [DeNora 2013a, p. 92]

At best the music therapists are working as Simon Procter (2013) suggests as a 'skilled facilitator', whose knowledge, experience and craft is not separated out from other participants, but rather works alongside them, albeit in a role with a special responsibility:

> [this] recasts the role of the music therapist away from the post-Freudian paternal figure of wisdom and authority which seems to underlie not only professional assumptions but also more general societal constructs of therapy, and towards a more skilled facilitator role – more like a yoga instructor than analyst.' […] The music therapist, even if they consider themselves to be working 'purely' musically, is in fact using gesture, space, timing and myriad other kinds of social work, all of which serve to permit music's affordances to be within reach of appropriation. (Procter 2013, pp. 12/3)

The project data is full of examples of Sarah and Gary reflecting on their facilitating role in relation to either the triumphs or troubles of the project. A single example will serve to illustrate this – from an early turbulent episode in the Band's history:

> Despite all the recent problems in the band Sarah reports that this week they've had as good musical experience together as they'd ever had. Robert's OT says that the band has transformed Robert's life – he says 'I'm in a band again', and it means everything to him.
>
> But there's a dilemma about the musical/personal problem with the membership direction of the band. What's right for whom? (or, more negatively formulated, what's *not* right for whom, and when and how do you intervene and help to find a solution?). These are questions for us without a previous map! There are some parallels in the early situation with Roger, where he didn't fit with the Band, it wasn't the right musical niche for him in the project. He accepted this, and has successfully joined the Singers. Is the situation now with Ella similar? It's both a musical and interpersonal problem – the seeds of possible destruction of the band are there. Partly it is musical territory thing too – the guys feel that Ella is pushing them in the direction that they don't want to go in terms of repertoire. So the questions are: what's right for Ella? What's right for the band as a whole? The therapeutic dilemma is how to intervene helpfully without disempowering anyone. How to mediate the situation, advocate for the needs of individuals, *and* for the ongoing survival of the group?
>
> Is this therapeutic dilemma any different from usual in music-centred work? That is, starting off with the needs of the music and the needs of the person/people as intimately related; trying to evaluate and understand what the situation is, what's leading to it, what's involved in it; then trying to intervene, as musically as possible, using what means you have. The personal/group developments, the growth and change ideally follow from the musical freedom and development … Illness and pathology are part of this whole situation, but

> must not dominate the situation, since the commitment to/need for musicking is still the vital motivating factor for all. [Gary's log, 1 May 2008]

The Therapeutic Skill of the 'Non-therapists'

Finally, an important part of this theme is how 'therapeutic action' is never in this project solely either the total responsibility of the professional therapist, or his/her unique expertise. Rather, as we've previously described above in Section 26 how one of our key findings in this research is how a basic 'therapeutic response' to others as they perform or learn music is somehow 'distributed' and shared across the 'audience' as a *collective* action of supporting, understanding and responding in a sensitive way. Sometimes (and this really is different from conventional music therapy) the members get on and do it for themselves when the therapists are not there …

> It's been 'do it yourself' at SMART. Neither Sarah nor I could get there last week. Staff say that they managed to keep the music going for the three groups – Amelia said it was great, first time that it really just did itself. On Thursday afternoon, the guys had gone in, set up and got on with it. It had lasted the usual time, with people being given space to do the usual different things.
>
> Our questions from this: how far is this a mark of (unconventional) music therapy success? What do Sarah and I do, as the 'expert therapists' when we *are* there that has made this possible after five years of this project? How also does this reflect on how SMART as a culture thinks of its members and their abilities – and the place of the mix of professional and lay expertise? [Gary's log, 22 April 2010]

45. Following the Music …

Gary and Sarah thought of their approach to this work at SMART as variously 'Community Music Therapy', 'music-centred music therapy', but also more informally as 'matter of fact music therapy' (Sarah), and 'everyday or common-sense music therapy' (Gary). You may remember that when Gary first approached SMART in 2005 they were nervous of 'therapy', and didn't really want 'music therapy' in their programme. Gary compromised by retaining his role as 'music therapist' but calling the initial group simply 'SMART Music'. In a sense this initial creative compromise has characterised the whole project, and shown its essential rightness for this setting. The members of SMART acknowledge and respect Sarah and Gary's professional role and skills, and acknowledge that these are often helpful for the music project ('You sort us out, musically and otherwise' says one member). But equally, Gary and Sarah quickly learn, and then find the deep wisdom in the fact that theirs is not the only music-therapeutic knowledge and skill in this community. As the project progresses there is a gradual uncovering of the ways that music can help (and sometimes heal); and there is a mutual learning of how best to let the music flourish, to sometimes intervene to deal with obstacles, and, equally how sometimes its best to let things sort themselves out, so that musical flow returns. There's a collective tacit learning that becomes more explicit through the research project that undergirding the development of musicking of this community is a number of ethical/aesthetic principles that link together an understanding of how music, people, illness and health relate:

> **Emerging 'ethical' principles**
> Sarah and I talk about a variety of recent incidents and triumphs in the project and realise how they somehow refract a set of more basic principles of this work, which are becoming clearer now. It's interesting that in relation to the specifics of practice and particular situations we often do end up talking about how ...
>
> 1. *The groups survive/the musicking culture survives* despite the ups and downs of people going in and out, despite people's initial scepticism and fears over whether we would be up to keep going, it has done so. There's a kind of testing as to whether it'll fall apart or can remain together. We've given our help as music therapists, developing the kind of confidence and resilience amongst the SMART musicians from which things are possible, despite ...
>
> 2. *Everybody is acceptable (both musically and personally):* deriving from a music therapy principle/attitude: we're there as therapists to balance the needs of people against the needs of music; to try to include rather than exclude; to try to make people feel good about what they're doing, and about each other. This acceptance aspect, which is mainly tacit, is both in regard to musical aspects (ability level, taste, ambitions, confidence) and health/illness/personality aspects. There's a level of mutual and collective understanding of this latter aspect, both from us, but also of members in relation to each other. People have bad times, don't turn up to planned gigs, but are then accepted back without excessive embarrassment or interrogation. The illness factor is accommodated, without losing focus on the music factor, or health factor.
>
> 3. *It's worth bothering!* Ella says to Sarah, 'most people wouldn't bother'. This in relation to working on music *and* collaboration at the same time, bothering to get things right, to make sure everyone is happy. Working on these things on Wednesdays in the smaller groups has improved them on Thursday too in the bigger session. It's an aesthetic aspect primarily, but a social one too.
>
> 4. *Changes and developments are happening*: people becoming more comfortable and confident to begin to be critical with each other, say what they do and don't want. This can involve a change in the traditional

balance of power in this micro-community (also for the therapists!), people have and do accommodate to the values and principles of making music together in this way.

5. *Individuals in a group/group of individuals*. Again, a classic music therapy value, thinking simultaneously about the musical life of the group, and also thinking about each individual – their problems, potential, circumstances, current state etc. Balancing this binocular vision in the service of musical/social development.

Is working on or from these 'principles' the real aim of the SMART Music Project?

[Gary's log, 26 September 2007]

***

In fact the project in its subsequent years became even more 'music-centred', following where people and music led. The 'real aim' of the project was not to work directly on anything like 'ethical principles', but rather on the simple but sometimes arduous process of 'good musicking'. All kinds of things follow subsequently from this …

Session 141, October 16, 2008

A visiting music therapist comments on how seriously people take making music at SMART Music. Several dimensions of this: people's preparation to come – bringing their own instruments (Roger, Michael, Jane), also their own music and preferences, and having prepared/rehearsed to do something (Jeremy, Jane).

There is an intention to make music, a seriousness and focus on 'good music' – which can be understood in a variety of ways. However, there's also not an expectation that the music, or people need to be perfect (e.g. today Helena sings badly out of tune, but nobody criticises her for this, Jane fumbles, Jeremy is out of time). So 'good music', 'good musicking' is a slightly paradoxical concept – there is a standard, but it's different from conventional performance standards. Rather, people help to *make something good of what's happening musically* – nobody is left to fail, there's nearly always a musical rescue. Other people contribute to someone's effort if necessary (with instruments, singing to support). [Gary's log]

***

There's a shared effort to keep music at the centre, because its collectively understood and acknowledged that following the music is what will really help …

Session 159, March 26, 2009

Today there's a playful and creative reciprocal musical relationship between people. Roger sings *When I fall in love,* and there's a sudden spontaneous turn to *how* we're playing together – in this case a change from a romantic, slow, legato idiom to – on a second go through the song – an up-tempo, swung style, seemingly initiated this time by Barbara with her tambourine! Cued by this change is then a playful interaction between me, the singers, the audience, with rhythmic play on percussion and piano. It is very noticeable how this playful latching-together of musical voices creates enjoyment, cohesion and a heightening of energy, attention and orientation. It counters the diffusion that sometimes invades this group at the moment.

A little later Barbara and a foreign lady with her head covered dance joyously in the aisle. This is the only way that Barbara can make coherent contact with people now. Poor Leslie is in full flight in a solo when his teeth partially dislodge, but he's quick to retrieve the situation, and the performance goes on with scarcely a pause!

By the middle of the afternoon it turns into quite a big group, all seats taken. Regulars, but also quite a few newcomers, as is a nice feature of this group – it naturally accommodates anybody.

Slightly comic situation when I see a suited young man sitting at the right-hand of the piano, looking rather awkward. Realise he'd been planted there by Amelia – they were doing interviews for a new staff post. Clearly she thinks that if he can cope with SMART Music, he can cope with anything!

Describing this group later to Sarah, tell her that one of her old patients in the hospital, Christine, surprised me by coming down to the group from the ward with a nurse, and both of them happily joined in. Because Sarah hasn't been in the hospital for some time some of her regulars are simply 'following the music' and coming down to SMART. How natural is that?

We talked about how this is one of the natural aspects of this project, and of music-centred music therapy in general: that, yes, people miss their therapists ... But most of all perhaps they miss *music* and musicking. Their primary therapeutic and healing relationship is somehow to music itself – and therefore when left to their own devices indeed they *follow the music* ... [Gary's log]

Part II
Continuous Outcomes

1. Self Evident?

> I remember on that *Music Matters* radio programme,[1] there were a couple of people who studied the scientific side of music therapy. It seems to me that we are trying to evidence things which aren't entirely evidence-able… because they are sort of…if someone goes away and they're smiling, on some level they're happy!
>
> And it seems self-evident that…as they were saying in the Alzheimers situation: where for that moment, people whose memory and communication skills were impoverished, for *that* moment with the music, there's no evidence of the condition. Their main presenting condition had vanished! Which I think is fascinating.
>
> Do you see what I mean? So, in a way, before we formulated all this highly intellectual stuff, which is beginning to not serve us very well, I feel, it gets in the way. And I feel that lots of people in the mental health services, and all levels of professionals and lay people, have tended to throw the baby out with the bathwater, and I think what you're doing has my backing – not financially at the moment, until I become a magnate [laughter]. It's absolutely worthwhile and it's self-evident, but how do we convince people? (Roger, interview with Gary, October 2008).

What came out of the SMART Music project during the 10 years we studied it? What continues to come out of it today? Whilst these are necessary questions, a tendency in the current scholarly and managerial culture of healthcare is to translate these into something more specific and precise: What was the *outcome?* Or, perhaps admitting there is more than one, What were the *outcomes?* But asking 'What came out of the project?' and 'What were the outcomes?' are subtly different questions. 'Outcomes' are reified consequences; processes turned into things that are expected to be discrete, definable, describable, observable, locatable and (ideally) measureable in some way. Even if acknowledged as 'complex outcomes' the hope is that such complexity can somehow be broken down into simpler components that *can* be accommodated within experimental 'outcome studies'. What is *not* welcome within this culture (of evidence-based practice, positivist science) is a suspicion that what comes out of such a project

[1] Roger is talking about the BBC Radio 3 programme on music and health that featured the SMART Music Project.

is really a heterogeneous, fuzzy, sometimes fused, overlapping, non-discrete, not always definable, not always locatable or measureable range of phenomena that come out of singular activity and situation.

And yet this is perhaps the more honest conclusion we can give of what came out of 10 years of the SMART Music project. Certainly there is much 'evidence' of the effectiveness of music and musical participation for the enhancement of the health and wellbeing for all concerned (members, staff and researchers alike). But as Roger comments, in a sense this evidence is 'self-evidence'; it is displayed on the surface of the activity, not 'underneath' it within hidden so-called 'underlying mechanisms'. And as the complex narrative of Part I of this book showed, this 'surface' is by its nature largely *not* differentiated, not cut up into individual people, individual sounds or individual trains of simple cause and effect that elucidate the impact of x (intervention) on y (problem). Neither is it conveniently limited either to determinate time or space, occasion or place (such as experimental models typically shoe-horn phenomena into). Rather it's often one undifferentiated and complexly connected whole, a joyously blooming, buzzing confusion of overlapping action and consequence. Individual benefits certainly emerge from this collective whole, but outcomes are often fuzzy, continuous, trans-temporal, trans-spatial and trans-personal.

This part of the book will explore some of the angles we've taken in relation to this question: *What came out of the project?*

2. An Attempted Professional Synthesis of Eight Findings

February 2014 – Sarah and Gary present the SMART Music Project at the *British Association of Music Therapy* conference in Birmingham. They wrangle with the dilemma of wanting to present the project and its positive outcomes in a professional way for a professional audience, but also wanting to portray the sheer individuality and uniqueness of this ongoing project (in the light of which it may not seem either entirely orthodox as either music therapy practice or as healthcare research!).

They settle on a presentation that attempts to synthesise the key findings and outcomes of the research to date in terms of its benefits for SMART as a community of people living with mental health challenges of various kinds. For each finding/outcome they identified a typical example:

The SMART music project – 8 findings

Finding 1 **– The music project accommodates variety and diversity, and works against segregation**: It works for a wide range of people in the SMART and broader mental health community; for people with a variety of different illnesses; for people with and without overt illness; over a range of states and severities of illness and of levels of recovery. It doesn't compartmentalise people up into either diagnostic groups or strictly segregated levels of severity /stage of illness.
Example – the population of SMART is diverse, with a typical cafe session including people under community recovery teams with long-term conditions; those using SMART as a short transition from illness back to work; inpatients from the nearby hospital; and those who don't identify themselves as mental health service users at all, although some of whom we know have various 'problems with living', and find that music helps...

Finding 2 **– The project is accessible and tolerant:** The access/participation criteria for the project are very simply that people want to come (and we know that they want to come first and foremost to *make music together)*. This is fairly unusual in both mental health and everyday culture – that 'membership' is not because of either illness or musical ability.
Example – the cafe session is open to the public, so anyone can turn up just how they are, and the session is managed and contained accordingly. The other music projects do require membership of SMART but are user-driven, with participants having direct influence on how things run. SMART Singers has a member who is a lawyer, and another who has mild learning difficulties, and they share a common focus of valuing singing for their wellbeing, knowing lots of pop songs and love to dance!

Finding 3 **– The project addresses needs flexibly and encourages recovery:** This ability to accommodate many and varying needs has benefits: it offers hope to people that recovery is possible (when they witness people as becoming better, and even take on some of the health that they may not yet feel personally); it also discourages 'illness behaviour' that comes from over-segregation of illness groups.
Example – One of the bands has skilled and able musicians, but they find it difficult to work together and make progress without facilitation from the music therapist. Over a period of a couple of years, they have been encouraged to make decisions, with the facilitator holding back at times, to the point that they now can meet sometimes together *without* facilitation. They've met outside SMART to rehearse in a studio, but the facilitated sessions are still there regularly to help them to come to conclusions and focus when gigs are approaching.

Finding 4 **– The project celebrates variety and generates new musical experience**: Where else would you find the sheer variety of music and musicking (both in a health or a regular cultural context)? It necessitates both tolerance and an opportunity to experience something new (musically/socially). People can learn to tolerate, enjoy and sometimes 'travel with' the various musical pathways (generating how things run. SMART Singers has a member who is a lawyer, and another who has for new

musical experiences, belonging in different ways to a community through how music paves the way...)
Example – a typical day in the project covers music of every genre and decade! One SMART Singer would sing songs from the 1920s and 1930s as this held important personal significance. Now, through the Singers group he is open to new music, listens to Magic FM for inspiration and sang Coldplay and Queen in the last gig. This has enabled him to relate to others better here-and-now, to take his focus away from ruminating on historical memories, whilst also giving him the opportunity to perform his own music and share/educate others in his particular genre and therefore fostering a mutual respect.

Finding 5 **– The project brings together key musical/social outcomes:** Musical/ social outcomes that derive from the above liberal and inclusive membership criteria:
hospitality – feeling welcome, being able to easily join in, being able to do something according to ability, illness state etc.
conviviality – the normalising effect of the natural blend of music, drink, food and good company.
musicality – feeling able and acknowledged to participate at any level that feels comfortable; toleration of different levels of musicianship and performance; feelings of achievement, self-esteem and empowerment etc. from a variety of levels of participation.
belonging to a musical enterprise that endures, changes, develops (as do the people who participate) – and lessening of isolation etc.
Example – Putting on an event/gig means a process of considering what we will play, how will we play it, who plays what, how will we achieve what we want to achieve in the time, what will be a measure of achievement – i.e., how good are we aiming for? How will we practically execute the event? (transporting kit, etc.) and how will we feel, how will we manage if someone doesn't show up? And so on. Musical outcomes are linked also with social aspects; with the teamwork that is fostered, the taking of responsibility for tasks and the 'buzz' of actually working together and making music everyone gets something out of collectively. This is also a normal thing that musicians do!

Finding 6 **– The project balances continuity of provision with immediate quality of experience:** The relationship between the 'long-span' and the 'here-and-now'. The project endures and develops, people belong and share experience over months and years. This helps with the 'creative maintenance' of a chronic illness and its accompanying psycho-social problems, not just through professional help, but via peer support. But there's always also the opposite of this long-termism going on – the focus on the musical here-and-now that affords mutuality, rapport, relationship, 'quickening', community (and which makes no distinction between members and therapists).
Example – SMART Singers work towards events, and are always thinking about how to improve the music, learning harmonies or words by heart etc. However, Sarah makes sure each session is an experience in itself, by watching we don't work on one song too long, for example, doing some fun warm ups, letting people chat as things spark off thoughts or memories, which can result in humour or reflection, but always drawing things back to music constantly, and to those of us present in the session.

Finding 7 **– The SMART project bridges sites and models of care, and experiences of illness/health:** music bridges physical sites of care (mental health unit/SMART); different treatment and care models (medical/social); transitions of care; experiences of illness/health... The means for this is the continuity of music therapist between the two sides of the bridge (which involves knowing about the person as a musician *and* having some understanding of how this interfaces with their illness/health). This means there's a continuity both of people and music...).
Example – the project assembled a series of 'pathway cases', examples of people who talked of using music as a 'hand to hold' or a 'bridge to cross' when they transitioned between the hospital and SMART, Sarah helping them 'over the road' with her personal and musical support. Members also helped each other over certain thresholds – for example, the steps across the cafe floor to do a first solo at the mic in public...

Finding 8 **– The project works with possibility and pathways of recovery:** Working with health/ability/ potential – the attitude is always 'What's *possible?*' – this is regardless of people's state/ability (or the mix of this). Therapists are helping (along with other members) to work for achievement through music; to find and cultivate what people can do. The aim is to maintain and develop health and wellbeing, not to directly treat a problem or symptom. The focus is on music, and where music leads for this person and this community. The musical pathways are pathways of recovery and possibility.
Example – Members reported that the project had been a crucial part of their recovery, through how it showed them the part of themselves that was still well, creative and able despite their illness; and which helped progressively to foster this wellness through active involvement in learning, playing and performing music in various settings, and being witnessed by others as being *musicians*, not just people with problems.

These eight themes are in their way an accurate summary of the key significant outcomes of the project. In the tradition of qualitative data analysis they synthesise the mass of complex naturalistic data through progressive abstraction, and because of this we can be relatively confident that emerging theory has been grounded through the progressive analysis of data. But nevertheless Sarah and Gary are somewhat dissatisfied with this formulation of outcomes. The problem is that it shoehorns the richness and complexity of the project into the usual professional mould of reporting outcomes and their significance. Their suspicion is, however, that one of the real outcomes of the project is that it is also telling us something about how we needed to understand 'outcomes' differently in relation to the complex ongoing process of the project over the 10 years.

3. The Problem With 'Outcomes'

As Roger says in the passage we quoted at the head of this chapter, a lot of the focus in research on mental health is on objective 'outcomes' and their quantitative assessment (think of RCTs, attitude and depression scales, brain scans, hormone assays and so on). These are generic measures, designed to produce 'generalisable' (read 'scientific') results, to offer statistical power and thus to provide a basis for large scale healthcare funding and provision. And yet, as Roger observes, outcomes 'don't really get measured when you look closely'. We take this to mean that there is not a good enough 'fit' between what counts as improvement or wellbeing from a 'patient' point of view and what counts as improvement from the more 'scientific', and more impersonal, point of view as assessed by standardized 'measures'. To continue the visual analogy, because such methods have such a narrow 'aperture' through which they attempt to see the 'when' and the 'where' of an outcome they tend to miss it at worst, or distort it at best.

In company with others, we have discussed these issues in some detail in other writings (Maratos et al. 2011; Ansdell and Pavlicevic 2010; DeNora 2013a, 2013b; DeNora and Ansdell 2014) and will not over-rehearse those arguments here too much, suffice to question:

- Why test what music therapy *doesn't* (primarily) do, just because this is what standard physiological or psychological tests can handle?
- Why demand evidence for what music therapy can't (primarily) achieve because that evidence best fits with standard medical model treatment?
- Why explore the 'epiphenomena' of music therapy rather than the focal phenomena? – that is, how music therapy can *uniquely* or specifically help people in particular situations …

A cautionary tale is the high profile 'MATISSE trial' of art therapy in the treatment of people with schizophrenia (Crawford et al. 2010), and the subsequent critical analysis of why it may have gone so wrong (Holttum and Huet 2014). In short, this large-scale RCT that was supposed to give acceptable evidence for art therapy practice with this client group ended up doing the opposite, with serious political consequences for the art therapy profession. Holttum and Huet's main point in their critique is that the research foundered on a crucial lack of alignment between theory, practice and research method. An outdated theory of what an art therapy intervention *should* do with this particular client group did not match either what the art therapists did in practice, or what was experienced and most needed as help by the particular people in the particular situation. The research method therefore did not have an accurate target for assessing beneficial outcome. From this muddled and negative experience it's clear that significant prior work is needed to get a better fit between theory, practice and method. In particular, detailed qualitative, naturalistic (and ideally longitudinal) exploration is needed of situations where a complex intervention such as an arts therapy is being evaluated.

In the case of music therapy such prior 'aligning work' is needed to give a precise report on:

- What music therapy best and primarily achieves in terms of individual and social benefits in a particular setting, with particular clients, with particular problems and challenges.
- How, when and where these benefits typically emerge and develop.
- How such benefits can be more formally 'shown up' with minimal distortion and maximal specificity and ecological validity.

A key aspect of the critique is to avoid 'black-boxing' the detailed process and ending up only with a too-simple input/output model, which by definition leaves out the 'how?' dimension, but also the complex and sometimes messy getting-*to* a benefit, or getting-*towards* something else paramusical at the other end of the temporal spectrum. We need a broader view than that provided by 'input/output' in order to capture the full variety and complexity of what comes out of something like the SMART Music project. As DeNora has written:

> If we do not attempt to open the black box of music's mechanisms, its 'active ingredients' (which may not be entirely or even mostly dependent on the actual musical stimuli per se) we are left with yet another blunt technology – the correlation, in this case between (on the one hand) an overly general conception of what music is and (on the other hand) an overly general conception of what wellbeing is and how to measure it. And instead of gaining insight into what music actually does, our focus is to narrow to two time frames – before and after the musical 'intervention', and two correspondingly, and seemingly static, health situations, before and after music. The middle time period (the phase of actual musical engagement and the phase where music 'gets into' how people are and what people do) is sidelined. (DeNora 2013b, p. 7)

Our aim in the present study of SMART has been to convert the black box into (at best) a 'perspex box', allowing us to see not just what happens inside it – *during* the process – but, as importantly, how 'before' and 'after' don't neatly connect to the box like two electrical leads, but rather how there's a more complex and messy process involved in what we commonly like to designate as 'intervention' and 'outcome', and how they relate to one another over time.

4. Varieties of 'Outcomes' in the SMART Music Project

On the basis of this critique of how 'outcomes' have been associated with the so-called 'effectiveness' of work such as we've presented in this book we have further explored the relationships between process and outcome in the SMART project – trying to find more 'fitting' ways of describing what 'outcomes' might mean in more indigenous terms, and how to 'bespoke fit' those concepts such that they are (a) intelligible to both SMART members and to academic and health-professional readers and (b) demonstrable through actual happenings and tales about those happenings at SMART, there, then, over time and space. And, lastly, if wellbeing 'outcomes' are robust – beyond SMART – out, back and into members' daily lives.

Analysing 178 'outcomes'

A final stage of analysis of the voluminous data from this project was to compile a summary analysis of all the logbooks and other material (compressed into FILES A–E). A final broad coding procedure followed this, enabling the writing of this book's narrative – through coding exemplary occasions, events and so on within the ten years of the logs. One of the ongoing codings was 'O' for 'outcome'. This code was used liberally, however, matching the spirit of our emerging theory that 'outcome' was not necessarily to be taken as it would in an experimental inquiry, to be a *point* of significance that would be (i) discrete, (ii) causally traceable to a precedent, (iii) directly measurable or definable. Rather, 'O' was designated to a variety of phenomena in the summary text – in fact to anything where there were signs of change, where 'something significant happened' and was notable – however and wherever it happened, whether it was traceable, or indeed immediately understandable.
One hundred and seventy-eight 'outcomes' of this kind were coded, then reduced to 69 which were exemplary in illustration of different types. These were then further coded in relation to an emergent schema that presented a continuity of eight sets of outcomes (Fig 10). We follow this schema with a sequence of illustrative examples.

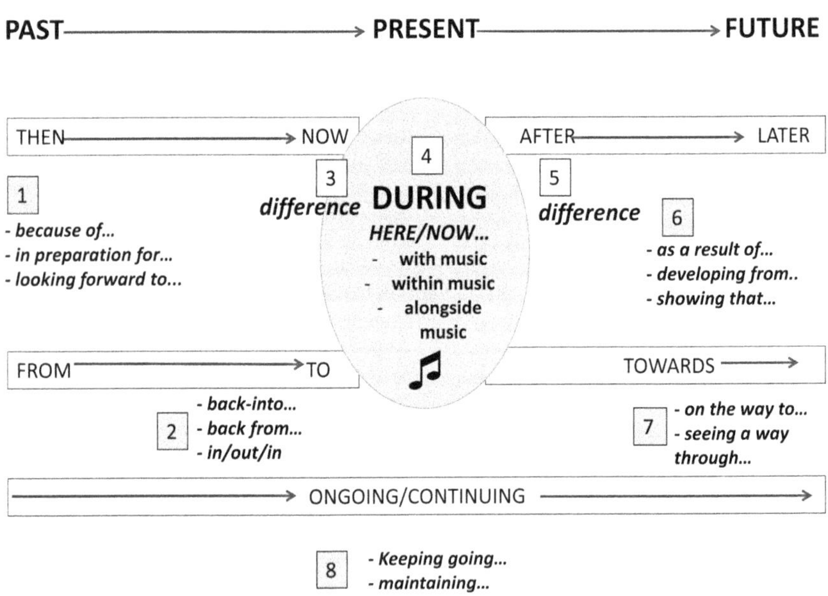

Figure 10 The continuity of outcomes

Outcome Set 1 – Because-of

i. Eloise has been away from SMART for some time, having experienced a minor crisis with panic attacks, unable to leave the house. She said that one of the motivating factors to get out again was to come to SMART Music, and this enabled her to make a tryout return today.

ii. Viv tells Sarah that she's been increasingly down, then told herself today 'come on Viv, get yourself along to the music!'. And she does, doing a nice duet today with another singer. Sarah asks Viv at the end of the afternoon whether it was worth coming today, and she says 'Absolutely! It motivates me to get out and see people...'.

iii. Michael's health is clearly worse, he says he nearly didn't come, but forced himself. He manages an Elvis number from the book, without guitar – and at the end comes up to me looking bright and happy. Says 'it bucks you up, this music – I feel good now'. And he looks it – quickened.

The 'because-of' category shows us how even the expectation of what music can/will do (if only one can get to it) is useful in overcoming debilitating effects of illness. Wanting to do something meaningful and pleasurable, and having something to go to (SMART Music) is itself part of what music 'does'. It is the catalyst that enables participants to move from 'there' (wherever 'there' is – apathy, anxiety, depression, lethargy) to 'here' (SMART). The remembrance of previous SMART Music Sessions and prior positive experiences, provides a basis for prospective thoughts about the music group such that there is a kind of 'looping' effect of after/before/after which enhances strength and redoubles motivation in a virtuous circle. We know that motivation and attendance are key factors in mental health services' attempts to help people, so anything that contributes to this is an important resource. And in group sessions, the exertion of individual agency (getting to the sessions in the first place, participating once there) is the catalyst for the benefits of what happens 'during' those sessions. The triple time form of before-during-after is circular and, over time, as the circle is reinforced, the 'benefits' of music participation take over the space that had previously been occupied by features of the illness. In this sense, getting well is, quite literally, replacing illness with musical activity. As the circle is repeated, the links between motivation, anticipation and participation grow ever stronger, making less room, or marginalising the feelings associated with being unwell. Key, then, to the design of any group activity is that it offers something reliable, that it will meet what is expected of it, time and time again ('if I can get there I won't be disappointed'). That reliability, and its circularity, is the first of our 'continuous outcomes'.

Outcome Set 2 – Moving back-into

i. Daniel says in his interview 'between 2001 in 2005 I played no music at all. The music sessions you run helped me rediscover music'.

ii. Bobby is back, after many months of being very sick both physically and mentally. He looks a lot better, and tells me he wants to sing. He sings *No Woman No Cry* – his signature song, re-introducing himself to the group musically. Lovely that he can 'come home' to this group on recovery, and find a warm reception and appreciation.

An outcome can be the process of getting-into. Many people like Daniel use the project to help them come *back-into* music again (both literally and symbolically). This involves forging a path back-into a place where playing happens in ways they can access, but also into the positive asylum and social relationships it affords which counteract the isolation they've often experienced in relation to their illness. Once the 'music space' has been established and they feel at home there it remains constant for people like Bobby and Daniel who may need to leave and come back at certain times. The continuity of the benefit is crucial.

For others the pathway is between mental health facilities, with music helping pave the way into, bridging transitions, entrances, shifts in belonging and presenting the self:

iii. Shirley is a new addition to the Singers. She's followed Sarah down from the hospital group, and also dared to come down to SMART Music today. She looks quite different at the end of the group.
iv. Robert's back and starts again after a long absence whilst he was ill. He went back to Sarah's music therapy group in the hospital – so a pathway back and forth between music in the two places. Today Robert sat himself in front of the conga and played well, and then got out his mouth organ to play Blues. When people clapped him for this his face softened and smiles for the first time, changing from its recent hangdog expression.
v. Mila – an example of a developing 'musical pathway' – someone who's graduated from Sarah's groups in the hospital to SMART Music. She's been increasingly coming forward physically in the last month – from sitting at the back to the middle of the cafe, joining in, picking a song this week, asking me questions about the group. I saw her first real smile today.
vi. Kerry has been building up her confidence for a few months, and had a breakthrough today – coming to the mic and singing two songs and a duet with Viv. People found this very moving – a good example of this group as a vehicle for personal development over fairly long scale (from 'I want to do this' to 'I can' to 'I did'). We have seen this progression of participation from the communal singing to individual performance, communally witnessed. Because it's a stable community of people, they know how much of a step that is for Kerry, and appreciate the significance. Later the staff said that they listened from their offices, and found it very moving.

Notice how in the three cases of Robert, Mila and Kerry the relationship between the meso-level of their musical pathways between services and health-identities, and the more micro-level of them moving into-and-around musical space: taking out a harmonica, moving physically forward in the group, up to the mic, coming into the musical here-and-now, into self-in-community.

People's individual musical presence (and their musical choices, repertoires and cultures) also moves into the musical situation – another form of pathway from and to. They actively inflect time and space by their intervention into a situation.

vii. Jeremy almost intentionally seems to intervene into this noisy atmosphere by singing in a quite different style *Some Enchanted Evening* – it's a welcome oasis, balancing out the music. At the end of it Daniel comments publicly 'Jeremy, your voice is getting stronger', and people agreed.

Outcome Set 3 – Before→During Difference

i. Will (SMART manager) talks about a lady we can see halfway back in the group, scribbling obsessively on a pad (seemingly nonsense). She evidently comes every day, but does nothing except this scribbling, seems utterly lost. Will saw her singing in the group, following the words, having temporarily stopped her obsessional writing session.
ii. Something emerged holistically from the Band today – a collecting together of what we had into something that really mattered. Mattered because so many of the people looked so battered – the difference was more apparent. This group feel is reflected in a shift of purely musical quality: for example, some good ensemble playing in an improvisation with flute, violin, drums... Bobby suddenly shifts to a lighter touch somehow through a shift in the playing as a whole. Ella says spontaneously 'it's beautiful'.
iii. Performance seems to turn some people on like a light bulb. Today the example of Luca, the man with learning disabilities who comes with his father. He becomes somebody else, or perhaps simply becomes himself!
iv. Peggy (87) has not been good over the past weeks, but today she says 'When I'm here in this group I go into another world – I feel good from [points] the top of my head to [points] the tip of my toes!'.
v. Leslie looks terrible when he came in today, but gives his all to his singing, and is appreciated, and suddenly looks better.
vi. Daniel who has perked up as the afternoon went on, says 'I feel *much* better now!'. It was like a revival! Struck by how tangibly music had moved his mood and wellbeing from one state to another. Bobby is also more co-ordinated today, he responds so transparently to good vibes in music, just gets more and more into it and smiley.
vii. Jonathan – a personal therapeutic transformation today. I'd noticed he was distressed at lunchtime, ranting about a benefit interview. The first half he hovered broodingly at the back, then suddenly late in the afternoon he joined in the song *Sailing*, conducting me. On the strength of that I get him up to sing at the mic, he does his trademark *Raindrops Keep Falling*, with

verve and character. Others join in on instruments, and it's a lovely but also personally symbolic finale for the day – transformation through music (by a person, *through* community, *for* community). Magic!

viii. Sarah reports that the band is changing the way it plays music. They improvise more freely, find a laid-back groove that is more jazz than rock/pop, and see where it goes, and it worked, it does go somewhere. There's a subtle reciprocal relationship between the style/type of musicking and a different quality of relationships between the members. The question of who leads or not, what space there is in the music for people, the opportunity for things developing in their own improvisational way, space for exploration, mutuality and collaboration...etc.

ix. Michael's often technically out of time, 'he seems to drop a beat' Antonia says. 'He often adds one too' Gary says, thinking of Daniel's description of Michael as the 'five beats in the bar man'. But Antonia has also noticed how the ensemble accommodates to his musical eccentricity, gets it together for him despite the problems. I explain to her the complex and tacit acceptance and co-ordination that this takes for musicians playing with him – how John for example watches Michael's guitar hand to predict his chord changes, and how we'll do our best to make the 'lurches' of his rhythm not a disaster for the music. This is true for the musical culture of SMART overall – how instead of people judging each other's performance as inadequate or wrong, they manage nevertheless to go with them, accommodate to the extrinsic eccentricities of their musicking, make them feel they belong, whatever they do, however they play or sing.

x. The outcome of the gig [the Singers performance at the older people's ward] is mutual respect, and mutual benefit – the musicians seem to grow six inches taller over the course of the hour. Henrietta comments that her voice gradually frees up and gets louder and she sings with the others and finds herself absorbed by the energy of the music and other people.

What happens *during* (the conventional time and space for an 'active ingredient') is shown up in this category particularly in relation to what came before. This 'before' might be a state of [mental or physical] health (Peggy, Daniel, Leslie, Jonathan), of being or aliveness (Luca), or behaviour (the 'writing lady'). These states might be individual or collective, and may be recognised 'externally' by others, or reported subjectively, or both.

The outcome represents a significant change between a past or prevailing condition and what happens 'during' the time of the session/the musicking – a shift or transition that matters or is of note. The qualitative difference that defines this outcome is not simply a contrast before/after, but between before-*during* – a getting *from* somewhere/something *to* somewhere else/something else – where having stepped into the process there's a transformation. But the transformation remains in the present tense: *feeling good/better* (Peggy, Daniel, Leslie), *being different* (Luca, the Singers), *behaving differently* (the 'writing lady', Jonathan, the Band guys), *sounding different/better*.

Such change may last after the music's stopped (for a minute, an hour, a day, a week, forever...), but this is not its chief reality. It may, however, only last whilst the music lasts – that is, during the conditions that support the change. The focus is rather on the arrival at here/now, and what this brings.

The examples stress how the specificity of the musical-therapeutic process underwrites these in-process outcomes. It's not just that something that happens 'in the music' changes something 'out of the music', but rather there's a more subtle relationship between musical change and paramusical change. When the Band guys step into music they change as the music changes (and vice versa). When Michael's co-players manage to accommodate to the idiosyncrasies of his playing both he and the situation changes. Through this relational and situational dimension (personal, but through community), a difference between 'before' and 'during' takes place *within and amongst musicking* such that outcome becomes process.

Outcomes are achieved 'over the course' of and 'inside' the event – not suddenly after it, as if the 'event' and its 'aftermath' are not part of the same weaving activity over time and place. The paramusical aspects might show up during or after, but are rightly part of the continuing flux of process once they've started...

Outcome Set 4 – During

> The telephone rings – someone holds up the telephone receiver, says 'listen, there's music here'.

It's an outcome in itself that music arrives, settles, establishes its world, its condition, its relationships. And along with this people settle down with and within music, and what it affords them just here, now in the musical present tense. With this category we are looking down squarely into the perspex box of ongoing musical and music-therapeutic process: on what can happen uniquely within and amongst musicking in this particular way, in this particular place:

i. A visitor comments on how relaxed people are in SMART Music, how natural the music making is, how generous people are – how willing to give music to others, and how there's a real spirit of music flowing through the place during this afternoon. It's just what we hoped SMART Music would be.
ii. Sadie says 'music brightens everything'.
iii. Viv says about music 'it takes me out of myself'. Claire says 'It moves you – moves your body, but also your feelings... you're in flow, you're here and now, not in the past or the future...'.

iv. Dave [SMART staff]: 'I'm still so emotional here on Thursday afternoons – we sit here blubbing'. The surprising events – people doing what they thought they couldn't do... they all have their own music, it connects to their past, they feel powerful when they do it in front of others. The music changes this place on Thursdays.'
v. The 'two ladies' bring a whole cake today, slice it up and pass it round. Conviviality!
vi. Margaret is too shy to request song, so Eloise does it for her – *Lady is a Tramp*. Daniel and Simon do it for her, and after Margaret says 'how lovely to have a song sung for me, it makes me feel so special'.
vii. Gemma does a spirited and characterful performance of *Cabaret*. She's smartly, even theatrically dressed up in black taffeta. She announces 'I *am* Liza', and indeed she is!
viii. Amelia [SMART Chief Exec] says before the session 'Thank God we've got the music this afternoon – it's one of the very few positive things here at the moment – it really helps unite the place'.
ix. Selima wanders in and out of the cafe, mostly attached to her flute. She looks distracted and worried, lost and acting rather like a three-year-old. Then suddenly she is 'in music', 'in the flute-playing' and as suddenly she is intentional, precise, focused, confident, oriented in space and time. And then she stops playing and she drops out of all of these qualities just as quickly. A great, if rather tragic, example of someone being totally different *inside* music – indeed her pathology seems suddenly to peel off, but it's also noticeable when the music stops that the pathology springs back. At present the musical solution is indeed very temporary!
x. Janice is shaking less today but her speech is difficult to understand. But she fully participates in the music – I think this is probably the only thing she joins in with now where her problem doesn't dominate for both herself and others. She sings a song with greater success than two weeks ago – *Say a Little Prayer* –, which again people almost instinctively sing-up as a way to try and help and support her. When the Blues guys start on the rock 'n' roll, Janice is suddenly up dancing at the back of the room – doing twists and turns, seemingly in balance, with no apparent shaking, and enjoying herself. At the end of the group when we're packing up she looks quite radiant – quickened – and says to me: 'makes you feel better, doesn't it?'.
xi. Late in the afternoon Anthony walks in, finely dressed in suit and tie, but disorientated. He greets Sarah who says 'Are you going to do a song today?'. He's casual and noncommittal, walks to the bar and talks to Leslie, who asks him 'Can you sing?', and then Anthony sings a snatch of *Long way to Tipperary*. I'm listening to this, catch and start playing Tipperary on piano, Roger and Selima on harmonica and flute join in, leading to Anthony singing a fragile and fleeting performance which fades as he exits to the garden, leaving flute and percussion segueing into an Irish jig. Dave

(staff) dances through the hall with Peggy... and the music finishes to roars of approval. Anthony returns from the garden to take the applause.

The here/now outcomes of musicking are often voiced as what music seems to *do*: to 'brighten everything', 'make me feel special', 'unite the place' and so on. It does some of these things through its collecting people into the musical present – 'you're in flow, you're here and now, not in the past or the future...'. But as we've constantly stressed (and we hope demonstrated through this book) what's happening here is not music *doing* things as some independent force, but rather people are doing things with music's particular helpful affordances, related to its eco-phenomenology (how it is /how it operates singularly *within* situation and action).

The musical 'present moment' sets the situation and the conditions for things big and small to happen: for 'the ladies' to slice up a cake in a moment of conviviality; for people to be taken out of themselves into a different qualitative experience of musical flow, companionship, community.

This quality of being musically in the here and now is the outcome, because this establishes the conditions for being different in some way – in state, in persona, in relationship and so on. Some of these outcomes are linked to a past, but they are not really about the past or the future. Rather the variety of outcomes *during* – personal, communal, – identity, belonging ... are present-moment states and happenings that matter to these people here and now.

'Feeling better' is also a case of here and now, whether this feeling transfers to the future or not. Symptoms do reduce – shaking lessens (Janice), orientation, awareness and focus increases (Selima); but sometimes only whilst the music lasts. But this is no less an outcome, both for the people who experience themselves differently for a few precious moments, but also for those who witness them being different and share hope for them.

As many of the examples above show these present moment outcomes are seldom the result of a single input, but rather the collective achievement of a shared, and sometimes widely distributed moment across time and space. For example, the musical here-and-now of 'Tipperary' is an amalgam of musical material, attuned musical consciousness from a variety of directions, and an unpredictably improvised course of musical development. Whose outcome is that? Whose benefit?

Outcome Set 5 – Before→After Difference

The traditional outcome – the clearly defined difference between 'before' and 'after' – is in fact the one least coded in the sequence of 69 vignettes. It is coded when people say, or it can be inferred, that there's a distinct 'after' when the effect is registered or noticed:

i. Sadie: 'I was feeling rotten this morning, but I forced myself to come. After the music I just felt better'.

ii. Jonathan sings *Raindrops* – first he looks awful, but after singing the song this face lights up. Transformation!

Whilst these examples conform to the grammatical formula they also resemble Sets 3–4 in their basic features. The way that this pattern is recorded in the data suggests sometimes that there's perhaps an attempt to fit the 'facts' into the required mould of outcome recording; to sculpt the narrative into a sharper before/after format:

iii. Jonathan is wearing a builder's crash helmet and dark glasses. When Amelia asks whether he's okay, he says is being assaulted by others' stupidity and feels he needs to wear special protection to keep himself safe. He's pressured and unhappy. I'm surprised a little later when he takes up my offer to sing, and does his trademark song *Raindrops Keep Falling On My Head*. He stays for the duration of the group, and it's one of those classic before/after music effects that I wish I could keep as the definitive evidence that this work really does make a rapid change to people: to their prevailing affect/mood; to their confidence and self-esteem; to diverting them away from obsessions of thought and behaviour – and, perhaps as important, to the shift in how other people see them, socially and interpersonally. By the end of the session people are no longer annoyed by the Jonathan who's been obsessively haranguing them that morning, but congratulating the Jonathan who sings with them, and entertains them this afternoon...

iv. Quite striking the difference today between a quite low beginning and where we got to in the end. The initial mood to do with the place as a whole, and individual people seeming ill and low. The musicking transformed both the mood of the place, and people's individual ability to do what they seemingly couldn't. Considering SMART Music as both a daily and a long-term process – some sort of ritual, transformational process. We mostly get *from* somewhere *to* somewhere, it's a road travelled.

v. The outcome of the gig [the Singers performance at the older people's ward] is mutual respect, and mutual benefit – the musicians seem to grow six inches taller over the course of the hour.

One of the issues is defining (and finding a way of showing up) the interval between 'it' happening and an outcome coming into shape – any 'after' being in theory from seconds to years. Perhaps this is why the more authentic expressions in this sequence seem to describe a logic that is more like 'before>during' and 'during' rather than 'before/after'. And then the next category – the 'as a result' presents a more realistic and complex following-on-from the musicking experience to other segments or sectors of life for people, or the place.

Outcome Set 6 – As a result of...

i. Henrietta has started to sing in the Dido performance at Kensington Palace press night last night. Ella's gig at Lighthouse last week seems to have gone well, a major achievement.
ii. Jeremy chooses a song from Jane's book and then sings one of his specials. Announces in his spiel that he's just bought a Walkman, and is now listening to all his CDs and songs. Found this moving – I know he doesn't have a TV and when I gave out CDs from the Atrium concert he didn't take one as he doesn't have a player. His home music life must have been the radio until now. Despite him going on about his age, his old songs, he's now getting the courage to try something new – not just new people, situations, songs, but new things such as the Walkman.

For some members things start to come out of their experiences in the SMART Music project, but at a distance (both temporally and spatially) from the initial experiences. They come as a result of, or a spin-off from, the music – but in various ways that are not direct, and not always directly linked to it:

iii. Ella recently said that she'd realised that singing in the SMART groups for her wasn't just about music; what she'd found through her musical renaissance applied to other difficult areas of her life. She'd found confidence, skill, aspects of role, self-image and esteem – other areas of life which music become a safe ground for rehearsal...

What happens next for people comes as a result of how their musical experiences at SMART are used in very individual ways as something that can be used *beyond* the time and space of the original experiences. These are the paramusical benefits of music therapy; sometimes defining something that members subsequently *have* done (such as Henrietta's performance), or alternatively *haven't* done:

iv. Eloise collars me after the end of the next and final SMART Music session for me. She says that she wants me to know 'I've not had mental lapse... *or a drink*... for 10 years now, and a major part of that is the benefit of music therapy!'.

Other 'results' reported or observed resulting consequences are to do with gains in skill, confidence, self-identity or self-esteem, motivation, focus and purpose linked to musical experiences in SMART but taken away and beyond (at whatever scale):

v. In the *Singers* Jeremy practices a song for Dr B's retirement. After Roger comments that he'd heard Jeremy sing now for many years and felt he'd greatly improved.

vi. Robert's OT says that the band has transformed Robert's life – he says 'I'm in a band again', and it means everything to him.
vii. Jane appears and sings *Close to You* well – she's centred, without any of the usual fussing. I compliment her later, and she says, 'Yes, I knew it was good today, because I felt good. You may not believe this, but I don't believe in myself much, and it comes out when I sing. When I do do well, then I believe in myself more...'.
viii. Roger returns to SMART Music. He says how valuable the music has been to him. His partner Penny told him she was very proud of him after the concert in the hospital – he said she'd not said that for seven years!
ix. A social worker tells us how shocked she is to hear Musei sing, she never knew that he did! She never heard something that was crucial to his life and expression. This is what Richard says that the music project does. It spreads and demonstrates hope.

A final aspect of 'results' is how a musical experience at SMART is taken in terms of some broader reality: how it can show, enact, or stand symbolically for something; can define or re-define, represent, or focus a stance – on the basis of which further action or reflection can happen:

x. Richard (hospital manager) has his retirement party in SMART Music, and makes a moving speech in which he said the best thing he'd seen from all his years in the NHS is our music groups. Said that the band get better and better, and how great it is to see service users achieving so much. A powerful speech, from a reticent but sincere man who really knows what he's talking about. Sarah writes 'another great example of music providing a service for an organisation and event, and the musicians too'.
xi. The *Singers* concert has some new repertoire, including the Coldplay song, *When I Ruled the World,* and *We are the Champions* at the end. Sylvie later links these choices to the fight they are all having at the moment with their everyday lives, with the new government benefit changes, and their struggle to manage. The songs they sang, Sylvie says, are all about power and strength. And in itself it's a performance of empowerment and strength in adversity (as it also is for many of the people in this hospital, patients, relatives and staff alike).

Outcome Set 7 – Towards...

All of the outcomes are implicitly carrying forwards towards some new state or possibility of action, but some are especially framed in this way, emphasising the temporal and spatial tendency towards a possible future and potentially new or altered social relation (where music can be understood, in Procter's (2011) sense as proto-social capital):

i. Mary says she's made a copy of the tape of the Willow Christmas concert to send to her sister in the USA as a birthday present.
ii. Henrietta says: 'Music and music therapy has been the support and driving force of my treatment and continuing recovery. The continuity, nurturing and support to my confidence and mental health have been key to where I am now. It has bridged and supported every step, to enable progress that no other therapy has managed in such an all-inclusive way.'
iii. Liliana said how she'd fallen into a severe depression a year ago, and that it's been the music that has lifted it. The Singers, and the musical company, but then through this her daring to get back to the piano, and then to now playing in a trio with other Polish people. Depression, she said, led back to music. This, she said, was what she thought the depression was about ultimately – to show her that music needed to be in her life again, or else she'd become ill.

Outcome Set 8 – Ongoing and Continuing...

Notwithstanding the previous emphasis on the forward-pointing nature of most of these outcomes, there's also an important message that the data gives about *not* emphasising particular segments of time and space, but rather stressing the ongoing, *continuing* nature of outcomes. What comes from keeping the music going month after month, year after year? The impact of this continuity is on how people are able to do certain things that require a longer-span: to inch into further participation; to find just how to play a tambourine in SMART Music; to develop a musical partnership or ensemble through its ups and downs; to find the group still there when you've had a bad time and had to be away for six months... and so on. For many people in this community maintaining the continuity of the musicking means helping maintain their health too. As Peggy says, it keeps her going...

i. After he's finished singing, Bobby says 'I love singing – I love music, it's therapy for me...'
ii. Mary is one of the people who fade and suddenly pop up again. She just says 'sorry, I've been ill'. I know from Sarah that she and Tim were briefly engaged, but then broke this off. But they sit together today, two damaged, but lovely people. Mary gets up to sing some of her standards – *Memory*, and later, *Clowns*. Her voice is strained and forced at times (I'm scared that this is what happens when she's getting ill), but perhaps not, as she is controlled and rather beautiful in *Clowns*. Simon plays a beautiful obbligato and it's magical. These songs are like a precious continuous thread in her harrowed, inconstant life. It's the way this music accompanies her across the difficult voyage of her life.
iii. 'The ladies' – a noticeable change here in recent weeks: their instrumental participation increasing. Especially Barbara on her tambourine – she looks at me intently for cues to play.

iv. Nice chorus of *Mama Mia*, with Dave and Sadie at the counter joining in at my request. Sadie is also participating much more in previous sessions. She clearly dresses up for the sessions, and makes more suggestions of songs to sing.

v. Mario does several Sinatra songs. His sister says he'd been talking about it all week, talked of preparing at home – not just the song, but practising in front of a mirror and listening to the original Frank Sinatra and his brand of 'American talk' after the singing. When he does the song, it's difficult for him to find the key at first, and getting him to listen to the ensemble trying to accompany him (me on piano, Stephen on guitar, Eloise on cymbal). But we get some sort of ensemble on *Strangers*, and then he does some bits of *New York*, then does the talk at the end, which amuses people. After he gets warm applause and looks very pleased with himself. His sister says 'it meant the world to him to do that'.

vi. Henrietta is temporarily back in hospital. She says, 'That's the great thing about the project, there's music in both places now... This morning I could dip into the music group on the ward with Sarah, which really helps... And I know that when I get out I can go back to SMART Singers – it's the continuity that matters... Music's still there, even when you have a blip, to hold your hand...'

vii. 'When I heard about Radio 3 coming to do a programme on music therapy in relation to health I was thrilled. I've always found music an integral part of me, but never thought of it as therapy until I started with the music group here at SMART. Meeting with people to work on something that we all share in common is an uplifting experience. Being able to tell part of my story, and how music therapy continues to support me, was important to help ensure that it will be there for people who will benefit from it in the future'. [Henrietta]

viii. At the *Singers* lunchtime concert in the main hospital I catch sight of an old lady with a shopping trolley – deeply involved and moved by the music. She looks wistful, and at the end I chat to her. She says the music's been lovely, has made her day. She's one of those people for whom music involves longing, and soon the story is out – her father and sister died in this hospital. 'I come most days – the music helps' she says.

ix. Jeremy says: 'I've not been feeling good for the last few weeks, but I've had my music – I go back to the music that means a lot to me – Jessie Matthews. I've been playing the CD that Dave, the last manager at SMART, gave me a few years ago... And I play and sing each of the songs, and I associate them with someone who means something to me, and that makes me feel better. And this afternoon I want to sing one of my favourite songs, *Dancing on the Ceiling.*'

x. Peggy is back after a bout of flu. She demonstrates her renewed health by getting up during a lively improvisation and dancing around the room, doing high kicks (at 87!), saying to a surprised audience 'I always did this when I was younger! Now it keeps me going!'.

5. A Continuity of Outcomes

This analysis has hopefully served to 'thicken' the sense of what 'an outcome' might look like for a project like this. To start with the obvious, it's clear that meaningful outcomes don't necessarily come only at the end of the process. We need to take a different view of both the temporal and spatial-relational fields in which we tend to think of what amounts to an outcome, benefit or result of such work.

Our view has focused on the 'middle period' (DeNora 2013a, p. 139) as the analysis in this section has shown. During the actual musical event certain causal strands stretch both backwards and forwards, creating as it were an 'extended present' across before>during>after in which music and musicking is effecting important change for people and places. Perhaps going a stage further, this might be thought of as a 'continuity of outcome', where outcomes are ongoing strands of process caught in action. Consequently we need to experience and conceptualise the holistic, dynamic and continuous coming-into-being of an effect, rather than trying to carve up the field into the static schema of before/after, or here/there. Thinking of 'continuous outcomes' rather than 'discrete and located outcomes' might alert us more to the on-the-ground reality of what's really important about this work: namely, that what comes out of it often continues within time and (relational) space – in ways that are difficult to capture through formal before/after methods.

A way of thinking and a method is needed (one that is naturalistic and ecological[2]) that can perceive and catch what's happening 'all the way along' – according to the natural timing, placing and scaling of micro- and meso-level events, and how these make sense of 'what matters' and what counts as transformative outcomes for people and places themselves, as well as (hopefully!) those who arbitrate 'effectiveness'.

A continuity of outcomes perspective entails thinking differently about:

- timing – is there really an exact 'when' an effect happens in musicking/music therapy?
- placing – is there really an exact 'where' such an effect happens?
- scaling – is a smile an adequate outcome?

For what the data shows is that this continuity of music-therapeutic outcomes affords variously a passage, a bridge, a pathway between physical locations of

[2] Such a philosophical and methodological perspective can be found in the tradition of Goethean science, and its approach of 'gentle empiricism' (Bortoft 2012; Pavlicevic & Ansdell 2010; Ansdell 2014).

care and between states of health/illness – not conforming to the false simplicity of before/after, because the situation isn't this simple. People's experiences of music, life and of their varying 'problems in living' are dynamically temporal, and fluidly spatial and relational. In this book we've portrayed the reality of outcomes in relation to social and material ecology. We've shown, that is, what can change for people given the right conditions that musicking supported by therapeutic attention can often afford. Our baggy list of outcomes has included a smile, a turn of a melody, an unexpectedly successful performance, the confidence to accept an outside gig, a decision to stop drinking, an improvement in negative symptoms, a way of imagining recovery.

The continuity of outcomes is the process of constructing the musical pathways that we've traced and witnessed (however short or long, transitory or forging...). 'Pathways' captures the sense of movement, and different routes away from the things that are linked with and taken to constitute illness, and toward those things associated with health and/or wellbeing. A path is by nature continuous...

Part III
Musical Recovery

Music triggered a healing process from within me. I started singing for the joy of singing myself ... and it helped me carry my recovery beyond the state I was in before I fell ill nine years ago ... to a level of wellbeing that I haven't had perhaps for thirty years ... .

[Ella, BBC interview]

It is the 'wellspring of wellness' within me, and consistently identifying with this that brought my recovery (with the aid and assistance of music and the catalyst of the expression of myself through singing that you provided - and which I still miss so much). I am now very well. I have been in remission for three years and have a normal life. See how the seeds of your music therapy brought me back to life!

[Ella – email]

Music and music therapy has been the support and driving force of my treatment and continuing recovery. The continuity, nurturing and support to my confidence and mental health has been key to where I am now. It has bridged and supported every step, to enable progress that no other therapy has managed in such an all-inclusive way.

[Henrietta – additional comment on checking interview]

I suppose I'm saying this now because you're both here: but this music here has been key to my recovery in the last years – I've dipped in and out of it, and it's always been here ... .

[Stephen, spontaneous comment]

Introduction

Many of the participants of the SMART music project have lived with mental health difficulties for a good proportion of their lives. During this time they've experienced different ways in which others have explained their difficulties or diagnosed their 'illness', and varying contexts in which help has been offered to them (or, occasionally, forced upon them): from the last days of the old-style asylums through to the early days of the community psychiatry movement, and now to the sometimes bewildering range of treatment and support options put in the shop-window of the latest UK government strategies and policies for mental health. These continual changes of theory and practice in the mental health sector have also meant that to some extent – as *patients / clients / service-users / customers* – they have also had to keep revising the stories they tell themselves and others about their lives, and their occasional or ongoing problems in living.

The complexity of this theoretical and political world of mental health provision (which we don't have space to go into any great detail about here[1]) points in turn to just how contested and slippery the notions of 'mental health'/ 'mental illness' are in the first place, and how this fuzziness seems at first so different from other medical and social problems. But equally, this is perhaps why this area is fascinating and important, in how it serves as a prism to help question and think about broader questions that concern us all, such as: *Can we really separate mental and physical health? Can we really separate psychological, social and cultural health? Can we be objectively sick but still flourishing as persons?* ***When*** *and* ***Where*** *are we healthy or flourishing? What supports our continued flourishing despite objective 'state of health'? How can we best help each other in sickness/health? Where and when do we best help and care for each other? How, and with what?*

Our particular focus in this book has been to consider these crucial if complex questions in relation to the relatively modest area of music, and the focal question: *How does music help?* Or, to be more accurate, we have listened and watched how music and musicking people show and tell us something important about the broader kinds of questions listed above.

To this point in the book we've mostly taken an inductive stance to the research: remaining 'theory-agnostic' during the process, allowing a gradual build-up of meaning in relation to our areas of interest within the specific setting of SMART. We have kept our attention local and specific; focusing on the micro- and meso-level detail of how music, people, and mental wellbeing relate and develop. In this final chapter, however, we will relax into a more abductive stance, by which we mean neither 'inductive' nor 'deductive' but the attempt to grasp knowledge somewhere in between the two. This means reaching out from our local indigenous understanding towards current thinking and practice in the mental health field and the broader area of health and wellbeing overall – looking for links, parallels, amplifications and confirmations of the key findings of this study.

'*Recovery*'

The four spontaneous comments from Ella, Henrietta and Stephen at the head of this chapter share a key word, and a similar attitude to the course of their mental health problems – *recovery.* As a word it comes from the Latin *recuperare,* and is one of those rich words in current English usage that has meanings and connotations

---

[1] Recent overview material on this complex area and its current perspectives and debates that we've found useful are: Tom Burns (2013) *Our Necessary Shadow: The Nature and Meaning of Psychiatry;* Richard P. Bentall (2009) *Doctoring the Mind: Why Psychiatric Treatments Fail;* James Davies (2013) *Cracked: Why Psychiatry is Doing More Harm Than Good;* Abraham Rudnick (2012), *Recovery of People with Mental Illness: Philosophical and Related Perspectives;* Larry Davidson et al. (2009) *A Practical Guide to Recovery-Oriented Practice;* Mike Slade (2009) *Personal Recovery and Mental Illness: A Guide for Mental Health Professionals.*

at many levels, amongst which are: *to get back, regain, restore, recuperate, return to, resume, reach, retrieve, repair, make good, get over, get better from, make up for, recycle, rehabilitate ...*

The three SMART members who use this word have all had at some point an acute episode of mental illness when they've been treated in a hospital setting according to the medical model. These episodes have in turn had considerable impact on their professional and personal lives, careers, living situations, relationships, ambitions and their ability at times to access everyday social and cultural resources. In short, for periods their lives have been severely disrupted by their illness and its treatment. Along with such acute episodes each person has also experienced an on-going process (sometimes over years) of coping with either the consequences of the acute episode, or with the on-going challenges of maintaining their mental health and quality of life.

But this is literally only half of the story! What we've also witnessed with these three people, and many others we've met through the project, is a quite different story when seen in the round. Not of illness, but of *recovery* – in all of the senses listed above: the on-going, challenging but hopeful process of getting things back, of restoring, regaining, resuming, retrieving many aspects of their lives. Restoring confidence and identity, relationships and social life, interests and skills, aspirations and vision. As each person points to in their own words, recovery is a process in time, something that comes about, something that is brought along with the person's engagement with life, something that is necessarily about the whole person and their lives, loves and aspirations. And importantly for these three people, recovery is something that can be helped along by music and music therapy – as has been the case for so many people in the SMART project.

Our three witnesses could also have been using the word 'recovery' as part of their thinking about themselves and their illness in relation to an increasingly common shared perspective (or philosophy, framework, vision, agenda – take your pick!) in international mental health theory, policy and service delivery. They have perhaps found a way of conveying their experiences in relation to the 'recovery approach'. Explaining this needs a level of comparison with what this approach critiques and sets itself up as an alternative to. This chapter is not the place for a detailed treatment of this subject, but it does need some level of attention at this point as our conclusions to the SMART project and this book will take 'recovery' as a point of departure.

***

A cartoon shows a woman onstage with a guitar and in front of a mic. She introduces her next song ' ... a sad little blues tune about love and pain that I wrote before I started taking Celexa!'. This sums up the practical dilemma that many people in the SMART project have told us about – that taking medication sometimes reduces symptoms, but at the cost of quality of life. The cartoon also symbolically introduces the theoretical and practical landscape of the current psychiatric critique, and its relationship to the recovery perspective.

The backstory of all this goes back to the earliest days of attempting to care more humanely for people with acute mental distress. The first asylums in the late eighteenth century offered respite from cruelty, and instead pursued 'ways of gentleness' through 'moral treatment' that attempted to remove people from distressing environments and encouraged natural healing through a benevolent social environment (Charland in Rudnick 2012). Sadly, by the mid-twentieth century this enlightened idea of asylum had become a cruel parody of itself in many countries, institutionalising patients and medicalising distress – and with this promoting a highly pessimistic view of mental illness as life-long and hopeless. The pendulum swung again from the 1960s onwards when old-style asylums were beginning to be closed and 'community care' developed, purportedly with the justification that the 'drug revolution' of a new generation of anti-psychotic medications allowed treatment and control of severe mental illness (SMI) 'outside'. A generation of patients has now passed through such combined medicalised hospital and community care provision, and longitudinal studies are beginning to produce worrying findings that are fuelling the rising critique of biomedical psychiatric theory and practice. This involves several key areas:

- **Diagnosis** – studies of successive diagnostic manuals (DSM III-V) show how many of the categories of SMI are culturally-dependent and established by expert consensus rather than scientific proof. Critiques of the latest DSM-V have re-fuelled the critique that psychiatry discursively 'manufactures' mental illnesses. When 'existing' such illnesses become disorders or deficits for the person diagnosed, with their accompanying stigma.
- **Aetiology** – what is the reality status of these 'mental illnesses' that are diagnosed? Are they brain or genetic disorders? According to the critics no strong evidence has ever been found that they are (Bentall 2009; Davies 2013). Rather illnesses are created that match what can be treated by medication, leading Darian Leader (2012, p. 27) to suggest that 'rather than seeing the drug as the key to the lock of the illness, the illness was defined as whatever would fit that key, rather like Cinderella's slipper'. The critique suggests that it is more likely that mental illness is not an illness in the traditional sense of a 'disorder' but more a set of understandable extreme responses to a complex set of bio-psycho-socio-cultural factors: an acute 'problem in living'.
- **Treatment** – So what then are psychiatric medications 'treating'? If they are not 're-balancing the chemical constitution of a brain', then what? Critics suggest that most medical drug treatments are no different from non-medical psychoactive drugs: that is, they temporarily *alter* mental states rather than treat an underlying illness. They may help dampen or mask symptoms, but perhaps much less so than is usually claimed. Longitudinal studies show similar continued prevalence of mental illness despite drug

treatment. And increasing evidence is coming to light of serious physical side effects of long-term use of psychiatric medication. The pharmaceutical industry has predictably defended biological and genetic theories and treatments of mental illness. The flipside of the dominant medical treatment of SMI has been that relational, social and cultural determinants (seen both as complex cause of mental distress and as possible site for interventions) have been severely underemphasised.
- **Prognosis** – from the early days of professional psychiatry there has been an unwarranted pessimistic view of SMI, a so-called 'myth of hopelessness', indicating that patients are unlikely to get better, and more likely to languish that flourish. This inevitably became a self-fulfilling prophecy within the contexts that people with SMI found themselves until relatively recently. Again the longitudinal evidence belies this professional belief: in fact a consistent number of people do recover from SMI, and recover their lives too ...

Overall, the critique is of the medical-model view of SMI being based on an inappropriate conception of mental illness that equates with other kinds of biological illness, and that is pessimistic overall in its view of people getting better. It also accords with a medical view that (i) medical authority and systems lead, (ii) there's an underlying biological cause to symptoms of mental distress, and that (iii) past personal experience, current relationships, context and culture are not significant factors either in the cause of the problem or its solution.

The recovery movement has challenged almost all of these assumptions and norms. An alternative image may help: a model of recovery that shows, and in ways that resonate with some of the classic health and illness research from second generation, 'Chicago-School' sociologists [Davis 1991 [1963]]) a pathway from crisis (where 'problems in living' overwhelm) through to recovery against a background of hope. And this is the key to this reorientation – that in contrast to the prevailing medical model, the recovery perspective takes a positive and hopeful vision of SMI.

As a movement 'recovery' has been developing in different contexts for the last 20 or more years, loosely allied to recovery theory in addiction, to user-led and survivor grass-roots activity in mental health circles, and in relation to academic critiques of traditional biomedical approaches to mental health. It has gained ground institutionally since the mid-1990s, being adopted gradually by many first world national health systems as a strategic direction to integrate with, and to reform traditional psychiatric care. More recently the critique of traditional psychiatry has also been echoed from within the professional establishment by 'critical psychiatrists'. A landmark article co-authored by 29 psychiatrists and published in *The British Journal of Psychiatry* (Bracken et al. 2012) is entitled 'Psychiatry beyond the current paradigm', and this critiques the dominant 'technological paradigm' which is based on a purely biomedical understanding of mental illness. It argues instead for a re-balancing towards 'the non-technical dimensions of our work such as relationships, meanings and values' (p. 430), and promotes the 'recovery approach', concluding:

> The evidence is becoming clear that to improve outcomes for our patients, we must focus on contexts, relationships, and the creation of services where the promotion of dignity, respect, meaning and engagement are prioritised. We must become more comfortable with cultural diversity, user empowerment and the importance of peer support (p. 432).

***

The most commonly cited definition of recovery in mental health is from Anthony:

> Recovery is a deeply personal, unique process of changing one's attitudes, values, feelings, goals, skills, and/or roles. It is a way of living a satisfying, hopeful, and contributing life even within the limitations caused by illness. Recovery involves the development of new meaning and purpose in one's life as one grows beyond the catastrophic effects of mental illness. (Anthony 1993, p. 17).

As this outline suggests, the perspective attempts to be both realistic and optimistic. It emphasises personal potential and sees recovery as an on-going *process*, a personal journey or pathway rather than a defined outcome to be achieved or not.[2] People talk about being 'in recovery' rather than 'recovering *from*' or 'being recovered'. It's possible to still have troubling symptoms but still be 'in recovery'; to be 'ill' but still register a level of wellbeing in relation to what's necessary and satisfying for a particular person in a particular context. In this sense the recovery model de-couples subjective wellbeing from objective illness and symptoms. As one service user puts it 'I am *not* my disorder' (Boevink, in Rudnick, p. 16). To go back to our opening image – the woman announcing her blues song – it might be that someone chooses to live with their symptoms rather than lose their creative spark through medication. The recovery model encourages individual choice, albeit guided by professional opinion and support at times. But the professional stance should be different from the traditional paternalistic and power-centred one of psychiatry's past, and instead be more based on a mutual and respectful collaboration, where both medical skill and knowledge, but also user's 'experiential knowledge' is respected and used. Another shift is from an exclusively 'needs-led' frame, where a patient is by definition passive, to a needs-and-*rights* perspective where issues of social justice and social critique are considered. Instead of the medical model process of 'getting back to normal' comes the more challenging question: What *is* 'normal'?

[2] Within the literature on recovery there's often a distinction made between *clinical recovery* (which is still within the medical model, describing reduction in symptoms and increase in functioning), and *personal recovery* – which is not an outcome to be achieved but a personal process to live through (and interpret subjectively and pragmatically).

In terms of the four categories that were critiqued above, the recovery perspective argues that: *diagnosis* be pragmatically linked to an acknowledgement that not enough is known about the root causes of mental illness to be definitive. In terms of *treatment* more attention should be given to a person's strengths (rather than their deficits), and to the relational, social, contextual and cultural origins of episodes of SMI; and that, conversely, help and support is seen to be individual and personal, but also social – providing therapeutic contexts where strengths are fostered, and good relationships, community support and access to cultural resources is possible. Given a suitable environment and resources the prognosis for a person with a SMI *can* be an optimistic one …

The aim of the recovery approach is to help a person live (once more) a meaningful life in the community as defined by the personal preferences and needs of that person, whilst attempting to reduce unnecessary distress and to maximise wellness (even if levels of illness remain). Whilst the approach attempts not to over-generalise and to keep attention on individual pathways, there is growing evidence of certain *core factors* that support good recovery from SMI. These include (from a user's perspective):

- Retaining your own voice, resourcefulness and wisdom within the recovery journey, and having these qualities acknowledged and respected by those helping you.
- Being guided by a hopeful attitude, focusing on wellness rather than illness as far as possible.
- Developing good coping strategies – that may at times involve traditional help (medication, therapy etc.) but within a different frame to the traditional medical model, where the emphasis is more on self-help or assisted help in collaboration with services (rather than old style paternalistic being 'looked-after').
- Establishing and maintaining a 'secure base' – physical, emotional, and social – to support and maintain recovery.
- Maintaining and sometimes rebuilding a sense of self – through experiencing oneself being known by others, developing a (new) identity, role, aims and aspirations – and through this counteracting the effects of stigma and exclusion by re-finding self-worth, self-esteem and confidence.
- Experiencing empowerment and inclusion – getting back self-determination, choice, control; feeling an equal part of how things happen, get sorted etc.
- Experiencing social connectedness, solidarity and belonging; being in community; contributing *to* community.
- Experiencing hope, meaning, purpose, spirituality, self-development. Becoming aware of the narrative of your recovery journey as potentially one of healing and transformation.

These 'core elements' are seldom established or experienced in a linear way, but are rather necessary parts of the landscape of a recovery path. The direction of this journey will be individual, even if shared; it will have its own style and tempo, and it will probably have progressive, static and recursive phases (as in life in general). As Wilma Boevink writes, 'Fundamentally, recovery is about daily life – something that all of us have in common' (in Rudnick, p. 27).

***

It's not our aim in this concluding section just to map our findings onto the recovery model. When writing a book it's usually a mistake to stand too closely to currently fashionable theories and policies for the obvious reason that they tend to change and date. There is, however, something about the notion of 'recovery' that transcends its current status in mental health policy and practice.[3] We aim to show rather where some of the close parallels between the results of our studies and the notion of 'recovery' perhaps point towards in a broader sense: to thinking freshly about the complex relationships between health/illness/wellbeing, environment and culture – whether this is within the particular area of mental health, or the broader remit of learning to live better with each other and our ever-varying states and possibilities of wellbeing – whatever our current 'problem in living' may be.

The following sections summarise what the SMART music project has led us to understand about a broad-based notion of 'musical recovery' – where 'musical solutions to living' are offered and taken up. We use the notion of recovery as a way of thinking about what the SMART Music project has been really telling us over its 10 years …

Recovering Music

Previous and emerging studies (Ansdell and Meehan 2010; Ansdell 2014b; Procter 2013; Solli 2014; Hense 2015) have shown how people with episodes of SMI often lose contact with the very resources that usually help them in everyday life. This can be because of a loss of motivation or confidence, or because something that previously helped has become problematic or entangled with illness. It can also be because of how special environments such as hospitals often involve cultural deprivation. Music is one of the personal/cultural resources that people can lose when illness sets in, severing a crucial resource for coping. For trained or serious musicians music has often been their main path in life before illness ('musicianhood'). For others it's not central but is helpful in many tacit ways. The SMART project shows how people can get back to music after illness has caused

[3] It's gratifying and reassuring to see how many national health and social care frameworks for chronic and enduring mental and physical illness are indeed converging on a recovery/wellbeing perspective. This bodes well for policy guiding service provision; the ability of this to incorporate non-medical therapies such as music therapy into a rationale for treatment; and a better alignment between user need, practice, theory and research in arts therapies.

a rupture in a previously helpful relationship. Music therapy, and the various activities that were spin-offs of this in the SMART project were often able to 'mid-wife' people back to a relationship with music again (or a more healthy relationship with it). Music became, in the language of recovery, a 'recovery ally' – something that helped build steps on a pathway away from illness and towards greater wellbeing.

Recovering Music's Help

> It's not magic; it's music! [Henrietta at SMART writing workshop, 5 March 2014]

But how did these musical pathways actually get built? As Henrietta says, it's not by magic! There's been a tendency in the popular story of 'music and health' in recent years to either suggest such a 'magical position', or in contrast to take a resolutely 'realist' experimental position where the musical material and the musical/personal/social process remains inside the 'black box' of an RCT, un-illuminated. In our research and this account of the SMART project we've tried rather to show-up this *how*-dimension. We start from the suspicion that music has little or no power in and of itself. Instead it offers its affordances (its possibilities within action and situation) and the help these affordances can in turn offer us – but only in relation to how, when and where they are taken-up, or appropriated. Music and people affect and transform each other reciprocally. So when trying to understand how music and people work together we always need to ask *who? where? when? how?*

This study has also been a manifesto for recovering a notion of the specificity and mediated power of music's affordances – for these are the cobbles, paving-stones, coloured mosaic fragments of people's recovery pathways, musically assembled. Musical help is given in relation to *how exactly* it's allowed to be taken-up into action (for example, laid down as a pathway, crossed over as a bridge). Like most forms of help, it can offer some things but not others; at some times but not others. How it helps is both unique and delimited. So what does music offer as seen through the evidence of the SMART music project?

Firstly, this question focuses light on just *how* music is, in and of itself, as a material medium and a practice. It has a basic 'ontological slipperiness' (DeNora 2013a) that is often handy in how it infiltrates and works implicitly, sideways, indirectly and modestly in situations (in comparison to the directness and explicitness of much speech/image). The 'stuff' of music has certain particular properties, qualities and tendencies (again, in comparison to speech or image) that enable it to do its building work. We call this its eco-phenomenology (Ansdell 2014). This phenomenological specificity as a medium shows up in exactly how music offers its particular help (in musical-personal forms of time, space, motion, combination, adhesion, diffusion, distribution etc.) and how people appropriate all of this within the situations of SMART musicking that we've followed in Part I.

We could sum up music's helpful affordances in this setting as helping people find a place and a pathway in music and musicking through:

- **'musical asylum'** – how musick(ing) offers a 'free space' in the two senses DeNora (2013a) has developed: asylum-*from* the negative aspects of mental illness, and asylum-*for* personal or communal creative play, which serves to 're-furnish' the social environment such that recovery and flourishing is possible: 'music as a way of making room for being well' (2013a, p. 62).
- **'musical personhood/identity'** – how musick(ing) offers a way of being positively recognised by others (as a musician, as musical, as courageous, playful or generous), and as a way of recovering and further developing a sense of self (as capable, talented, resourceful, social etc.)
- **'musical relationships/community'** – how musick(ing) offers ways of cultivating intimate non-verbal relationships and building community together.
- **'musical transcendence'** – how musick(ing) offers experiences of flow, joy, pleasure, spirit, beauty, meaning and hope.
- **'musical pathways'** – how these aspects working together can afford both a direction of travel but also the means whereby to move forwards – the pathway-making material.

It will be clear that these 'continuous outcomes' of the SMART project map almost perfectly onto the list of core factors that have been widely demonstrated to foster recovery in illness and life crisis (see bullet list above, p. 219).

Recovering Music Therapy

> Several people have come up to me in the last few weeks to say how much SMART music has helped, or is helping them – in ways that seem to mirror our idea of what we're trying to do – or, alternatively, because people have taught us what we need to do! [Gary's log, October 2010]

A professional debate that's been fermenting in the international music therapy community in the last decade mirrors the critique the recovery model makes of the medical model and its practice in psychiatry. Music therapy, as with many paramedical practices and disciplines, has historically become entangled with the medical model – through treatment contexts, and through borrowing medically-based theories of treatment for guidance, legitimation and prestige (Bunt and Stige 2014; Procter 2013; Rolvsjord 2010). Whilst there are currently (mostly in the US) directly biomedical models of music medicine/medical music therapy (Dileo 1999), so too are behavioural or psychological 'clinical' approaches to music therapy strongly determined by the assumptions, practices and values of the medical model. A growing critique suggests, however, that the medical model has been over dominant in music therapy and does not fit well with how music therapy fundamentally works, what it can best do, and how this can be best evidenced (Rolvsjord 2010; Ruud 2010; Aigen 2014; Stige and Aarø 2012; Procter 2013; DeNora 2013a).

Paralleling the recovery critique, the music therapy critique has pointed out that the natural picture music therapy practice presents, and the frame that the medical model provides do not align well. Medicalised theories and practices of music therapy are typically expert-led, pathology and deficit-focused, individualistic, non-contextual and 'internalist'. The treatment logic stemming from this meta-frame involves locating and diagnosing an individualised problem (preferably based on a biological cause), then treating localised symptoms and evaluating effectiveness on the basis of symptom remission and function returning to normal.

In comparison, other music therapy models such as music-centred music therapy (Nordoff and Robbins 1977/2007; Aigen 2005, 2014), resource oriented music therapy (Rolsvjord 2010) and Community Music Therapy (Ansdell and Pavlicevic 2004; Stige and Aarø 2012; Wood 2016) have mirrored the recovery model's alternative perspective and practices: to give access to 'musical help' that involves expertise (on both sides, music therapist and client) but is fundamentally collaborative; that is strengths-based, balancing needs with rights; is less interested in symptoms or diagnoses, but rather 'problems in living'; that acknowledges that both problems and help are not just individualistic, but relational, communal, environmental and political; that therapy is not just 'internal' but involves the whole inwards-and-outwards ecology of people's life worlds; and lastly that effectiveness of a therapy does not necessarily mean removing illness, or returning a person to 'normal' functioning. Ken Aigen (2014) helpfully sums up the logic of this perspective:

> In this [music-centered] framework, music therapy is conceptualised as a specialised application of music (specialised only in the sense that some of the implicit functions of music are rendered more explicitly) rather than as a specialised medium of therapy. Hence, the practice of music therapy cannot be subsumed to a medical model because many of the uses to which music is put – both in therapy and outside of therapy – are not addressing the problems that can be accurately described by a medical framework. They cannot be conceptualised by an illness ideology that requires the action of an authoritative professional who bases the intervention on a particular problem, illness, or condition. (Aigen 2014, p. 238)

The SMART Music project began with the principles and practices of the music-centred Nordoff Robbins approach, and has matured during the last 10 years in step with some of the recent psycho-sociocultural approaches such as Community Music Therapy and resource oriented music therapy that have been developing during this period. The evidence from SMART shows how these more recent approaches to music therapy make practical and theoretical sense, and fit with parallel current developments in other parts of health and social care such as the recovery model.

More recently a direct discussion and use of the recovery model is beginning to emerge in music therapy literature, practice and research (Solli, Rolvsjord and Borg 2013; Solli and Rolvsjord 2014; Solli 2014a, 2014b, 2015; Hense 2015), echoing and confirming previous studies that were leading in a similar direction (Ansdell and Meehan 2010; Procter 2011, 2013; Hooper and Procter 2013; Rolvsjord 2010; Jampel 2006).

Together, this represents in our view something of a recovery of the core of music therapy practice, theory and research itself. As we wrote in Part II, one of the continuing problems with medical-model outcome research in music therapy has been the lack of alignment between a theory of change for music therapy that matches the needs and aspirations of clients, and a suitable methodology for evidencing whether practice in particular contexts is successful and useful. Medical model assumptions and practices of much music therapy have distorted this enterprise for some of the reasons outlined above. It could be that an alternative logic based more on the idea of 'musical recovery' might in turn help bring about a recovery of music therapy more generally in terms of its ability to more successfully align practice, theory and research.

As the quotation at the head of this section from Gary's log illustrates, finding such an alignment is often helped by reflections coming from qualitative/ethnographic studies such as we've done with SMART – where engaged, long-term study of 'natural practice' (rather than 'ideal practice' guided only by extant theory or previous research models) can help anchor a more realistic practice-led theory which can then be more systematically assessed for effectiveness by a variety of evaluative methods.

Recovering a Notion of Musical Wellbeing

Underlying this 'new' perspective for music therapy is a 'new' developing perspective on health/illness, wellbeing and care in general – which is to an extent recovering something lost through the extensive medicalisation of everyday life (Frank 2004). We are at the beginning of a gentle revolution in thinking about what it means to be ill or well, to be able or disabled, to be flourishing or languishing. Again this perspective is aligned with recovery thinking, but has been developing in relationship to a specific focus on how culture, health and social action fit together beneficially. It could apply, we would argue, to any situation where we consider the nature, practice and effectiveness of music's help in relation to health/illness, ability/disability, potential/limitation.[4]

---

[4] This section is based on material we've previously developed in Ansdell and DeNora (2012), DeNora (2013a), Ansdell (2014), DeNora and Ansdell (2014) relating to the notion of 'musical wellbeing'/ 'musical flourishing'.

The medical model, and its influence on broader thinking and practice tends to operationally define health and illness as discrete binary opposites: for its practical purposes we are either 'well' or 'ill'. It tends also to define states of ill health mostly biologically (usually in terms of deficits, disorders or diseases), individualistically, and independently of immediate or ongoing context, social relationships, material and cultural resources, or fluctuations over time. 'Health' on the other hand tends to be under-defined – there's only one form of health (often negatively described as the absence of disease or dysfunction). In contrast, we champion an ecological perspective that tries to see health and illness more on a fluid continuum, heavily dependent on all of these crucial psycho-sociocultural variables that surround and influence our purely biological functioning. This perspective sees health/illness as a non-binary, complex, ever-fluctuating phenomenon that is multidimensional, context-dependent, materially mediated and richly temporal. It concentrates on the questions we posed earlier: ***When*** *and* ***Where*** *are we healthy or flourishing? What supports our continued flourishing despite objective 'state of health'? Can we be objectively sick but still flourishing as persons?*

The language of 'wellbeing' is increasingly used for talking about physical and mental health (Vernon 2008). It both enlarges and problematises the medical model, asking simply 'What counts as a good life?' regardless of the objective state of health or ability we might find ourselves in. A wellbeing or wellness perspective derives from a social model of health and disability, influenced by philosophical concepts such as Aristotle's *eudaimonia* (literally, 'well-spirited' – the root of 'wellbeing', originally meaning a holistic form of 'flourishing' through living a balanced physical, mental and ethical life[5]). Importantly, a wellbeing perspective takes people's subjective experience and preferences seriously, adding a first-person 'user perspective' to objective evaluations of health, asking people what makes them feel better or flourish – and importantly, where and when, and with what and whom. This perspective usefully re-frames some of the priorities of health and social care, as the authors of *A Practical Guide to Recovery-Oriented Practice* helpfully articulate:

> ... if we begin with describing the processes involved in minimising deficit, disability, and dysfunction, we may never arrive at a process of maximising the person's health and everyday life. Beginning with the person's everyday life and his or her efforts to live with the illness, on the other hand, naturally extends to efforts to minimize the illness as disrupting or posing barriers to that life. In brief, minimizing illness is not the same as maximising health, and our model must incorportate both. (Davidson, Tondora, Lawless, O'Connell and Rowe 2009, p. 34)

---

[5] In current thinking 'wellbeing' is taken to stand for the positive flourishing of identity, relationship and community (Vernon 2008; Carel 2008).

An ecological perspective such as we've outlined in this book helps balance attention on everyday wellbeing, and on maximising it, even within relatively severe illness or psycho-social challenge. The focus on people with mental health problems has highlighted the key fact of the recovery/wellbeing connection – that a broader conception is needed of what it is to be well, and along with this suitable political action to change attitudes, and social action to make available the necessary resources and support to help people be and stay well in this broader sense.

We've explored in particular that maximising health needs attention being paid to more than individuals, but also to contexts and resources – especially cultural resources. Recovery is said to be a personal achievement, but a social phenomenon. The same could be said for wellbeing. In this book we've traced the interdependence between musical people, musical things and musical situations in the service of greater wellbeing. We've seen how wellbeing and recovery are personal, emergent and are 'performed' in time and place – they are not abstract, context-free phenomena. We've seen how people's health and wellbeing is dependent on where they are, who they are with, what resources they have to work with, how other people see them and collaborate with them, and what kind of possibilities and pathways open up for their future. For all these broad needs it seems that for many people music offers a very particular kind of help.

***

Three over-arching concepts have emerged during the writing of the three-book triptych that characterise and support a particular understanding of musical wellbeing and recovery: how *music's help* represents a continuity between everyday and specialist uses in affording *musical asylum* and *musical pathways.* The detailed account of the SMART Music Project in this third volume has confirmed how these could be seen as key practical and theoretical tools for musical flourishing.

Musical asylum stands for how music can afford 'a way of making room for being well', 'a place and time to flourish' (DeNora 2013a, pp. 62, 1). Practically it can at times be a more private refuge, taking us away from states of distress or illness, offering something to cling onto or to retreat into. But equally musical asylum can represent the 'furnishing' of a creative social space for performing health through musicking. In the SMART project we've seen how members and therapists worked with and through music in these two senses to variously create niches, spaces, venues, stages, corners and positions for being well and flourishing – musically imagined and enacted. The idea of musical asylum nicely reframes the long term critique of the old-style discredited mental asylums, restoring the idea back to its original aim and achievement – the 'gentle way' of 'moral treatment' that encouraged recovery through a benevolent social environment.

Musical pathways stands for how music and musicking together can then afford a concrete way of moving forward through providing physical and symbolic steps, passages, inroads, trails, directions, aims, trajectories, bridges and purposes – musically imagined and enacted. The idea of 'care pathways' has for several decades now been part of the policy and bureaucratic scheme of healthcare delivery in many countries. Our idea of musical pathways echoes this but goes beyond the literal – showing how music lifts off from the purely practical, and 'lends' qualities of life, movement, direction, purpose and development to people and situations.

Together these two ideas work to imagine and enact a place and a path for wellbeing and recovery: helping us move both away from and towards; allowing us to be both 'lost and found in music' (Clarke 2014) – reminding us that wellness and recovery (in single moments, in a whole life) are always processes in time and situation, and never simply an outcome (Davidson, in Rudnick 2012).

Recovering Hope Through Music

Music is a hopeful means of travel.[6] As an art of time it naturally leans towards the future, its energy and purpose calling us into its hopeful space, time and motion. These qualities help people form pathways into the future, into recovery: through perhaps a beautiful moment in a song, a moment of interpersonal contact or support during a performance, a shared moment of appreciation or sympathy when listening together to an evocative song. In these, and a score of other ways, music provides 'a way of making room for being well' that can initiate a pathway towards future wellbeing. Of all the factors supporting mental health recovery hope is the key. Richard Bentall (2009) tells of a person who said 'We were able to begin recovery only when we felt we could connect and borrow someone else's hope until ours returned' (p. 278). Music is interesting in being a 'thing' that seemingly has hope to lend – albeit intertwined with the musical people and musical situations that we've witnessed throughout this book.

Ella, Henrietta and Stephen describe in their quotes at the head of this chapter various images of recovery in relation to music. For each of these people this has been a longish and complex, winding path during which they've used music variously to trigger, catalyse, support, drive, accompany, bridge and nurture an ongoing recovery process. Although these pathways are certainly individual to an extent, there's also a shared pattern of them recovering aspects of their lives before illness: talents, resources and ambitions. Ultimately the process is one of recovering hope that there is something beyond the significant challenges of mental illness.

Something of the same 'pathway narrative' has been told many times during this book by so many of the members of the SMART community. 'Pathways' seems to be a natural metaphor for recovery experiences as personal and hopeful

---

[6] See Ansdell (2014) Chapter 20 – *Musical Hope* – for a more detailed account of the ecophenomenology of musical hope. In short it's argued that hope is above all about time, and as music gives a non-verbal way of experiencing and (re)thinking time it also gives a template for the parallel complexities of hope and hopefulness.

journeys – working *towards,* being on the road to somewhere known or new. The idea of 'musical pathways' blends musical stories (the love of music, the need for music) with recovery stories – echoing something of the age-old symbolism (think the Orpheus myth) of music leading, of people responding and following, finding themselves somewhere quite different, finding themselves changed.

These musical pathway narratives in turn become part of the making of a recovery path. They turn into what recovery theory calls a 'new story' that helps shape a more hopeful future. Musical recovery is supported by an ecology of hope that emerges from how we help each other become and keep well together through our collective efforts: furnishing a shared space for being musical together … taking our part in good musicking … keeping the performance going …

Coda –

Sarah Wilson (December 2014)

This book is an extraordinary journey through memories and events: some chapters are interesting reminders of times forgotten; other vignettes are a pleasing or emotional re-reading of vivid experiences. Additionally I found it a thought-provoking process to read what is mostly other peoples' interpretation of my experiences and of events that have been a big part of my professional and personal life over the past 10 years. The project has been a unique and humbling opportunity to share pathways with people, and to be present alongside a spectrum of music making, time, space and health.

It is clear SMART music doesn't totally fit one predefined model or format; it draws from several and currently aligns with two predominantly (the Community Music Therapy model and the recovery model) but equally performs as its own special blend of people, time and place. Reflecting on how SMART Music is today, crucially the fundamental ethos remains: the belief that music can meet people where they are at, can mould to the time, people, place and mood and that music is an agent for change. We still don't aim to 'fix' or 'cure', but it is continually evident that what we offer people consequently enables them to cope better, at least some if not all of the time.

Practically, the project has expanded, (as at November 2014 SMART Music has increased to two days): the cafe drop-in session still happens weekly; the Singers is still going strong; we have more band musicians now, playing gigs in-house and in the community plus we run music courses and workshops. We are constantly evaluating and instigating new musical opportunities, directed largely by our members. In 2014 we saw the inaugural SMART Festival and member-led drumming tuition, both initiated by members' feedback and enterprise.

An overriding theme that emerges when reflecting on the current project is 'expectation'. Firstly, there is an expectation that SMART will have music. Many of the members written about here still use the music project, to a greater or lesser extent, but new members now join an organisation that has music as an intrinsic part of its programme and ethos; there are no question marks or debates about its worth anymore.

It is still evident that the skills and training of being a music therapist are needed to craft the project in the way it works: the knowing when to step in and out, lead or allow, perform or listen, teach or learn. But significantly, music now often still happens, albeit in a different way, if I'm away. Members run an acoustic session in the cafe themselves, and have to experience for themselves negotiating each other's musical variances, preferences and nuances!

There is an expectation that members will get involved. Rather than music put on *for* them, the culture is that we work with them, towards a collective and inclusive goal. It also means that everyone is expected to help do what it takes to make sessions happen; that's everything from moving instruments, chairs etc., to bringing sheet music or recordings along for the groups to help them learn new songs.

There is also an expectation of 'quality'. The book refers to 'good musicking', and my sense is that the culture of SMART Music is one of knowing that the music played, performed and received is of a quality which supports talent and/or also embraces enthusiasm and musical passion in equal measure.

The definition, in music, of a Coda is a 'passage which brings a movement or piece to a conclusion through prolongation'. SMART Music hasn't stopped, it continued from the very next day after the data collection for this book was completed. Therefore the purpose of *this* Coda is to conclude the project to the current position, whilst highlighting that the music plays on.

Instead I prefer to pause on an anacrusis (*definition* - a 'pickup note' or 'upbeat' …)! SMART Music is an ongoing, ever changing vibrant entity that has multiple influential factors and features, but a solid core that is music and people. We work in the musical moment, as well as with individuals and groups, and influence the organisation as a whole. Sometimes we have aims and an overview that direct the project over the coming months; other times the work is instinctive, intuitive and impromptu and changes minute by minute, day to day. Hence there is always an upbeat to the next moment in the life of SMART Music … .

Appendix A
About Method: How We Wrote This Book

... the ambition, at least, is to tell 'my story' about 'their story' through the fullest conceptual bringing out of 'their story'.

Paul Willis (2000, p. xi), *The Ethnographic Imagination.*

It's only words, and words are all I have ... Da da da da da da ... .

– The Bee Gees

In this book, we have written a series of stories about music and musical activity and what music can do for wellness and wellbeing. Here we describe what we did to make those stories, where they came from, how we sought to 'see', how we went 'about' the task of writing 'about' music. And so it is with the word 'about' that we begin this, our final, story.

We are naturally aware that, to paraphrase the Bee Gees, we are using words to convey a process that not only greatly exceeds those words, but also takes shape in reference to the words we use. However, as the song reminds us, 'words are all [we] have' and we continue to use them albeit imperfectly, understanding that in so doing we are doing things with words. To agonise excessively about the ethnographer's bias, construction of the field, or metaphysical pathos is *de trop*. As one highly distinguished ethnographer has put it, the task is or should not be to engage in solipsism and extended autobiographical reflection, nor is fieldwork the place for, 'exhortation to researchers to be "reflective practitioners", and capable of understanding their own actions as social researchers' (Atkinson 2015: 26). On the contrary, and here we concur with Atkinson that, '[t]he fundamental principle of reflexivity is an essential part of social research. It is an unavoidable feature of it ... .Reflexivity is the condition whereby any social research inevitably helps to constitute the phenomenon under investigation ... we are inevitably and inextricably implicated in what we study' (Atkinson 2015: 26). The point is, in other words and given this inevitability, we need to get on with research, not to waste time and attention upon our own role(s) within the research process, so diverting attention away from the actual members of the field and their own reflexive accounts. (Marshall Sahlins' joke about the 'native' who said to the postmodern anthropologist, 'enough about you, let's talk about me' is, we think, ever-apt.) Indeed, throughout our focus on accounts 'about' experience have been less concerned with the use of accounts (e.g., interview transcripts) as 'data' than as media by which certain things come to be performed (recipes, exemplars, glosses, holding forms), and we have described the importance of music and talk in tandem (DeNora 2013c) in the previous chapters (for example in our account of Mary and her micro-narratives of 'this f*****g life' and 'that's better'. As Atkinson observes, there is no time out from the performative features of narrative – and for everyone who is implicated in the research process.

So we saw our own methodological challenges as being about the using and choosing of our words so as to make stories that can hold and convey complexity and, in the case of this book, that pick out or illuminate pathways for and to wellbeing to show how they were made. In one sense, then, what we did with our stories was didactic ethnography or the crafting of stories in such a way that their protagonists could demonstrate some of the ways that pathways to wellbeing are crafted, step-by-step, in and through reference to musical activity. Underlying this vision, our aim has been to fix the tales we offer in terms of their grounding in the practices and experiences and life events of SMART members such that they will recognise themselves 'in the act'.

Our Methodological Values

We have written elsewhere, together (Ansdell and DeNora 2012; DeNora and Ansdell 2014) and separately (DeNora 2013a; 2013b; DeNora 2014; Ansdell and Pavlicevic 2010; Ansdell 2014) about our mutual interest in – as we've often put it – *opening the 'black box' of musical engagement*. As we describe in the body of this book, too much research on music and wellbeing tends to ignore the question of what music does in real time. Attempts to measure music's benefits, for example, offer before and after comparisons and focus on specific variables so as to measure change. But they rarely address what actually occurs when people and music come together. That question, and its associated 'music-led' perspectives (Aigen 2005) are what we wanted to illuminate. It is also the question that unites our respective research disciplines of music therapy (specifically *Community* Music Therapy) and music sociology which, at least for us as we've worked together for now over 11 years, are very intertwined.

Along with this 'black-boxing', and attempts to open such boxes, comes the question of *ecological validity*. In our accounts about how music helps we wanted to ensure that our stories would be commensurate with SMART members' actual, real-world practices, experiences and accounts, that they would not only recognise themselves when looking into the mirror of our stories, but that our stories would themselves mirror, or be grounded in, actual, worked examples from lived experience. Part of the quest of ecological validity involves a concern with members' practices, their own 'ethno-methods' of making do and getting by and this user-centred, person-centred focus was another of our touchstones. That focus in turn has been linked to an interest in 'lay expertise' that is in what SMART members themselves have to say about how they are and what they need – to get and remain well.

The pursuit of ecological validity can be demanding, problematic. To have any chance at achieving it the researcher needs to tread carefully. The process is rather like cooking from scratch, it takes time and care and a feeling for ingredients. It shies away from 'one size fits all' accounts of how music works (we hope we never again get asked 'which kind of music should I play to help [fill in the blank with an ailment here]?'). And it cannot afford to sidestep details, the seemingly 'small' things that sometimes turn out to be of magnitude. We have described all this in some detail through the prisms of two methodological strategies that we regard as complementary (indeed the first was an important influence on the second). These are *'gentle empiricism'* (Ansdell and Pavlicevic 2010) and *'slow sociology'* (DeNora 2014).

The former (gentle empiricism) calls attention to the ways that researchers can and ought to work like attendants, supporting, quietly questioning, not butting in, closely observing, dwelling with but unobtrusively and always ready to abandon any notion if it fails to mesh with what can be traced in actual observation. The latter (slow sociology – itself inspired by Ansdell and Pavlicevic's promotion of the gentle empiricism concept) reminds us not to rush things and not to cut in too quickly or too deeply 'all at once'. At its core, this slow and gentle form of enquiry involves takes care not to make too hasty identifications between what it thinks it knows and what there is to know. Here it follows what we have come to call 'Hennion's dictim' – namely that 'it must be strictly forbidden to create links when this is not done by an identifiable intermediary' (Hennion 1995, p. 248, quoted by DeNora 2000, p. 4). Thus, as we described early on in the body of this text, we have tried to offer stories that tell by showing, and that follow actors as they link, and come to be attached, to music, objects, places, people and occasions and as those attachments resulted in some change – in social connection, sense of self or presentational skills, musical skills and repertoires, moods and occasions, customs and values. To what extent, in other words, can music be seen, and in grounded ways, to 'get into' change, in this case change in wellbeing status and how, simultaneously, do those changes accrue so as to alter and define the realms of action where they occur? This dual question points to our key concern throughout with music in action. And here lies the kernel of what we explore when we speak, as in Part I Section 10, of an *ecological perspective* and a focus on gatherings and concatenations, tinkering and patterning within musical worlds. That is what we tried to capture in our writing 'about' music.

Data Collection

As we have described, the research arm of the project ran over six years. It gathered data through a variety of means, some of them quite conventional forms of qualitative and ethnographic research and some of them more specifically linked to musical research. The former included dual and three-handed Participant Observation at both ends of the classic continuum (full participant and nearly-full observer) with Ansdell and Wilson (and for a short time Rob Szymanek) as full participants and DeNora as part-time observer (she attended, sang along, helped out but never sang a solo). These observations included regular SMART Music sessions and special occasions as we have described. As supplement to these observations, Szymanek and Ansdell conducted two full rounds of interviews with regular SMART members, some of whom we have presented in the body of this text as 'pathway cases'.

The more specific musical data was collected through audio-recordings (50 of the approximately 200 SMART Music Sessions were recorded and most of these 'indexed' – see below – with time-based description and commentary by Ansdell). In 2005–6 four whole sessions of SMART Music were video recorded as were a selection of special events, in and out of SMART, that involved the SMART Singers and the SMART Band, between 2005–11. Some of these sessions were also indexed. Finally, there are a few recordings (audio/visual) of routine Singers groups.

Techniques of Analysis

Studying musical action ecologically is not only time consuming, it also involves specific analytical techniques if the project of mapping out traces, links, attachments and their adjacent practices is to be described, and if that process is to be depicted in all its subtle and rich ecological complexity, then the mechanisms by which music comes to work as an 'active ingredient' are to be made traceable. Our techniques varied from those that were primarily heuristic to those that were devoted to real time and a highly detailed form of content analysis. Their purpose was to help us pinpoint, with as much precision as possible, what, about people and ecology, changed over a temporal interval and how that change was made.

The first analytical tool sits on the borders between theory and method. It is the notion of the 'musical event' (DeNora 2003; 2013a; 2013b; Ansdell 2014; Stige et al. 2010; Stige and Aarø (2012). Used as a grid for observation, the musical event logs connections made by actors themselves between musical and extra-musical matters and in ways that highlight music's role as an agent of short and longer-term change. This log examines three interconnected time periods: **Time 1**: what do participants bring to musical engagement *before* engagement begins (e.g. musical/biographical memories, embodied musical pre-dispositions, self-perceptions of physical state, emotional orientations, psycho-social concerns) and how are these matters linked by participants to the musical engagement (e.g. through talk during music about music, or through expressed connections between features from Time 1 and the present moment)? **Time 2**: what do participants do *during* musical engagement? These practices are often minute, for example, quiet humming, micro facial expressions, gestures, fragmented commentary). **Time 3**: what do participants do, say, feel or think after the moment of musical engagement and how can that engagement be seen to incorporate traces of Time 2 and in ways that inform subsequent action (e.g. reorientation, narrative accounts of the Time 2 experience, changes in emotional orientation, self-perceptions of physical state, comportment or gesture, reminiscence, music-associated forms of motivation, expressed aspiration, forging of new acquaintances or the discovery of shared values)?

The musical event implies questions about how things come to be arranged, concatenated, linked together. It is an historically-grounded schema, one focused on music 'in action' and one that requires us to know a great deal about the background to any real time musical activity such that what any individual or group comes to do can be considered in terms of how they make connections between the here-and-now and the there-and-then, a two-way process that allows for the present and the past to influence each other. It is probably obvious but worth underlining that the concern with historical connection in this way is something that is normally sidestepped by more positivistic and reductionist accounts that seek to measure music's 'effectiveness' in health-related settings. Here, by contrast, we have been concerned with the meanings and resonances of present-based music practices in what has come before – biographically, institutionally, culturally and – in terms of SMART Music – collectively. Thus, one of the key features for us was to map the 'music history' of SMART over time, understanding that music history in terms of the music practices that were most prominent, more marginal, segregated, inclusive and – over time – transitional. Various further tools and techniques assisted the process of understanding how people, and SMART Music itself, moved over time from A to B, from B to C, etc. in ways that laid down musical pathways toward wellbeing.

One of these was mapping. By thinking about SMART Music's terrain in terms of 'common' and well-hewn territory versus 'niche' territory we were able to understand individual musical strategies and attachments in terms of how they were pulled out from the collective and (differentially) shared territory of what was known and done in SMART, and thus how they contributed to the modification of that territory over time. So, for example, as we have described, Jeremy was very firmly ensconced in a subset of SMART Music terrain for many years but, gradually, and with encouragement from Sarah and from other SMART members, his musical attachments broadened; he was drawn on to other parts of the musical space and thus also into new musical occasions, new musical forms of expression and new forms of participation, such as the SMART Singers. As his musical world expanded, so too (to some extent) did his social network widen, the ties to others more solidified. Similarly, we examined all of the log books and coded according to emerging themes. These themes highlighted space, furnishing activities, objects, repertoire, events, people, occasions, celebrations, identities and musical skills. Through this coding we were able to identify trends within SMART Music, even extremely small changes, such as Eloise's increasing participation and confidence with her cymbal playing and the cymbal's shift from periphery to centre over time.

Another technique involved grounded thematic analysis of interview transcripts. We did this both separately and together and, on one occasion, drew together a panel of ourselves, Sarah, Amelia, Dr John Meehan, consultant psychiatrist, Simon Procter and Mercedes Pavlicevic who each presented and discussed two transcripts over the course of a day at the Nordoff Robbins Centre, London. The interview transcripts were – as we conceived them – simultaneously data and strategic action. This is to say that they were informative about SMART members' histories, tastes, concerns and self-perceptions and, simultaneously, as we have described earlier in this appendix, they were forms of discourse, ways of using words to make attachments to things, to define situations and to effect forms of change, in self and others. So, for example, when at one stage Gary asks Ella to talk about musicking and what it's done for her, she turns to metaphors such as driving a car and getting warmed up. It's at points like this that we think we can begin to see how music gets converted into things paramusical, such as accounts, how music is connected imaginatively and metaphorically to other aspects of self and world, and thus how music functions as an agent of change. Ella's talk refers back to her musicking activities (examples of Time 2) and projects forward into sketches of how she is and what she is like. The interview, in other words, and its accounting procedures, makes an arch between before and after as it describes the 'during' musicking.

It is this 'during' however, that is of great interest and thus we also needed methodological techniques for viewing and making sense of what transpires there. For this we turned to the music-therapeutic 'index'. The 'index' is a staple documentary and analytic/reflective technique in music therapy (Nordoff and Robbins 1977/2007). It consists of a detailed real-time chart of multi-channel musical and paramusical action in real and often split-second time, usually with parallel columns for different communicative channels (e.g. music, talk, gesture, concurrent events and the movement or use of objects). The index is expressly devoted to exploring the 'inside' of the 'black box' we spoke of earlier. It is a way of providing a record of musical action in terms of its social distribution and paramusical dimensions. Indexing allows us to dwell not only on 'what' was performed and by whom, when, but what that performance consisted of in real time, understanding performance to be a multi-media endeavour that includes forms of embodiment, musical inflection, talk, interruption, direction, variegated participation and levels of intensity. More specifically, indexing musical events allows us to see what was drawn into the vortex of a musical event, when and how and with what consequences *during* that event.

And so the point of these stories is to join up the triple time of musicking – the complex tale of where musicking comes from (its local history), the rich and varied occasioning of actual musical events, and the knock-on effects that it fosters. Pulling these strands together was how we made the materials from which our tales were spun (we thought of the book as akin to macramé). We know our stories could have been different and we know we were also protagonists in them (though we have not engaged in autoethnography as a deliberate strategy here because our aim was to showcase what SMART members did). As we are very aware, in our respective fields of music therapy and music sociology, music is never 'about' people any more than people can write 'about' music. Rather, in both cases, music and social life get put together, arranged, in different ways with different consequences. Telling about this process is, in other words, itself a form of musicking. The general point, as we hope we have begun to illustrate, is that music – put together with other things – can make something happen and in particular it is possible to trace the ways in which music can be used to help to make us 'well' in the rich and varied meanings of that term. We like to think that this tracing, via the journeys of the SMART members whom we describe, might be useful pedagogically to others for whom music might be helpful and to others whose work is devoted to being helpful through musical means.

Appendix B
How We Negotiated the Ethics of this Project

> ... ethical experience begins with the approval of a demand, a demand that demands approval. Ethical experience is virtuously circular.
>
> Simon Critchley (2012, p. 39)

The philosopher Simon Critchley (2012) describes ethics as 'infinitely demanding', and indeed this long research project and the book based on it has made great demands on many people in relation to its ethical aspects. And it needed to. For the focus of this study is on people in varying states of illness and health, and their often very personal experiences and musical stories – told, sung, played and performed – and then often recorded, documented, analysed, compared, and so forth. These stories are rich, but also sometimes fragile in how they take in people's whole lives: their experiences of illness and health; their blend of strengths and vulnerabilities, triumphs and troubles, experiences of stigma and courage. How, then, have we responded to the rightful demand to take care of these people and their stories whilst communicating as full an overall story as we can in this book from our perspective?

Ethics was our very first priority from the inception of the project. Indeed managing the ethics could be thought of as yet another one of the key 'pathways': an ongoing, not always straightforward, but also illuminating and satisfying 10-year journey. As the authors we've learned so much from reflecting on this area with SMART members and colleagues, and through engaging as creatively as we could with what emerged. What follows in this Appendix is both a factual account of this 'ethics pathway', but also some brief reflections on aspects of the demands of research ethics in such a project, and how we have 'navigated' the sometimes choppy waters of this vital area.

***

Seen from a research ethics angle the project had four main phases, each one of which included formal and informal ethical processes, issues and negotiations:

PHASE 1 - PREPARING AND PILOTING (2006)

Although a particular aim of the project was to study peoples' musical pathways between sites of care, we decided not to extend the study directly into any medical NHS premises as this further complicated UK statutory ethics procedures (especially given that ethnographic methods were viewed sceptically at that time in these circles). Instead we studied people from the outside door of the hospital as they then moved towards and into SMART, and then out further into the community in various ways.

We made formal applications for the pilot project to the Chief Executive and Trustees of SMART, and an ethics application was scrutinised by the Nordoff Robbins Research Ethics Committee (NRREC). An ethics formulation was also part of an ESRC application made at this time (which was well reviewed but did not achieve funding). These ethics applications included an outline of methodology and methods, and samples of participant information and consent forms for interviews. Meanwhile we introduced the SMART community to the research project by preparing an accessible project description and briefing the Chief Executive who put the project to the next Members' Meeting, asking for feedback and concerns. The members were keen for the research to happen and asked good questions about practical aspects, which we then tackled in the early months when initial data gathering took place. For example, Gary made an announcement every time he made an audio recording of a SMART Music Session, and when these were occasionally filmed this was preceded by negotiating how those who didn't want to be filmed could still participate (sit on one side of the room with the camera operator suitably briefed). The other part of the pilot was research assistant Rob's two-month sustained fieldwork at SMART doing 30 short ethnographic interviews with members about their everyday use of music and their early experiences of SMART Music. Rob's research journal charts how he negotiated the research ethics of these interviews in a way that was most respectful and 'safe' for each member. Every interviewee signed a consent form.

PHASE 2 – FOCUSING (2007–10)

The pilot stage had identified a group of key participants of the various music groups who were willing to help us understand more about their various 'musical pathways'. Detailed ethnographic interviews were planned with a set of participants, tracing their music-health/illness pathways within and beyond the music project. A second ethics application was made to both SMART and Nordoff Robbins ethics committees in relation to this phase, its aims and methods. The then Chief Executive of SMART wrote: 'I've had the chance to review the research proposal and I think the research design looks good and, importantly, safe for our members' (14 February 2008). Participants were given clear information about the purpose and format of the interview, and the future use of the material within both the research process and potential future publication in scholarly articles and a book. Interviewees were judged to have capacity to give signed consent. These interviews were fully transcribed and the transcripts returned to the interviewees to correct, edit and then sign their further approval of this material. All complied with this.

Parallel with this data source we continued to collect ethnographic data from participant observations of sessions, rehearsals and events and to build a bank of audio-visual material of these. All such data was scrupulously coded to maintain anonymity and confidentiality of sites and people involved. The Chief Executive of SMART was able to provide informal monitoring of the organisation and its members' ongoing trust and satisfaction with the research process. Gary, Sarah and Tia attempted to keep an ongoing conversation about the transparency of the project, 'keeping their ears to the ground' for any discomfort or confusion.

PHASE 3 – REVIEWING AND CONSULTING (2011–12)

The end of 2010 marked the end of the formal data gathering. The music groups and events continued after this, and we continued to study what happened, but collected no further systematic data. As we collated and started analysing the considerable volume of data we had collected we also organised what we saw as the next stage of the ethics process, to reviews and consult SMART and its members about what we thought we had understood, and how to convey this as the 'results' and dissemination of the research project.

This round of ethics consultation was partly spurred by us picking up some nervousness about the consequences of writing up the research – both for the organisation and individual members. These concerns could be summarised as:

1. Should SMART be identified in such publications directly? Or should a pseudonym for the organisation and its location be used? What are the advantages / disadvantages?
2. What is the relationship between anonymity of the place and anonymity of individual members?
3. What are the ethics of individual representations of members and their activities within the study data? Should we (after suitable anonymisation / disguise) under-report aspects that the organisation or individuals in it may not like? Is this helpful to the integrity of the research as a whole?

We decided to make this an open and transparent conversation at all levels, to address concerns, but also to creatively explore dilemmas and possibilities. Firstly, we informally gathered members' opinions and concerns and wrote-up a paper for the SMART Board of Trustees [*Outline of Research Ethics Consideration for Phase 4*], reviewing the whole process (including all ethics processes) to this point, outlining a range of current views, and asking for advice on how to bring the project to a conclusion in the fairest, safest and most beneficial manner for all concerned.

SMART recommended a general final briefing to the whole organisation about where the project had arrived at, coupled with an individualised process for 'pathway cases' to check final content of the write up. We compiled a members' update – *Researching the SMART Music Project: News, Questions and Answers* – which was made available to attendees of SMART. For those participants who had individually contributed through interviews (2006/2009) personalised letters were sent inviting them to a closed meeting at SMART. Members were asked to read the update and, if they wanted, to forward any particular questions (anonymously) for the meeting through Amelia. This meeting was held at SMART in July 2011, and included most of the relevant contributors, Amelia, Sarah, Gary and Tia. A lively discussion balanced an overall support for the writing-up stage of the project, with some clear and well-expressed opinions and concerns as to how members would or would not like SMART or themselves to be represented in future publications. Minutes from the meeting were circulated to members present and absent, and submitted to the SMART Board of Trustees. These phases highlighted ongoing considerations and concerns to take into account during the final writing-up stage:

- If 'SMART' as an organisation was identified as the research site would this compromise individual members' confidentiality and anonymity? If it was not identified would a chance for the advocacy of a positive and successful mental health service model be lost?
- How would the story of the project be told in a way that balanced the overall success with the acknowledged ups and downs of aspects of it? In the words of a participant 'How to tell it, worts and all, but still make sure people know it's been brilliant?'
- How to reconcile the need to use as much of the research data as possible in the write up, but also ensure that members are happy with any representations of them in the final manuscript.

These issues were considered through a final phase of the ethics process:

PHASE 4 – CHECKING (2013–14)

As the writing-up stage was delayed more than we'd hoped we decided to do a final 'checking-in' session with SMART and the key project members in 2013. The practical project was still happily ongoing, and members frequently asked 'When is the book going to be ready?', philosophically listening to Gary's excuses. But we also took their impatience seriously, in case the enthusiasm also included some anxieties about the conclusion of the research arm. After consulting Amelia and Sarah we decided to have a final meeting for key participants, inviting their last thoughts about the project, briefing them about how we'd manage checking the final manuscript, but also thinking together creatively one last time about how to 'tell the story' of the music project. SMART invited an expert in story-telling workshops to help us with this. This event was reassuring and illuminating in equal measures. There was a space for us all to tell our version of this long story we'd all been involved in, and to experience directly how we inevitably told it in different ways, with different emphases, and so on. It became clear that Tia and Gary's 'research story' was one of many angles. Another aspect of this meeting was that certain key formulations naturally emerged (for example, Henrietta's 'It's not magic, it's music!').

In terms of the concerns about publication a consensus developed that almost everyone wanted SMART to be explicitly identified as the organisation, and the priority was that this decision had minimal impact on the few members who considered personal anonymity to be important for them.

The main text of the book was ready by the summer of 2014 for members to check (by autumn 2014). Two aspects of checking from an ethical point of view happened at this stage. Amelia and Sarah read the whole draft manuscript to check that the overall representation of SMART, its members and staff, and the music project was not unfair, damaging or detrimental to anyone's dignity or wellbeing. Secondly, as agreed, we would share with individual members those passages in the manuscript that referred directly to them, or that quoted from any interview material with them. Sarah and Amelia, who invited people to 1:1 meetings with them to ask how they wanted to check their material, mediated this process.[1] Some members asked to read the text and return with any comments, corrections or concerns; others asked Amelia and Sarah to read out the text during the meeting. The publication process was explained, and any potential negative impacts for themselves were highlighted. Members were given the option to withdraw their material from the book, to correct any inaccuracies, to redact any passages that they were now uncomfortable with, and finally to choose a pseudonym and to change any aspect of their identity in order to fully disguise themselves in the text. All SMART members portrayed in the final text of the book were seen this way. Two people requested and chose their own pseudonyms, the rest were happy to retain their own names. Small factual corrections were made, but overall members found the representations of themselves within this project to be acceptable, and no redactions were requested. Several members did not want to engage in detail with this checking process, they said that they trusted Gary, Sarah, and the process.

***

These, then, are the 'facts' of a research ethics process that we have tried to make as systematic, comprehensive and sensitive as we could in the circumstances. This process follows what's taken to be current 'best practice' in academic research ethics, which sometimes has a tendency to assume that procedure will suffice to ensure good ethics. There is, however, a sub-plot to the research ethics process

[1] Two ex-members of SMART in the category of, 'pathway cases' who had moved on, were contacted by email and the member-checking process was done this way.

of this project, which became something else that we discovered from our long-term immersion in this culture[2]. We'll begin with two small stories that come from Gary's logs (which we told earlier in the book, but we'll remind you of here):

> Jeremy is signing a consent form to be interviewed on the first stage of his musical pathway. I've known J for many years and know he trusts me. He understands what the project is about, what we're asking him to consent to, and I thought he was happy to participate. With his pen poised over the consent form he hesitates and looks distressed. I ask him what the matter is, and he says: 'I'm perfectly happy to sign, but I just had a flash-back – the last time I signed one of these was thirty years ago, for ECT treatment – it was ghastly!'. A research ethics moment that no amount of preparation or committee approval could have prepared me for.
>
> Near the end of the study we make one final round of informing participants how we would end the study. I'm sitting in the Centre cafe talking to some of the members about this topic and see a member's puzzled face. 'Research *ethics?'* says this man who'd been involved in the project for five years – 'I think that must have passed me by!'. I swallow my shock and discomfort, and start again with the research ethics process, right there and then with this person. He's suitably reassured at the end, and says 'I'm sorry, I forget lots of things – it's the medication'.

Here are two examples of real-world research ethics, where the relatively easy answers of tick-box proceduralism come against the face-to-face reality of real people in real time and real situations. At these times we were confronted with a different level of ethical demand that was often unexpected, and sometimes shocking. These situations typically involved the dissonance between what was technically right according to 'compliance research ethics' (get signed consent, inform people fully etc.) and what was humanly right within a face-to-face situation.

We learned from these examples how to think about ethics in what the doctor-philosopher Raymond Tallis (2013) calls 'the real mess of the real world' (p. 202). 'Messy ethics' comes about when there's a conflict between abstract procedure and the face-to-face demands of real-world human situations. Tallis' advice is that 'if they are in conflict you must choose an overriding principle, and doing this involves consultation and the deployment of your imagination' (p. 204). Our recourse during this project has been to two such overriding principles: face-to-face responsibility to the individual whilst also 'doing justice' to something often broader than that individual.

Our face-to-face responsibility to a person is in the present moment: in the relationship, in the situation – something that parallels the immediacy of the music therapy situation itself. The ensuing demands of the moment – ethical, relational,

[2] The following section draws on Ansdell (2014b).

aesthetic – trump more abstract formulations or rules, whilst also attempting to align with them.[3] The core ethical question is then: 'What is good, here and now, with this person? What then should I do?'. Ethics seen this way consequently becomes part of ongoing creative work, eliding neat distinctions between creative practice and research, between personal and professional, individual and communal. A second useful formulation of modern ethics in relation to musical situations we've found helpful comes from Cobussen and Nielsen (2012) – their idea of 'doing justice' to a person, a work of art, a situation – or the multiple relationships between these. One of the key ethical dilemmas we've faced as researchers of the SMART Music project is how to do justice to the complex story of the work as a whole, whilst not compromising individual wellbeing or trust. This has involved negotiating how to tell a story that is not 'air-brushed', but is also just and respectful.

It's not of course for us to gauge whether we've succeeded in squaring the circle between ethics and research, but we can say that we've tried our best to be both rigorous and creative with the many ethical demands that have emerged from this project.

---

3 The principles of research ethics are based on medical ethics and its meta-principle of *Benificence* – 'first do no harm!'. Following this the key principles of research ethics are: autonomy and choice; justice; respect; truthfulness and honesty.

Bibliography

Aigen, K. (2005). *Music-Centered Music Therapy.* Gilsum, NH: Barcelona Publishers.

Aigen, K. (2014). *The Study of Music Therapy: Current Issues & Concepts.* New York: Routledge.

Aldridge, D. (2004). *Health, the Individual & Integrated Medicine*. London: Jessica Kingsley.

Ansdell, G. (2002). Community Music Therapy and the Winds of Change – A Discussion Paper. *Voices: A World Forum for Music Therapy*, Vol. 2, No. 2 (2002). Retrieved 4 August 2013, from https://normt.uib.no/index.php/voices/article/view/83/65

Ansdell, G. (2014a). *How Music Helps: In Music Therapy and Everyday Life.* Farnham: Ashgate.

Ansdell, G. (2014b) "Infinitely demanding": the creative work of research ethics. Preface to Farrant, C., Pavlicevic, M. & Tsiris, G., *A Guide to Research Ethics for Arts Therapists & Arts & Health Practitioners*. London: Jessica Kingsley.

Ansdell, G. (2014c). A prevailing breeze: a retrospective evaluation of 'Community Music Therapy and the winds of Change'. *International Journal of Community Music*, 7(1).

Ansdell, G. and DeNora, T. (2012). Musical Flourishing: Community Music Therapy, Controversy, and the Cultivation of Wellbeing. In: R. MacDonald, G. Kreutz and L. Mitchell (eds), *Music, Health, and Wellbeing*. Oxford: Oxford University Press.

Ansdell, G. and Meehan, J. (2010). 'Some Light at the End of the Tunnel': Exploring Users' Evidence for the Effectiveness of Music Therapy in Adult Mental Health Settings. *Music and Medicine*, 2(1), pp. 41–47.

Ansdell, G. and Pavlicevic, M. (2010). Practising 'Gentle Empiricism': The Nordoff–Robbins Research Heritage. *Music Therapy Perspectives*, 28(2), pp. 131–9.

Ansdell, G. and Stige, B. (2016). *Community Music Therapy*. In J. Edwards (ed.), *The Oxford Handbook of Music Therapy.* Oxford: Oxford University Press.

Ansdell, G., Davidson, J., Magee, W., Meehan, J. and Procter, S. (2010). From 'This ****ing Life' to 'That's Better'… in Four Minutes: An Interdisciplinary Study of Music Therapy's 'Present Moments' and their Potential for Affect Modulation. *Nordic Journal of Music Therapy*, 19(1), pp. 3–28.

Atkinson, P. (2006) *Everyday Arias: an Operatic Ethnography*. Lanham, MD: AltaMira.

Atkinson, P. (2010) Making opera work: bricolage and the management of dramaturgy. *Music and Arts in Action*, 3:1.

Atkinson, P. (2013) Blowing Hot: the ethnography of craft and the craft of ethnography. *Qualitative Inquiry,* 19, 3, pp. 397–404.
Atkinson, P. (2015) *For Ethnography*. London: Sage.
Banner, M. (2014). *The Ethics of Everyday Life: Moral Theology, Social Anthropology, and the Imagination of the Human.* Oxford: Oxford University Press.
Barthes, R. (1991). 'The Grain of the Voice', In: *The Responsibility of Forms.* Berkeley: University of California Press.
Bateson, G. (1985). *Mind and Nature: A Necessary Unity*. London: Flamingo.
Becker, H. (2000). The Etiquette of Improvisation. *Mind, Culture, and Activity*, 7(3), pp. 171–6.
Benson, B E (2003). *The Improvisation of Musical Dialogue: A Phenomenology of Music.* Cambridge: Cambridge University Press.
Bentall, R.P (2009). *Doctoring the Mind: Why Psychiatric Treatments Fail.* London: Penguin.
Bithell, C. (2014). *A Different Voice, A Different Song: Reclaiming Community through the Natural Voice and World Song.* New York: Oxford University Press.
Bortoft, H. (2012). *Taking Appearance Seriously. The Dynamic Way of Seeing in Goethe and European Thought.* Edinburgh: Floris Books.
Bourdieu, P. (1984). *Distinction: A Social Critique of the Judgement of Taste.* (Trans. R Nice). Cambridge, MA: Harvard University Press.
Bracken et al. (2012). 'Pyschiatry beyond the current paradigm'. *British Journal of Psychiatry*, 201, 430–34.
Bunt, L. and Stige, B. (2014). *Music Therapy: An Art Beyond Words*, 2nd Edition. London: Routledge.
Burns, T. (2013) *Our Necessary Shadow: The Nature and Meaning of Psychiatry.* London: Penguin.
Carel, H. (2008). *Illness*. London: Acumen.
Charmaz, K. (1997). *Good Days, Bad Days*: *The Self in Chronic Illness and Time.* New Brunswick, NJ: Rutgers University Press.
Charon, R. (2008). *Narrative Medicine: Honoring the Stories of Illness*. New York: Oxford University Press.
Clarke, E. (2005). *Ways of Listening: An Ecological Approach to the Perception of Musical Meaning*. Oxford: Oxford University Press.
Clarke, E. (2011). Music Perception and Musical Consciousness. In: D. Clarke and E. Clarke (eds), *Music and Consciousness: Philosophical, Psychological, and Cultural Perspectives*. Oxford: Oxford University Press.
Clarke, E. (2014). Lost and found in music: Music, consciousness and subjectivity. *Musicae Scientiae*, Vol. 13(3), 354–68.
Cobussen, M. and Nielsen, N. (2012). *Music and Ethics.* Farnham: Ashgate.
Cook, N. (1998). *Music: A Very Short Introduction.* Oxford: Oxford University Press.

Cook, N. (2003). Music as Performance. In: M. Clayton, T. Herbert and R. Middleton (eds), *The Cultural Study of Music: A Critical Introduction*. New York and London: Routledge.

Crawford, M.J., Killaspy, H., Kalaitzaki, E., Barrett, B., Byford, S., Patterson, S., . . .Waller, D. (2010). The MATISSE study: A randomised trial of group art therapy for people with schizo-phrenia. *BMC Psychiatry*, *10*, Article 65. Retrieved from http:// www.biomedcentral.com/1471-244X/10/65

Critchley, S. (2013). *Infinitely Demanding: Ethics of Commitment, Politics of Resistance.* London: Verso.

Darnley-Smith, R. (2013). What is the Music of Music Therapy? An Enquiry into the Aesthetics of Clinical Improvisation. Durham theses, Durham University. Available at Durham E-Theses Online: http://etheses.dur.ac.uk/6975/

Davidson, L., Tondora, J., Lawless, M.S., O'Connell, M.J., and Rowe, M. (2009). *A Practical Guide to Recovery Oriented Practice. Tools for Transforming Mental Health Care.* New York: Oxford University Press.

Davies, J. (2013). *Cracked: Why Psychiatry Is Doing More Harm Than Good.* London: Icon Books.

Delamont, S. and N. Stephens (2008) Up on the Roof: The Embodied Habitus of Diasporic Capoeira. Cultural Sociology (2:1), pp. 57–74.

DeNora, T. (2000). *Music in Everyday Life.* Cambridge: Cambridge University Press.

DeNora, T. (2011a). *Music-in-action: Selected Essays in Sonic Ecology*. Farnham: Ashgate.

DeNora, T. (2011b). Practical Consciousness and Social Relation in *MusEcological* Perspective. In: D. Clarke and E. Clarke (eds), *Music and Consciousness: Philosophical, Psychological, and Cultural Perspectives*. Oxford: Oxford University Press.

DeNora, T. (2013a). *Music Asylums: Wellbeing through Music in Everyday Life*. Farnham: Ashgate.

DeNora, T. (2013b). 'Time after time': A Quali-T method for assessing music's impact on well-being. *International Journal Qualitative Studies of Health & Well-being* 2013, **8**: 20611. http://dx.doi.org/10.3402/qhw.v8i0.20611

DeNora, T (2013c). Music and Talk in Tandem: The Production of Micro-Narratives in Real Time. In: L Ole Bonde (ed), *Musical Life Stories. Narratives on Health Musicking*. Oslo: NMH-publikasjoner.

DeNora, T (2014) *Making Sense of Reality: culture and perception in everyday life*. London: Sage.

DeNora, T. and Ansdell, G. (2014). 'What can't music do? Shedding different kinds of light on music and health enquiries'. *Psychology of Well-Being: Theory, Research and Practice* 2014, 4:23. http://www.psywb.com/content/4/1/23

Dileo, C. (1999). *Music Therapy and Medicine: Theoretical and Clinical Applications.* Silver Spring, MD: American Music Therapy Association.

Fine, G.A. (2010). *The Sociology of the Local: Action and its Publics Sociological Theory* 28/4, 356–76.
Finnegan, R. (1989/2007). *The Hidden Musicians: Music-making in an English Town.* Middletown, CT: Wesleyan University Press.
Frank, A.W. (2004). *The Renewal of Generosity: Illness, Medicine, and How to Live*. Chicago, IL: University of Chicago Press.
Godlovitch, S. (1998). *Musical Performance: A Philosophical Study*. London: Routledge.
Goffman, E. (1959/1990). *The Presentation of Self in Everyday Life*. London: Penguin Books.
Hagberg, G. (2011). Jazz Improvisation and Ethical Interaction: A Sketch of the Connections. In: Garry Hagberg (ed.), *Art and Ethical Criticism*. Chichester: Wiley-Blackwell.
Hense, C. (2015). Musical Identities of Young People Recovering from Mental Illness. Unpublished doctoral dissertation, Dept of Music Therapy, University of Melbourne.
Holttum, S. and Huet, V. (2014). The MATISSE Trial−A Critique: Does Art Therapy Really Have Nothing to Offer People With a Diagnosis of Schizophrenia? *SAGE Open* 2014 4: DOI: 10.1177/2158244014532930
Hooper, S. and Procter, S. (2013). Less Comfortably Numb, More Meaningfully Occupied. In: L Ole Bonde (ed), *Musical Life Stories. Narratives on Health Musicking*. Oslo: NMH-publikasjoner.
Jampel, P. (2006). Performance in music therapy with mentally ill adults. Doctoral dissertation, New York University.
Law, J. (2004). *After Method: Mess in social science research*. London: Routledge.
Leader, D. (2012). *What is Madness?* London: Penguin Books.
MacDonald, R., Kreutz, G. and Mitchell, L. (eds) (2012). *Music, Health, and Wellbeing.* Oxford: Oxford University Press.
Malloch, S. and Trevarthen, C. (eds.) (2008). *Communicative Musicality: Exploring the basis of human companionship*. New York: Oxford University Press.
Maratos, A., Crawford, M. and Procter, S. (2011). Music for Depression: It Seems to Work, But How? *British Journal of Psychiatry*, 199(2), pp. 92–3.
Midgley, M. (2014). *Are You an Illusion?* Durham: Acumen.
Newman, F. (1999). A Therapeutic Deconstruction of the Illusion of Self. In: Lois Holzman, *Performing Psychology: A Postmodern Culture of the Mind.* London: Routledge.
Noë, A. (2010). *Out of Our Heads: Why You Are Not Your Brain, and Other Lessons from the Biology of Consciousness*. New York: Hill & Wang.
Nordoff, P. and Robbins, C. (1971/2004). *Therapy in Music for Handicapped Children*. Gilsum, NH: Barcelona Publishers.
Nordoff, P. and Robbins, C. (1977/2007). *Creative Music Therapy*. Gilsum, NH: Barcelona Publishers.
Pitts, S. (2004) Everyone Wants to be Pavarotti. *Journal of the Royal Musical Association* 129(1), 143–60.

Procter, S. (2011) Reparative Musicking: Thinking on the Usefulness of Social Capital Theory within Music Therapy, *Nordic Journal of Music Therapy* 20(3), 242–62.

Procter, S. (2013). 'Music therapy: what is it for whom? An ethnography of music therapy in a community mental health resource centre'. University of Exeter Doctoral thesis, available online at http://hdl.handle.net/10871/11101

Rolvsjord, R. (2010). *Resource-oriented Music Therapy in Mental Health Care.* Gilsum, NH: Barcelona Publishers.

Ruud, Even (2010). *Music Therapy: A Perspective from the Humanities.* Gilsum, New Hampshire: Barcelona Publishers.

Rudnick, A. (2012). *Recovery of People with Mental Illness: Philosophical and Related Perspectives.* Oxford: Oxford University Press.

Sennett, R. (2004). *Respect: The Formation of Character in an Age of Inequality.* London: Allen Lane.

Sennett, R. (2007). *The Craftsman.* London: Allen Lane.

Sennett, R. (2012). *Together: The Rituals, Pleasures and Politics of Cooperation.* London: Allen Lane.

Slade, M. (2009). *Personal Recovery and Mental Illness: A Guide for Mental Health Professionals.* Cambridge: Cambridge University Press.

Solli, H.P., Rolvsjord, R., and Borg, M. (2013). Toward understanding music therapy as a recovery-oriented practice within mental health care: a meta-synthesis of service users' experiences. *Journal of Music Therapy*, 50(4), 244–73. doi: 10.1093/jmt/50.4.244

Solli, H.P. and Rolvsjord, R. (2014). 'The opposite of treatment': a qualitative study of how patients diagnosed with psychosis experience music therapy. *Nordic Journal of Music Therapy* 24(1), 67–93.

Solli, H.P. (2015). Battling illness with wellness: a qualitative case study of a young rapper's experiences with music therapy. *Nordic Journal of Music Therapy* 24(3), 204–32.

Small, C. (1998). *Musicking: The Meanings of Performing and Listening.* Hanover, NH: Wesleyan University Press.

Small, C. (2010) 'Misunderstanding and Reunderstanding', *Peace & Policy*, 15, 4–12

Stern, D. (2010). *Forms of Vitality: Exploring Dynamic Experience in Psychology, the Arts, Psychotherapy, and Development.* Oxford: Oxford University Press.

Stige, B., Ansdell, G., Elefant, C. and Pavlicevic, M. (eds.) (2010). *Where Music Helps: Community Music Therapy in Action and Reflection.* Farnham: Ashgate.

Stige, B. and Aarø, L. (2012). *Invitation to Community Music Therapy.* New York: Routledge.

Tallis, R. (2013). *Reflections of a Metaphysical Flâneur & Other Essays.* Durham: Acumen.

Turino, T. (2008). *Music as Social Life: The Politics of Participation.* Chicago, IL: University of Chicago Press.

Turner, V. (1982). *From Ritual to Theatre: The Human Seriousness of Play*. New York: PAJ Publications.
Vygotsky, L. (1978). *Mind in Society: The Development of Higher Psychological Processes*, ed. M. Cole, V. John-Steiner, S. Scribner and E. Souberman. Cambridge, MA: Harvard University Press.
Willis, P. (2000). *The Ethnographic Imagination.* Cambridge: Polity Press.
Wood, S. (2016). *A Matrix for Community Music Therapy Practice.* Gilsum, NH: Barcelona.
Zembylas, T. (Ed). 2014. *Artistic Practices: Social Interactions and Cultural Dynamics*. London: Routledge.
Zuckerkandl, V. (1956). *Sound and Symbol: Music and the External World.* Princeton, NJ: Princeton University Press.
Zuckerkandl, V. (1973). *Man the Musician.* Princeton, NJ: Princeton University Press.
Žižek, S. (2014). *Event.* London: Penguin.

Index

For Product Safety Concerns and Information please contact our EU
representative GPSR@taylorandfrancis.com
Taylor & Francis Verlag GmbH, Kaufingerstraße 24, 80331 München, Germany

www.ingramcontent.com/pod-product-compliance
Ingram Content Group UK Ltd.
Pitfield, Milton Keynes, MK11 3LW, UK
UKHW020013200926
475702UK00014B/1855
* 9 7 8 1 1 3 8 5 0 4 8 8 2 *